Advances in Operative Dentistry

Advances in Operative Dentistry

Volume 2: Challenges of the Future

Edited by

Nairn HF Wilson, PhD, MSc, BDS
Professor, Chairman
Unit of Operative Dentistry and Endodontology
University Dental Hospital of Manchester
Manchester, United Kingdom

Jean-François Roulet, Prof Dr Med Dent
Professor, Chairman
Department of Operative and
Preventive Dentistry and Endodontics
Charité, School of Dental Medicine
Humboldt University of Berlin
Berlin, Germany

Massimo Fuzzi, DMD
Private Practice
Bologna, Italy

quintessence
books

Quintessence Publishing Co, Inc

Chicago, Berlin, London, Tokyo, Paris, Barcelona,
São Paulo, Moscow, Prague, Warsaw, and Istanbul

Library of Congress Cataloging-in-Publication Data

Advances in operative dentistry : contemporary clinical practice /
edited by Jean-Francois Roulet, Nairn H.F. Wilson, Massimo Fuzzi.
    p. ; cm.
Includes bibliographical references and index.
  ISBN 0-86715-402-0 (hardcover)
  1. Dentistry, Operative.
  [DNLM: 1. Dentistry, Operative. WU 300 A2445 2001] I. Roulet,
Jean-François. II. Wilson, Nairn H.F. III. Fuzzi, Massimo.
  RK501 .A36 2001
  617.6'05--dc21

                                                        2001001460

quintessence
books

© 2001 Quintessence Publishing Co, Inc

Quintessence Publishing Co, Inc
551 Kimberly Drive
Carol Stream, Illinois 60188
www.quintpub.com

Lithography: S & T Scan, Berlin
Printing and Binding: Jütte Druck GmbH, Leipzig

Printed in Germany

ISBN 0-86715-403-9

Contents

Contents

Contributors

Javier Garcia Barbero, PhD, MD, DDS
Department of Conservative Dentistry
Faculty of Odontology
Complutense University
Madrid, Spain

Fanny Basset, DDS
Department of Biomaterials
Faculty of Dental Surgery
University of Paris V
Montrouge, France

Julien Bijaoui, DDS
Department of Biomaterials
Faculty of Dental Surgery
University of Paris V
Montrouge, France

Denis Bouter, DDS, MS, PhD
Department of Restorative Dentistry
Faculty of Dental Surgery
University of Paris V
Montrouge, France

Douglas Bratthall, Odont Dr
Department of Cariology
Faculty of Odontology
Malmö University
Malmö, Sweden

Paul A. Brunton, BChD, MSc, PhD
Restorative Dentistry
University Dental Hospital of Manchester
Manchester, United Kingdom

Carel L. Davidson, PhD
Department of Dental Materials Science
ACTA, University of Amsterdam
Amsterdam, The Netherlands

Michel Degrange, DCD, DSO, DEO
Department of Biomaterials
Faculty of Dental Surgery
University of Paris V
Montrouge, France

Didier Dietschi, DMD
Department of Cariology,
  Endodontics, and Pedodontics
School of Dentistry
University of Geneva
Geneva , Switzerland

E. Steven Duke, MSD, DDS
Department of Restorative Dentistry
School of Dentistry
Indiana University
Indianapolis, Indiana, USA

Reinhard Hickel, DDS, Prof Dr Med Dent
Department of Restorative Dentistry and
  Operative Dentistry
Ludwig-Maximilians University
Munich, Germany

Laila Hitmi, DDS, MS
Department of Biomaterials
Faculty of Dental Surgery
University of Paris V
Montrouge, France

Norbert Hofmann, Dr Med Dent
Department of Operative Dentistry
  and Periodontology
Julius-Maximilians University of Würzburg
Würzburg, Germany

Peter R. Hotz, Prof Dr Med Dent
Department of Preventive, Operative,
  and Pediatric Dentistry
Bern University
Bern, Switzerland

Burkhard Hugo, Priv Doz Dr Med Dent
Department of Operative Dentistry
  and Periodontology
Julius-Maximilians University of Würzburg
Würzburg, Germany

W. Rory Hume, DDS, PhD
University of California, Los Angeles
Los Angeles, California, USA

Samuel Gonthier, DDS
Department of Biomaterials
Faculty of Dental Surgery
University of Paris V
Montrouge, France

Bernd Klaiber, Prof Dr Med Dent
Department of Operative Dentistry
  and Periodontology
Julius-Maximilians University of Würzburg
Würzburg, Germany

Ivo Krejci, DMD, PhD
Department of Cariology, Endodontics,
  and Pedodontics
School of Dentistry
University of Geneva
Geneva, Switzerland

Paul Lambrechts, DDS, PhD
Department of Operative Dentistry
BIOMAT
U.Z. St. Rafaël, Catholic University
  of Leuven
Leuven, Belgium

**Adrian Lussi, Prof Dr Med Dent,
  dipl.chem.ETH**
Department of Operative, Preventive,
  and Pediatric Dentistry
School of Dental Medicine
University of Bern
Bern, Switzerland

Felix Lutz, Prof Dr Med, Dr Med Dent
Clinic of Preventive Dentistry,
  Periodontology, and Cariology
School of Dentistry
University of Zurich
Zurich, Switzerland

Juergen Manhart, DDS, Dr Med Dent
Department of Restorative Dentistry
  and Operative Dentistry
Ludwig-Maximilians University
Munich, Germany

Jorge Perdigão, DDS, PhD
Division of Operative Dentistry
Department of Restorative Sciences
University of Minnesota
Minneapolis, Minnesota, USA

Gunnel Hänsel Petersson, DDS
Department of Cariology
Faculty of Odontology
Malmö University
Malmö, Sweden

Alphons J.M. Plasschaert, DMD, PhD
Department of Cariology and
  Endodontology
College of Dental Science
University of Nijmegen
Nijmegen, The Netherlands

Jean-François Roulet, Prof Dr Med Dent
Department of Operative Dentistry,
  Preventive Dentistry, and Endodontics
Humboldt University (Charité)
Berlin, Germany

James C. Setcos, BDS, MSc, DDS, PhD
Restorative Dentistry
University Dental Hospital of Manchester
Manchester, United Kingdom

Roberto Spreafico, MD, LMD
Private Practice
Busto Arsizio, Milan, Italy

J. Ramanathan Stjernswärd, DDS, PhD
Department of Cariology
Faculty of Odontology
Malmö University
Malmö, Sweden

Fabio Toffenetti, MD, DDS
Private Practitioner
Gallarate, VA, Italy

Guido Vanherle, MD, PhD
Department of Operative Dentistry
BIOMAT
U.Z. St. Rafaël, Catholic University of
  Leuven
Leuven, Belgium

Bart Van Meerbeek, DDS, PhD
Department of Operative Dentistry
BIOMAT
U.Z. St. Rafaël, Catholic University of
  Leuven
Leuven, Belgium

Emiel H. Verdonschot, DMD, PhD
Department of Cariology
  and Endodontology
College of Dental Science
University of Nijmegen
Nijmegen, The Netherlands

Nairn H. F. Wilson, PhD, MSc, BDS
Unit of Operative Dentistry and
  Endodontology
University Dental Hospital of Manchester
Manchester, United Kingdom

Stefan Zimmer, DDS
Department of Operative and Preventive
  Dentistry and Endodontics
School of Dental Medicine
Humboldt University (Charité)
  Berlin, Germany

Preface

Most dental care continues principally to comprise operative dentistry, which is the most widely practiced discipline in dentistry. Operative dentistry has been transformed in recent years and is expected to undergo further and far-reaching changes in years to come. This is the attraction and fascination of operative dentistry as a core element of the past, present, and future of oral health.

This book, the second of two volumes to emanate from the highly successful inaugural ConsEuro meeting held in Bologna in 2000, captures the state-of-the-art views and approaches of present-day European opinion leaders in the field of operative dentistry. Each chapter includes a vision of things to come in the hopes of enticing the next generation of operative dentists to continue the tradition of innovation, scholarship, and scientific endeavor, underpinned by expertise and skill in preserving and restoring the form, function, and esthetics of teeth. At the same time, it is hoped that established practitioners, teachers, and researchers, together with students at all levels, will find this text to be a unique source of quintessential information of immediate practical interest and application. It is only through complete knowledge and understanding of what can be achieved today that it will be possible to realize the dreams of tomorrow.

Conceiving, planning, and editing this volume of *Advances in Operative Dentistry* has been an enriching and even fun experience. We hope that browsers, readers, and all those who studiously digest the contents of this book will be enlightened, enthused, and encouraged to join in the quest to discover new horizons in the pursuit of excellence in the practice of operative dentistry. Please enjoy and put to good use the thought-provoking contents of this unique and invigorating book; new opportunities in clinical practice stem from an understanding of future challenges in oral health care provision.

N.H.F. Wilson, J.F. Roulet, and M. Fuzzi
Manchester, Berlin, and Bologna

Introduction

E. Steven Duke

Readers of the text *Advances in Operative Dentistry: Challenges of the Future* will find themselves challenged to deal with the novelty of the approaches to patient care presented. In contrast to the historical texts of operative dentistry in North America, which have changed very little in context over the past century, the present European collection of manuscripts addressing operative concepts is a dramatic move toward focusing on the patient's interests, rather than dentist's interests.[3] Balanced with a wealth of scientific references, restorative approaches are offered as alternative interventions to deep-seated modes of treatment that have been the core of dental education in many countries around the world. Maximum benefit to the reader can only be realized with an open mind to innovation and a resistance to the historical pattern of "tradition without question." This is not to suggest that one should not question issues and approaches forwarded in the text. The text itself is based upon a foundation of exploring new avenues for improving the oral health of the public. As health professionals, we are obligated to this end, regardless of the potential bias that has been inherent to our profession over the years.

The present text deals in great depth with risk assessment and decision making in operative dentistry. This refreshing approach to patient treatment planning has only recently emerged in North American educational programs.[4] With the exception of some Canadian dental schools, only a handful of institutions have integrated dynamic concepts such as dietary habits, social status, ethnic background, and oral hygiene practices as principal components in decision making in operative dentistry. Such critical assessment is focused directly at the patient with the aim of providing treatment that is optimized for the individual patient. In addition, treatment options for aging patient populations are presented in a format that is evidence-based and focused, regardless of the economic or educational level of the patient.[1] These concepts will eventually become a vital aspect of treatment options presented to the patient.[2] Once completely informed, the patient becomes intimately involved in the decision-making process regarding their oral health problems and possible resolutions.[5]

The novel concept of "refurbishment" procedures is presented as conservative management of previous interventions.

While there will be very little question in educated circles regarding the benefit of such an operative approach, its endorsement by traditional educational programs will be resisted. Previous concepts of "patched-up" treatments are at risk of overshadowing the novelty of true refurbishment, or restoring restorations to their original state. For many years clinicians have repaired teeth, why not consider the more conservative approach of repairing restorations?

While the text is not a dental materials text, ample scientific evidence is presented in support of the treatment options presented. Again, such integration of materials science, patient factors, and skills of the clinician are a modern, patient-centered focus to care. Maximum benefit to the patient is the primary focus of care delivered. With an emphasis on esthetic options complemented with form restoration, great emphasis is placed on how to achieve optimum results with new adhesives, ceramics, and polymeric-based restorative procedures. These new techniques are presented comprehensively so that the reader will appreciate the complexity and the need for care when embarking on such a course of oral health care. The issue of maintenance and modifications unveils the concept of maximizing results with follow-through of care, rather than an isolated, short-sighted treatment option.

Prevention is present throughout the text, from early diagnostic factors to treatment decisions that prevent early failures. While there remains controversy surrounding the individual technologies presented for early caries diagnosis,[6] there is overwhelming agreement on the concept worldwide. To see this concept recognized as an integral component of operative dentistry is a major step forward in patient assessment and ultimately final decision making. An extensive chapter of the text deals with restoration longevity. A comprehensive review of the literature on all operative options is presented. The significance of this material becomes evident when the final factors relating to the individual characteristics of the patient are considered. What becomes apparent is the multifaceted approach to treatment, in which there may be several options, all potentially equal in outcome if all factors are weighed into the decision process.

"Evidence-based" clinical decision-making concepts and "problem-based learning" approaches to education in North America are highlights of the advances that have been made as we move into the 21st century. *Advances in Operative Dentistry: Challenges of the Future,* the collective effort of a number of European scholars, is a major step in this direction.

References

1. Gordon M. Problems of an aging population in an era of technology. J Can Dent Assoc 2000;66:320–322.

2. Hirano H, Ishiyama N, Watanabe I, Nasu I. Masticatory ability in relation to oral status and general health on aging. J Nutr Health Aging 1999;3:48–52.

3. Meskin LH. Patients first and always. J Am Dent Assoc 1997;128:138–140.

4. Reich E, Lussi A, Newbrun E. Caries risk assessment. Int Dent J 1999;49:15–26.

5. Robbins JW. Evidence-based dentistry: What is it, and what does it have to with practice? Quintessence Int 1998;29:796–799.

6. Stookey GK (ed). Early Detection of Dental Caries. Indianapolis: Indiana Univ School of Dentistry, 1996.

Part 1

Prevention and Diagnosis

Chapter 1

Prevention of Dental Caries

Peter R. Hotz

Introduction

In many populations, oral disease, especially dental caries and periodontitis, is a widespread problem with considerable biologic, physical, economic, social, and psychologic consequences. Oral health is an important aspect of human well-being and quality of life. There is scientific proof that dental caries and periodontal disease can be managed and, to a large degree, completely prevented. A substantial improvement in oral health status in some segments of the European population has been achieved over the last two to three decades. Consequently, the effects of caries and periodontal disease have been reduced. Nevertheless, the burden of oral disease is still excessive for many individuals; therefore, increased preventive efforts remain necessary.

In two documents,[21,22] the World Health Organization postulates that oral health services and the education of personnel will need to be transformed. More emphasis will have to be placed on such skills as diagnosis, pathophysiology, disease risk assessment and management, and communication.[14] A group of experts identified 12 guiding principles, including:

- Oral health is an essential part of human function and quality of life.
- Oral health status should be improved and maintained in the most economical manner consistent with quality and access.
- Prevention is preferable to treatment as a general rule.
- Caries and periodontal diseases can be prevented and controlled.
- Individuals should do as much as possible for themselves to achieve and maintain oral health.
- Community methods of prevention should be supportive of individual and personal care, and in some situations are more efficient.

Caries prevention programs can be instituted on three levels:

- Preventive programs for the community
- Preventive programs for the dental office
- Preventive programs for home care

As health professionals and experts, dentists are obliged to support and practice dental prevention on all three levels.

Preventive Programs for the Community

The principal requirement for the conception of cost-effective preventive strategies for the entire population is the availability of epidemiologic data regarding distribution patterns and intensity of the disease.[8] Dental caries data for various European countries are available. They have been collected over the past one to four decades, especially among children and adolescents. A clear-cut decrease in caries has been observed, although it was of variable extent for different countries. The reasons for this decrease have been discussed extensively in the past. In a "review of the reviews," Pettersson and Bratthall[16] indicated that most authors tend to believe that the use of fluorides in various forms has contributed significantly to the decline in the prevalence of dental caries. In addition to the fluoridation of public water supplies, the main measures mentioned in the various reports were the widespread use of fluoride toothpastes, fluoride mouthrinsing programs, and dietary fluoride supplements. A number of other factors and hypotheses were mentioned, including: increased dental awareness, availability of dental resources, decrease in sugar consumption, dental health education programs, professional oral prophylaxis and fissure sealants, preventive approaches in practice, the widespread use of antibiotics, changes in diagnostic criteria, and other currently unknown factors. The observed decline in caries must under no circumstances be interpreted as the final solution to the problem. There is increasing evidence that while caries levels have declined in developed countries during the past decades, there continues to be a large "at-risk" group for which caries remains a major problem. Perhaps the most widely reported at-risk group comprises those individuals of lower socioeconomic groups among whom higher caries levels are consistently reported.[20] Preventive programs for the community, such as water fluoridation, salt fluoridation, availability of low-cost fluoride toothpastes, and oral health education programs in schools, are more likely to benefit these groups of the population than individual dental health education and efforts to alter lifestyles. What is the role of the dental practitioner? He must reemphasize the importance of collective prophylaxis programs and defend at all times the impact of fluorides on the prevention of dental caries. An increasing percentage of the population tends to believe that, in view of today's reduced caries incidence, fluorides may no longer be necessary. In spite of studies indicating that a reduction of the fluoride supply will not immediately be followed by a new increase in caries,[13] this important element in the prevention of dental decay must not be discarded. Additionally, the widely reported decline of the prevalence of dental caries in children and adolescents over the past decades may produce an adverse effect on future public financing of oral health education programs in schools. Therefore, we must remain vigilant in order to prevent caries from regaining its former spread and prevalence. Today's reduced levels of caries are a result of planned, appropriate prophylaxis. Any reduction in these efforts will disturb the subtle equilibrium between attack and defense, and caries will inevitably return.

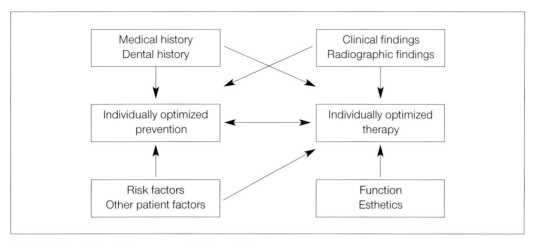

Fig 1-1 Interrelations between prophylaxis and therapy.

Preventive Programs for the Dental Office

Prevention of dental disease is the dentist's most noble task and obligation. Therapy without concomitant prophylaxis makes no sense. Costly reconstructed teeth have a very limited life expectancy in a neglected oral environment.

An individual program of prophylaxis is based on clinical findings, the individual's risk of disease, and other patient factors such as willingness to cooperate (comply) and general health problems with likely effects on the oral system (Fig 1-1).[12]

Dental prophylaxis starts with an exact medical and dental history, followed by an appropriate clinical and, where indicated, radiologic examination and diagnosis.

The dental examination must comprise the following elements:
- Oral hygiene status
- Dental caries, clinical, and radiographic analysis
- Noncarious changes in dental hard tissues
- Gingival and periodontal status
- Tooth vitality/endodontic status
- Condition of restorations, presence of secondary caries
- Actual preventive measures, professional and patient applied
- Attitudes and expectancies regarding prophylaxis and oral health

The extent of the examination varies with the individual. For a caries-inactive subject with adequate individual prophylaxis efforts, the above scheme will be sufficient. However, if the oral hygiene is judged to be insufficient, the extension of dental plaque will need to be recorded by means of a simple index such as the "plaque control record"[15] and the degree of gingival inflammation will have to be documented according to, for example, the "bleeding-on-probing" index.[1] In cases in which there is more serious periodontal involvement than just localized gingivitis, appropriate diagnostic and therapeutic measures have to be introduced. However, these are not the subject of this chapter.

When new lesions appear in the dental hard tissues, their etiology needs to be carefully evaluated using the following additional diagnostic measures:

- Detailed analysis of the general health status, including the ingestion of medications
- Saliva/oral fluid assessment (flow rate, buffering capacity)
- Microbiological analysis of plaque (mutans streptococci, lactobacilli)
- Dietary history
- Sociocultural history

The dental team must be aware of all illnesses with possible effects on the dentition and the oral cavity as a whole.

The most common cause of xerostomia is the use of xerogenic medications. Several hundred drugs, some of them in common use, have the potential to cause salivary gland hypofunction,[19] thereby inducing oral dryness. These drugs include:

- Anticholinergic drugs
- Antihistamines
- Antidepressants
- Antipsychotics
- Antihypertensives
- Antiparkinsonian drugs
- Diuretics

Generally, low doses of the above drugs do not damage the structure of the salivary glands. Therefore, their effects are reversible.

Other principal causes of salivary gland hypofunction are therapeutic irradiation, systemic diseases (rheumatoid conditions, dysfunction of the immune system, hormonal disorders), and aging as a contributory factor. In most patients subjected to therapeutic irradiation, the reduction of the function of the salivary glands and the resultant xerostomia are irreversible. The type of prophylaxis selected must take this consideration into account. Determination of the stimulated salivary flow rate is simple. The patient is asked to chew sugar-free gum or a cube of paraffin wax for 5 minutes and to collect the oral fluid produced during the time in a cup. Secretion rates of over 1 mL/minute are considered safe. Lower readings give cause for concern because they are considered to increase the risk for dental caries.[18] Kits are commercially available to readily determine salivary flow rate and buffering capacity (Dentobuff, Orion Diagnostica, Espoo, Finland). Furthermore, there are relatively simple chairside methods for gaining information as to the microbial composition of the oral flora and the plaque population, especially regarding the mutans streptococci and lactobacilli count (Dentocult SM and Dentocult LB, Orion Diagnostica). Unfortunately, there is only limited correlation between microbial findings and clinically observed increments of caries. Nevertheless, such tests have value in cases in which no clear-cut cause-and-effect relationship can be established. In addition, microbiologic testing may be of help to check patient compliance and to test the effects of a particular prophylaxis program.[6] Even when considering dental caries to be of multifactorial etiology, fighting the infection has become an important issue in any modern concept of prophylaxis against dental caries.

Regarding dietary habits, gathering information by direct personal interview is typically inadequate and unreliable. Usually it is better to ask the patient to record in detail over a period of 4 days all ingestions of food, drink, and drugs by quality, quantity, and time of day. It appears useful to record in detail all oral hygiene habits at the same time. Dispensing a questionnaire including recommendations and instructions as to how to use a dietary and oral hygiene diary has been found successful.

Precise information about dietary and oral hygiene habits of an individual allows the formulation of customized recommendations for a personalized dental prophylaxis program.

Social and cultural factors may have an important impact on the development of dental prophylaxis plans. Language-based communication difficulties, lack of awareness and understanding of the benefits of appropriate dental health, as well as lack of compliance must be considered. It may well be that successful personal dental prophylaxis may be achieved only after an intensive initial boost to incentive by professional care.

Another important challenge and obligation for the dental team is the creation of conditions that allow for the best possible effects of any personal efforts toward good oral hygiene. The measures necessary to achieve this goal include the removal of hopeless teeth and retained tooth fragments, excavation of all decay and obturation with well-adapted temporary restorations, removal of overhangs in fillings and crowns, and removal of supragingival and subgingival calculus, dental plaque, and stains.

Caries Prevention by Individual Home-Care Procedures

Individual prophylaxis offers preventive measures adapted to individual needs. The dentist is responsible for the prophylactic concept and its implementation by the dental team. The prime requirement for effective and efficient individual prophylaxis is in-depth knowledge of the patient's history, the clinical situation, and the etiology of and risk level for the disease. The patient is informed about his or her condition and the possibilities, goals, and concept of the preventive plan. Motivation and instruction are delivered simultaneously. Preventive efforts must be optimized by clinical monitoring and untiring motivation. With children, the involvement and cooperation of the parents is a must. Mentally challenged patients depend entirely on the willingness and capabilities of the caregivers in their immediate environment. Such personnel must, therefore, be convinced of the importance of carrying out the prophylactic procedures. Success with prophylaxis is most likely if all possibilities for intervention are deployed (Fig 1-2).

Oral Hygiene

Only plaque-free tooth surfaces are protected from caries. Bacterial plaque therefore must be removed as completely and regularly as possible by appropriate oral hygiene procedures. Clinical experience has shown that special attention needs to be given to interproximal surfaces. The use of every aid considered appropriate for the situation must be instructed meticulously and its correct application checked regularly. The ultimate criterion of efficiency is neither the number nor the price of the

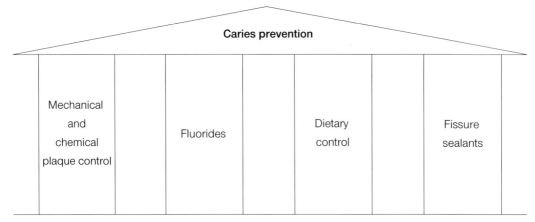

Fig 1-2 Factors contributing to the prevention of caries.

various instruments and devices used, only the number of plaque-free tooth surfaces achieved and maintained.

In addition, care should be taken to ensure that the methods and instruments used (perhaps wrongly) will not damage either hard or soft tissues by giving rise to either noncarious cervical lesions or gingival injuries. Toothbrush, toothpaste, and cleaning technique must be adapted to each other and fine-tuned in order to achieve an optimum cleaning effect while avoiding detrimental side effects.

Plaque removal to the extent necessary for effective caries control is difficult for many patients. It has been shown that plaque removal by toothbrushing without fluoride-containing toothpaste may not be effective against caries.[3] Today, the use of fluoridated toothpastes is widespread and a correlation between the quality of oral hygiene and the incidence of dental caries has been observed in recent investigations.[11] One of the reasons for the significant difference in oral hygiene as it relates to dental caries between pre-fluoride- and fluoride-era studies may be found in the fact that small to moderate amounts of plaque in prefluoride times were cariogenic. Therefore, the use of fluoridated toothpastes is unreservedly recommended. Also, avoiding rinsing the mouth with water after brushing teeth with a fluoridated toothpaste may increase the protective effect.[5,17]

Chemical Plaque Control

Unfortunately, there is still no antibacterial agent that can be used efficiently and safely over extended periods of time in the battle against caries. Several chemical compounds have been evaluated. No other antimicrobial agent has received the experimental attention directed at chlorhexidine. Best results have been observed in patients severely infected with mutans streptococci. Chlorhexidine provides the means to reduce substantially and rapidly mutans streptococci in patients with high counts of the bacteria and/or high caries activity. The most persistent reduction of streptococci has been found with the use of chlorhexidine gel in custom-made trays or when applied as a varnish. The application of chlorhexidine gel by toothbrushing or chlorhexidine in a mouthrinse also have beneficial effects.[7] Because antimicrobial therapy with chlorhexidine only reduces the number of organisms, the effect is reversed after the treatment is stopped. Therefore, treatments must be repeated as required, usually at intervals of 1 to 3 months.

Diet

The patients must be informed about the relationship between diet and dental health. Dietary assessment and counseling are crucial to the success of preventing caries and erosive lesions. The complexity of the etiology of caries and the fact that the net outcome of a cariogenic challenge may be simultaneously influenced by several factors make it impossible to furnish firm recommendations as to a "safe" number of food (sugar) intake. For some patients, a habit (eg, frequent consumption of chocolate or sugar-containing lozenges or snacking at night) may explain their caries activity and may be easily corrected. For others, very complex eating patterns may be found. It must be noted that it is not only common sugar that is detrimental to the teeth. All readily soluble monosaccharides and disaccharides, as well as boiled starch, can be metabolized glycolytically by plaque microorganisms to form organic acids. Therefore, all these substances are to be considered cariogenic. The cariogenicity of a diet is not determined by absolute amounts of ingested fermentable carbohydrates, but rather by the frequency of their intake. The practical consequence for dietary counseling is, therefore, the need to reduce the number of intakes of cariogenic snacks to a minimum, with special emphasis on the elimination of cariogenic snacks at night. Caries is not the only diet-linked phenomenon meriting attention in the course of diet counseling. Dietary erosion requires attention to the ingestion of acid-containing foodstuffs and drinks.

Fluoride Prophylaxis

Caries is not a fluoride deficiency disease. The caries-protective effect of fluorides is considerable and documented well by countless studies and investigations. The methods and intensity of application are geared by need, ie, by the individual patient's risk for dental caries.[10] Drinking water– and salt-fluoridation are recommended methods of collective supply. Additionally, the appropriate use of fluoride-containing toothpaste is to be secured as part of the mechanical cleaning of teeth. More intensive uses of fluorides are governed by individual needs and possibilities. Fluoride tablets may be appropriate for infants, providing there is no other source of systemic fluoride. The preeruptive effect of fluoride seems to be limited, especially in children with relatively low caries risk. It seems that the preeruptive contact of the tooth surfaces with fluoride may reduce the susceptibility of erupting molars to fissure caries.[9] Fluoride-containing mouthrinses, gels, and varnishes are indicated for high caries risk patients. Because the posteruptive cariostatic effects of fluoride are correlated with fluoride concentration and total exposure time, a combination of various fluoridation methods is appropriate for patients with high caries risk. It should be noted that the effects of the various methods are different when combined according to the concentration of fluoride and the frequency of application.

Sealing of Fissures

Most primary caries lesions in children and adolescents are found in fissures. In countries with high levels of oral hygiene, 80% of all caries in children and adolescents between 5 and 17 years of age is found in pits and fissures.[4] The reasons for this phenomenon are most likely the morphology of the surfaces and the reduced efficacy of fluorides in plaque-filled fissures. Hence these surfaces, especially those in permanent molars, require special attention and preventive care. Fissure sealing is a proven method for the prevention of caries in these locations.[2] However, it makes sense only for patients at an increased risk of caries and when used in conjunction with preventive measures for all other surfaces.

Sealed fissures must be checked at regular intervals. Lost and partially lost sealants must be replaced. Appropriate indications are an important factor in achieving a reasonable cost-effect ratio.

Quality Management of Dental Prevention

Oral health makes an important contribution to general well-being and quality of life. Therefore, oral health must be a goal for the entire population and must be accessible to all age groups and social strata. It is a proven fact that caries and periodontal disease can be managed and even prevented. Offering preventive services should not be at the discretion of the dental team. Patients have the same right to optimum preventive care as to restorative treatment. Achieving the goal of prevention of dental disease is a challenge for the entire dental team, led by the dentist. Prime requisites for successful individual prophylaxis are: diagnosis, documentation, individual prophylaxis, and the cooperation of the patient. Swiss Dental Association guidelines for quality management in preventive dentistry[12] recognize three categories of management: good (A) to excellent (+), unsatisfactory (faulty, but correctable) (B), and insufficient (poor, not correctable) (C). The categories B and C are to be avoided whenever possible.

Diagnosis

It is necessary for all oral diseases to be diagnosed correctly, recognizing the reasons for the disease and further risks. Diagnosis of caries includes radiographic analysis where and when needed (A to +).

Insufficient or faulty clinical diagnosis of caries (B and C) is unacceptable, as is the unsatisfactory determination of the etiology and further risks of the disease.

Documentation

Clinical findings (diseases of the teeth, oral hygiene, etc) as well as recommendations for prophylaxis are to be documented as completely as possible (A to +). Insufficient or lacking documentation is classified as B or C.

Individual Prophylaxis

"Excellent performance" is accorded to an individually adapted optimum prophylaxis program comprising oral hygiene, fluoride prophylaxis, dietary control, chemical plaque control, and fissure sealing as necessary. Recall visits are adapted to individual needs with regard to intervals and professional services to be delivered.

On the other hand, inadequate information, insufficient or faulty preventive efforts that do not respect the individual needs of the patient, and the absence of an organized recall are unacceptable (B).

Cooperation of the Patient

It is evident that optimum prophylaxis results can only be achieved given adequate patient compliance and cooperation. The "good to excellent" patient is most interested in oral health. He or she practices fair to good oral hygiene, follows individual recommendations to a large extent, and is interested in regular professional care.

Only limited success can be expected in patients with little interest in oral health, regardless of care. Such patients follow advice in part, exhibit plaque deposits, etc. Of course, catagorizing patients is not a primary goal. However, if the dentist views prevention as an obligation, the patient also has a part to play. Should the patient be unwilling to do this, proper documentation will help to weaken and invalidate allegations of inadequate preventive care.

Conclusions

Since dental caries is an avoidable disease, all dentists are called upon to show their patients how to achieve good oral health and to accompany them on the road to this goal. Prevention is an integral and indispensable part of the dental care of every individual. However, patients are ultimately responsible for their dental health. The dental team assesses all aspects of the clinical situation, the reasons for the disease and the likelihood of further risks. Individually adapted programs of prophylaxis tailored to specific needs of the patients help to achieve the desired goal—good oral health.

References

1. Ainamo J, Bay I. Problems and proposals for recording gingivitis and plaque. Int Dent J 1975; 25:229–235.

2. Axelsson P. An Introduction to Risk Prediction and Preventive Dentistry. Chicago: Quintessence, 1999.

3. Bellini TH, Arneberg P, von der Fehr FR. Oral hygiene and caries: A review. Acta Odontol Scand 1981;39:256–265.

4. Bowden JW, Cohen DW, Collier DR, et al. Consensus development conference statement on dental sealants in the prevention of tooth decay. J Am Dent Assoc 1984;108:233–236.

5. Chesters RK, Huntington E, Burchell CK, Stephen KW. Effect of oral care habits on caries in adolescents. Caries Res 1992;26:299–304.

6. Einwag J. Möglichkeiten und Grenzen häuslicher Prophylaxe. In: Professionelle Prävention in der Zahnartzpraxis. München: Urban und Schwarzenberg, 1994:77–118.

7. Emilson CG. Potential efficacy of chlorhexidine against mutans streptococci and human dental caries. J Dent Res 1994;73:682–691.

8. Fejerskov O. Strategies in the design of preventive programs. Adv Dent Res 1995;9:82–88.

9. Groeneveld A, Van Eck AAMJ, Baker-Dirks O. Fluoride in caries prevention: Is the effect pre- or post-eruptive? J Dent Res 1990;69(special issue):751–759.

10. Hotz P. Anwendung der Fluoride in der Zahnmedizin. Dtsch Zahnarztl Z 1996;51:649–654.

11. Hotz P. Dental Plaque Control and Caries. In: Lang NP, Attström R, Löe H (eds). Proceedings of the European Workshop on Mechanical Plaque Control. Berlin: Quintessence, 1998; 35–49.

12. Hotz P, Imfeld T, Lussi A, Menghini G, Meyer J, Minnig P. Präventivzahnmedizin. In: Qualitätsrichtlinien für zahnmedizinische Arbeiten. Stämpfli: Schweizer Zahnärztegesellschaft, 1999;7–24.

13. Künzel W, Fischer T. Caries prevalence after cessation of water fluoridation in LaSalud, Cuba. Caries Res 2000;34:20–25.

14. Murray JJ. Oral Health for the 21st century. In: Murray JJ (ed). Prevention of Oral Diseases. Oxford: Oxford Univ Press, 1996:275–276.

15. O'Leary TJ, Drake RB, Naylor JE. The plaque control record. J Periodontol 1972;43:38–39.

16. Pettersson HG, Bratthall D. The caries decline: A review of reviews. Eur J Oral Sci 1996; 104:436–442.

17. Sjögren K, Birkhead D, Ruben J, Arends J. Effect of post-brushing water rinsing on caries-like lesions at approximal and buccal sites. Caries Res 1995;29:337–342.

18. Saliva: Its role in health and disease. Working Group 10 of the Commission on Oral Health, Research, and Epidemiology (CORE). Int Dent J 1992;42(4, suppl 2):287–304.

19. Sreebny LM. Xerostomia: Diagnosis, management and clinical complications. In: Edgar WM, O'Mullane DM (eds). Saliva and Oral Health. London: British Dental Association, 1996.

20. Whelton H, O'Mullane DM. Public health aspects of oral diseases and disorders. In: Pine CM (ed). Community Oral Health. Oxford: Wright, 1997:75–92.

21. World Health Organization. Alternative Systems of Oral Care Delivery. [Technical Report Series 750]. Geneva: World Health Organization, 1987.

22. World Health Organization. Recent Advances in Oral Health. Report of a WHO Expert Committee [Technical Report Series 826]. Geneva: World Health Organization, 1992.

Chapter 2

Prevention—Practical Aspects

Jean-François Roulet and Stefan Zimmer

Introduction

In an ideal world everyone would enjoy oral health. There would be no caries and no gingivitis. Periodontitis would not exist.

Is this possible? From a theoretical viewpoint, the answer is yes. Axelsson and Lindhe[1] have demonstrated in a controlled prospective clinical study that caries and periodontal disease can be prevented almost completely. They treated 555 patients and divided them into two groups. The control group patients (n = 180) were advised to see their dentist on an annual basis. The experimental group (n = 375) was subjected to a customized, need-related professional tooth-cleaning regimen by a dental hygienist approximately four times per year. After 6 years, the results were overwhelming. While the control group had accumulated on average more than two new caries lesions per year, the experimental group remained essentially caries free (Fig 2-1). This corresponds to an odds ratio of 70, meaning that without professional preventive care the risk of caries was 7,000% higher than in the experimental group. The prevalence and progression of periodontal disease was assessed by monitoring attachment loss and similar results were found (Fig 2-2).

Based on these data, one would conclude that it is possible to virtually eliminate caries and periodontal disease by providing professional prevention services to the entire population. Assuming this conclusion to be true, its realization would lead to a "horror scenario." Let us apply it to Germany.

If the 80 million inhabitants of Germany each require four 1-hour sessions of individualized prevention per year they would consume 320 million hours of prevention. If it is assumed that this preventive care were to be delivered by auxiliaries (dental nurses or dental hygienists, depending on the patient's risk of disease), and assuming that these auxiliaries work the hours worked by dentists (1,800 per year), 177,778 auxiliaries would be needed to deliver the necessary care. Such a workforce is not available and there are not the facilities to train such a large number of auxiliaries. If half of the dental schools were converted into schools for training auxiliaries, it would take approximately 90 years (based on a 1-year curriculum) to develop the necessary workforce.

Such a scenario is therefore no more than an illusion and can be set aside.

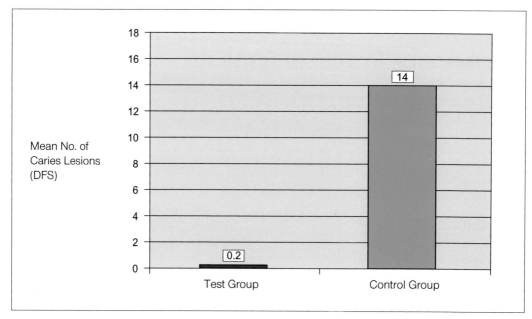

Fig 2-1 Mean number of caries lesions detected per participant over course of 6-year experiment. The test group received personalized professional prevention therapy.[1] DFS = Decayed and filled surfaces.

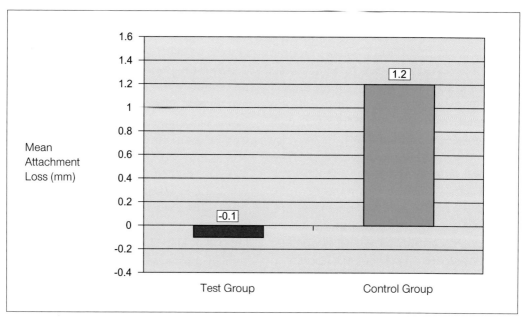

Fig 2-2 Mean attachment loss per participant in same study as Fig 2-1. The graph illustrates the dramatic effect of personalized prevention therapy on periodontal disease.[1]

DMFT at different age classes

	Age 8	Age 10	Age 12	Age 14
1974	2.27	4.22	6.84	11.53
1979	1.98	3.07	4.98	7.79
1983	0.74	2.13	2.93	5.28
1987	0.49	1.20	1.64	3.22
1992	0.33	0.66	1.10	2.35

Fig 2-3 The effect of fluoridated table salt on caries prevalence in Switzerland 1974–1992.[17]

Hierarchy of Needs

According to Maslow,[15] humans organize their lives according to a need hierarchy. Primary needs are physiological needs, such as food, housing, clothes, and the need for security. The need for security includes the absence of fear (fear of unemployment, war, etc) and the need for law and order.[15] Secondary needs include self-fulfillment, hobbies, sport, travel, and health care. Health issues are ranked low in the need hierarchy as long as individuals feel healthy. When acute pain occurs (eg, toothache), then health becomes a primary need. In essence, secondary needs only become important when all primary needs have been met. For example, the need to attend a dental hygienist is not a primary need if you have just been informed of your dismissal. However, when all primary needs are fulfilled, teeth possibly may become extremely important to the individual. This is one of the reasons why prevention does not erode the dental economy; in contrast, it improves it. With healthy teeth, new demands are created, including orthodontics, esthetic dentistry, and more sophisticated reconstructions.

Systemic Prevention

It is widely accepted that fluoride is the most effective caries-preventive agent. The profession should, therefore, advocate its use. For many years fluoridation of drinking water (1 ppm F) has been known to be very effective and inexpensive in the prevention of caries, especially if it is applied in large cities with treatable water supplies.[25] If the caries prevalence is high, a caries reduction of approximately 50% can be expected.[20] The fluoridation of table salt (250 ppm F) is a valuable alternative to water fluoridation, as data from Switzerland have clearly shown[17] (Fig 2-3). A reduction in caries in the same magnitude as the one obtainable with fluoridation of water may be expected. The use of

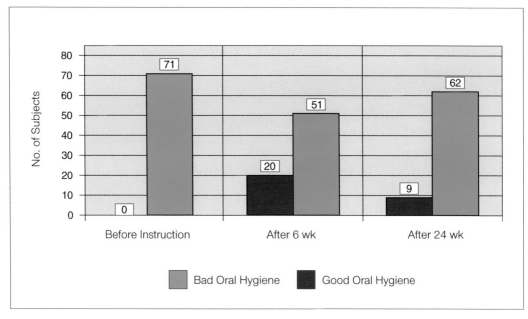

Fig 2-4 The efficiency of oral self-care after oral hygiene instruction.[24]

fluoridated table salt is, however, highly dependent on its price. In Switzerland, where fluoridated salt is sold for the same price as nonfluoridated salt, approximately 90% of the salt sold is fluoridated (Fischer A, personal communication, 2000). In Germany, where fluoridated salt is more expensive (a few cents per kg) than non-fluoridated salt, only 49% of the salt sold is fluoridated. State subsidy of fluoridated salt may therefore be found to be a cost-effective caries prevention measure.

Oral Self-Care

For a health system, eg, a sickness insurance scheme, the delivery of oral self-care is free of cost. Authorities responsible for the provision of oral health care therefore actively promote self-care.[5]

In contrast to popular belief in the population and among dentists, toothbrushing per se has relatively little effect on the incidence of caries. Many studies have demonstrated that unsupervised toothbrushing has no effect on caries incidence.[4] Even supervised toothbrushing, eg, in schools, has little, if any, effect.[2] Furthermore, oral health instruction has only a short-term effect on the quality of plaque removal[24] (Fig 2-4). It would, however, be wrong to conclude on the basis of these data that patients should not be advised to brush their teeth. There are two important reasons for toothbrushing:

1. Because most toothpaste sold is fluoridated (> 90% in Germany), toothbrushing is an effective method of fluoridation. In contrast to the studies cited above, Matthiesen et al have shown that

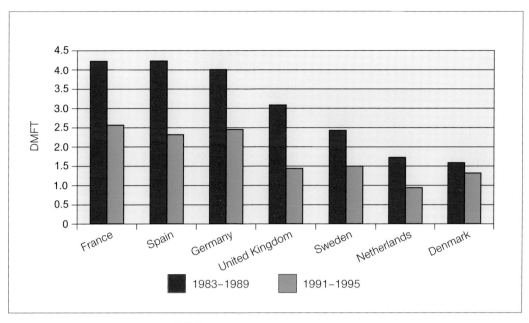

Fig 2-5 Caries decline in Europe.[12,21,22]

oral hygiene has an important caries-preventive effect if performed with fluoridated toothpaste.[16] The worldwide decline in caries can best be explained by the use of fluoridated toothpaste[11,12] (Fig 2-5).

2. The best means of preventing periodontal disease is the prevention of gingivitis. Gingivitis is strictly plaque-dependent. Therefore, thorough plaque removal once a day should keep the soft tissues healthy.

It may therefore be concluded that patients should be advised to brush with a fluoridated toothpaste. However, patients should be advised against excessive frequency of tooth brushing, notably after every meal. Apart from being unrealistic to expect patients to brush their teeth after, for example, a meal in a restaurant, the like-

lihood of compliance is low,[18] except possibly among dental personnel.

Improvements in toothbrush manufacturing technology have opened a new field for toothbrush designs with enhanced efficiency. Such developments may offer practical improvements in oral health. In a recent study, Zimmer et al[27] tested the effectiveness of a novel toothbrush design (Fig 2-6). The effectiveness of the Superbrush (Denta Co AS, Minde/Bergen, Norway) was compared with that of a standard manual toothbrush (Elmex super 39, GABA, Lörrach, Germany) and a powered toothbrush of the newest generation (Braun Plaque Control, Braun AG, Frankfurt am Main, Germany). A double-blind crossover study was performed with 36 healthy volunteers in three age groups: children (6 to 12 years old), students (23 to 35 years old), and adults

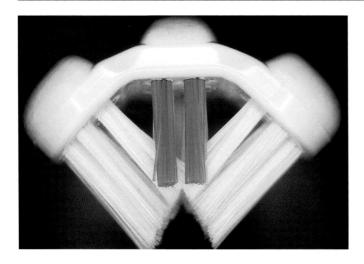

Fig 2-6 Superbrush.

(37 to 60 years old). A baseline status was established by professional tooth cleaning. The volunteers then cleaned their teeth with the experimental toothbrush for one week. Following a further week the procedure was repeated until each participant had used each type of toothbrush. The quality of their effort was measured using the Quigley-Hein plaque index (PI)[23] and papillary bleeding index (PBI).[19] In all age groups, the use of the Superbrush resulted in a significantly better outcome than the other two brushes (Figs 2-7 and 2-8).

In another clinical study, the effectiveness of two sonic toothbrushes, Water Pik Sonic Speed (Teledyne Water Pik, Fort Collins, CO) and Sonicare (Optiva Corp, Bellevue, WA) was compared to a manual toothbrush (Elmex Super 39).[29] Thirty-six healthy volunteers between 13 and 69 years of age participated in this single-blind crossover study. They were randomly assigned to three groups (A, B, C) with 12 participants each. Two weeks after a screening examination, a baseline examination was performed for each participant, followed by professional tooth cleaning. Three indices were recorded to assess the oral hygiene status: the PBI,[19] the PI,[23] and the approximal plaque index (API).[9] After 2 weeks the indices were recorded a second time. Following a further 2 weeks, the procedure was repeated until each participant had used each type of toothbrush. Compared to the manual toothbrush, the Sonic Speed and the Sonicare were more effective in removing plaque and preventing gingivitis (Figs 2-9 and 2-10).

Both studies[27,29] demonstrate that newly developed toothbrushes may contribute to significant improvements in oral hygiene.

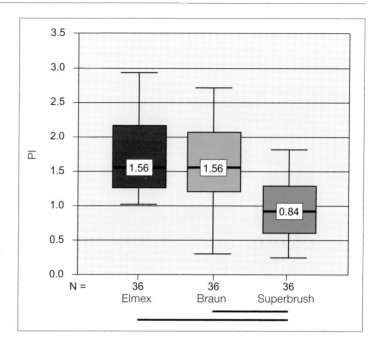

Fig 2-7 PI after brushing teeth for 1 week with three different toothbrushes (Elmex = manual toothbrush; Braun = powered toothbrush). The horizontal bars indicate statistically significant differences ($P < .01$).

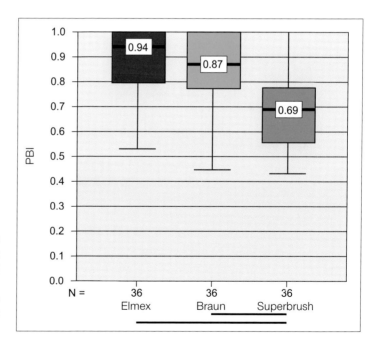

Fig 2-8 PBI after brushing teeth for 1 week with three different toothbrushes (Elmex = manual toothbrush; Braun = powered toothbrush). The horizontal bars indicate statistically significant differences ($P < .01$).

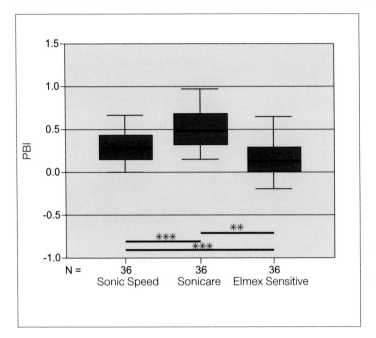

Fig 2-9 Median changes of the PBI between baseline and final examination. The horizontal bars indicate statistically significant differences (**$P < .01$, ***$P < .001$).

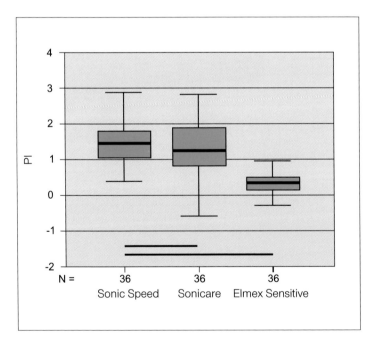

Fig 2-10 Median changes of the PI between baseline and final examination. The horizontal bars indicate statistically significant differences ($P < .01$).

Personalized Professional Prevention

Personalized professional preventive care is by far the most effective approach,[1-3] but also the most expensive given the high personal costs. Patients with low risk of dental disease may have their oral health maintained using basic preventive measures only. In contrast, patients with high risk of dental disease may require personalized professional care to maintain their oral health. Dentists therefore must be able to perform a risk assessment in order to offer their patients appropriate treatment and an effective maintenance program. This is not an easy task because it requires considerable knowledge and clinical experience. First the dentist must determine the risk factors.

Risk factors for caries in children include:

- *Stained fissures.* It is known that a stained fissure in a child has a much higher risk of developing caries than a nonstained fissure.[8,14] Stained fissures are an indication for fissure sealants to reduce the risk of caries.[13]
- *Initial lesions.* The presence of an initial lesion is indicative of disease progression. It is therefore apparent that the prevalence of initial lesions is the best predictor of susceptibility to caries.[8,26] However, this is age-related. The initial lesion is clearly an alarm signal in children and adolescents. However, this may not be the case in adults, since pre-cavitated white spot lesions can be arrested or even remineralized.[7]
- *New cavitated lesions.* The presence of new cavitated lesions is indicative of active caries. In such cases, everything should be done to limit disease progression (prevention = causal therapy).

- *Poor oral hygiene.* Since plaque is an important etiologic factor in caries and periodontal diseases, individuals with poor oral hygiene are considered to be at high risk.[6]
- *Saliva parameters.* Saliva plays a key role in the remineralization process. Individuals with xerostomia are high–caries risk patients. The microorganisms present in saliva (mutans streptococci and lactobacilli) may indicate high caries risk. However, saliva testing methods presently available lack sufficient predictive value.[26,28]
- *Fixed orthodontic appliances.* Such appliances are excellent plaque-retention sites and are very difficult to clean. It is therefore wise to classify all individuals with fixed orthodontic appliances as high–caries risk patients.

Risk factors in adults (for caries and periodontitis) include:

- *New cavitated lesions.* As already stated, new cavitated lesions are indicative of active caries.
- *Exposed root surfaces.* A root surface is more susceptible to caries than enamel because denuded roots are difficult to keep clean. Therefore, individuals with exposed root surface should be considered to be risk patients, even if the loss of periodontal attachment is only a weak predictor of root caries.[10]
- *Poor oral hygiene and salivary parameters.* Conditions such as xerostomia are risk factors at any age.
- *Loss of periodontal attachment.* Loss of attachment means that the patient has suffered periodontitis in the past. Patients with loss of attachment are considered to be risk patients because areas where loss of attachment has oc-

curred are always difficult to clean and are usually associated with exposed root surfaces.

- *Active pockets (> 4mm + bleeding on probing).* Such pockets are indicative of active periodontitis. Such periodontitis should be treated to decrease the overall risk of further disease (causal therapy = prevention).
- *Increased mobility.* This is very likely to be an indicator of progressive periodontal disease.

The frequency of the recall should be determined based on the assessment of the risk factors This is one of the most important and challenging responsibilities in contemporary clinical practice.

Because there are no clear-cut predictive criterias for different recall programs, in reality, the recall interval is determined on the basis of clinical experience. For the majority of patients, the recall program should be set at 2 to 6 sessions per year. Depending on patients' personal circumstances, the recall interval may be maintained, shortened, or increased.

Case Report

The patient, born in 1936, presented in April 1988 with severe pain associated with a periodontal abscess in relation to the left mandibular first molar. As an emergency measure, the tooth was extracted. After initial healing, the patient was entered into a comprehensive care regimen. A careful assessment of the patient (Figs 2-11a to 2-11d) helped to define the treatment plan. Following numerous hy-

giene sessions, the patient was reconstructed in two phases: first extractions were performed, followed by long-term provisional fixed partial dentures, together with essential periodontal and endodontic therapy. A long healing phase followed, after which the patient was reconstructed with definitive fixed partial dentures in 1989 (Figs 2-11e to 2-11h). Between 1989 and 1993 the patient participated, somewhat irregularly, in a recall program, attending 14 appointments in this time. The status in 1993 was virtually unchanged (Fig 2-11i) from that established in 1989. From then on he attended the recall program on a regular basis (four visits per year). In 1999 the situation was stable (Fig 2-11h). This success is not attributed to the quality of the materials used or to the skills of the dentist, but to the preventive nature of the care and the patient's involvement in the recall program.

Conclusions

From this review, it may be concluded that:

- Prevention = causal therapy. Oral health care must therefore be preventatively oriented.
- Dentists must:
  - Recommend oral self care
  - Assess risk factors
  - Offer personalized professional prevention

With such an approach, oral health care may offer compliant patients the opportunity of a lifetime for healthy teeth and supporting tissues.

Figs 2-11a to 2-11k Patient who presented with a periodontal abscess related to the left mandibular first molar in April 1988.

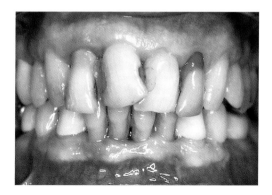

Fig 2-11a Anterior view in 1988, following the initial hygiene phase.

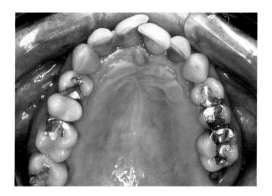

Fig 2-11b Occlusal view of the maxilla (1988).

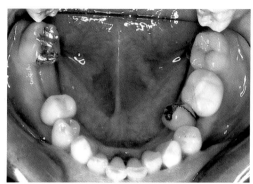

Fig 2-11c Occlusal view of the mandible (1988).

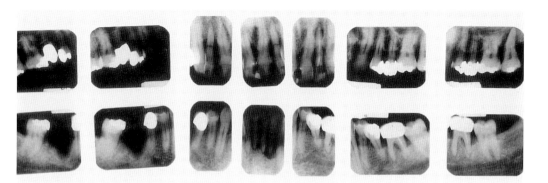

Fig 2-11d Radiographic status (1988).

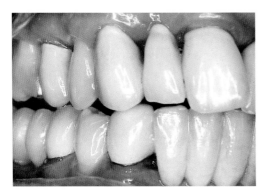

Fig 2-11e Buccal view of first and fourth quadrant following reconstruction in 1989.

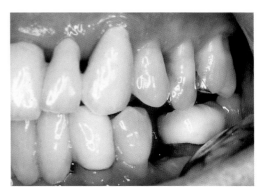

Fig 2-11f Buccal view of second and third quadrant following reconstruction in 1989.

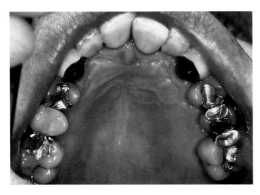

Fig 2-11g Occlusal view of the maxilla after reconstruction in 1989.

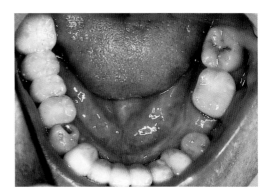

Fig 2-11h Occlusal view of the mandible after reconstruction in 1989.

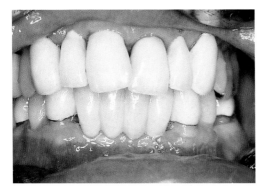

Fig 2-11i Recall appointment (1993).

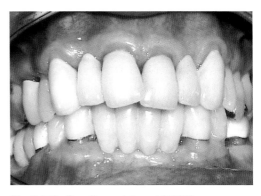

Fig 2-11k Recall appointment (1999).

References

1. Axelsson P, Lindhe J. Effect of controlled oral hygiene procedures on caries and periodontal disease in adults. Results after 6 years. J Clin Periodontol 1981;8:239–248.

2. Axelsson P, Lindhe J. The effect of a preventive programme on dental plaque, gingivitis and caries in schoolchildren. Results after one and two years. J Clin Periodontol 1974;1:126–138.

3. Axelsson P, Lindhe J, Nystrom B. On the prevention of caries and periodontal disease. Results of a 15-year longitudinal study in adults. J Clin Periodontol 1991;18:182–189.

4. Bellini HT, Arneberg P, Von der Fehr FR. Oral hygiene and caries. A review. Acta Odontol Scand 1981;39:257–265.

5. Deutscher Bundestag. Sozialgesetzbuch, 5. Buch, §22. München: Beck-Texte im DTV, 1993:122.

6. Dominguez-Rojas V, Astazion-Arbiza P, Ortega-Molina P, Gordillo-Florencio E, Garcia-Nunez JA, Bascones-Martinez A. Analysis of several risk factors involved in dental caries through multiple logistic regression. Int Dent J 1993; 43:149–156.

7. Grube M, Binus W, Bredy E. Untersuchungen über die Remineralisation von Initialkaries. Stomatol DDR 1986;36:204–209.

8. Helfenstein U, Steiner M, Marthaler TM. Caries prediction on the basis of past caries including precavity lesions. Caries Res 1991;25:372–376.

9. Lange DE, Plagmann HC, Eenboom A, Promesberger A. Klinische Bewertungsverfahren zur Objektivierung der Mundhygiene. Dtsch Zahnärztl Z 1977;32:44–47.

10. Locker D. Incidence of root caries in an older Canadian population. Community Dent Oral Epidemiol 1996;24:403–407.

11. Marthaler TM. Changes in the prevalence of dental caries: How much can be attributed to changes in diet? Caries Res 1990;24(suppl 1): 3–15.

12. Marthaler TM. The prevalence of dental caries in Europe 1990-1995. Caries Res 1996;30: 237–255.

13. Marthaler TM. Zahnmedizinische Gruppenprophylaxe in der Schweiz. Beobachtungen und Schlüsse für die Vorbeugung in Deutschland. DAZ Forum 1995;14:211–215.

14. Marthaler TM, Steiner M, Bandi A. Werden verfärbte Molaren-Fissuren innerhalb von vier Jahren häufiger kariös als nicht verfärbte? Schweiz Monatsschr Zahnmed 1990;100: 841–846.

15. Maslow AH. Motivation und Persönlichkeit. Reinbek: Rowohlt, 1999:395.

16. Mathiesen AT, Ögaard B, Rölla G. Oral hygiene as a variable in dental caries experience in 14-yearolds exposed to fluoride. Caries Res 1996;30: 29–33.

17. Menghini G, Steiner M, Marthaler TM, Bandi A. Kariesbefall bei Schülern des Kantons Glarus in den Jahren 1974 bis 1992: Wirkung der Salzfluoridierung. Schweiz Monatsschr Zahnmed 1995; 105:467–473.

18. Micheelis W, Schroeder E. Sozialwissenschaftliche Daten und Analysen der drei Alterskohorten. In: Zahnärzte IdD (ed). Dritte deutsche Mundgesundheitsstudie (DMS III). Köln: Deutscher Ärzte Verlag, 1999:433–455.

19. Mühlemann HR. Patientenmotivation mit individuellem Intensivprogramm für orale Gesundheit. In: Peters S (ed). Prophylaxe. Ein Leitfaden für die tägliche Praxis. Berlin: Quintessenz, 1978.

20. Murray JJ (ed). Appropriate use of fluorides for human health. Geneva: World Health Organization, 1986.

21. Pieper K, Deutschen Arbeitsgemeinschaft für Jugendzahnpflege. Epidemiologische Begleituntersuchungen zur Gruppenprophylaxe 1994. Bonn: Eigenverlag, 1995:1–61.

22. Pieper K, Deutschen Arbeitgemeinschaft für Jugendzahnpflege. Epidemiologische Begleituntersuchungen zur Gruppenprophylaxe 1995. Bonn: Eigenverlag, 1996:1–73.

23. Quigley GA, Hein JW. Comparative cleansing efficiency of manual and power brushing. J Am Dent Assoc 1962;65:26–29.

24. Weinstein P, Milgrom P, Melnick S, Beach B, Spadafora A. How effective is oral hygiene instruction? Results after 6 and 24 weeks. J Public Health Dent 1989;49:32–38.

25. World Health Organization Expert Committee on Oral Health Status and Fluoride Use. Fluorides and Oral Health. Geneva: World Health Organization, 1994.

26. Zimmer S, Bizhang M, Jochimski P, Roulet J-F. Ermittlung von Faktoren zur Kariesrisikorestimmung. Oralprophylaxe 1998;20:87–93.

27. Zimmer S, Didner B, Roulet J-F. Clinical study on the plaque-removing ability of a new triple-headed toothbrush. J Clin Periodontol 1999; 26:281–285.

28. Zimmer S, Dosch S, Hopfenmüller W. Kariesrisikobestimmung durch Speicheltests. Dtsch Zahnärztl Z 1995;50:806–808.

29. Zimmer S, Fosca M, Roulet J-F. Clinical Study on the Effectiveness of two Sonic Toothbrushes. J Clin Dent 2000;11:24–27.

Chapter 3

Methods for Caries Detection

Adrian Lussi

Introduction

The onset of caries is characterized by the surface demineralization of dental hard tissues. A change of diet or oral hygiene habits in combination with optimal fluoridation may stop the progression of a lesion and possibly allow its remineralization. The aim of modern dentistry must be a preventive approach rather than an invasive repair of defects. This is only possible if the remaining structural organization of the attacked tissue will still allow *restitutio ad integrum*, assuming early detection and preventive measures. Some of today's diagnostic tools are not sufficiently sensitive to detect the early onset of caries. Therefore, in many cases remineralization or stabilization is no longer possible at the time of detection, and restoration is inevitable. This, in turn, is the start of the downward spiral of restorative therapy, given the limited life expectancy of all restorative materials (Fig 3-1).

The purpose of this chapter is to compare the methods used by dental practitioners for the detection of caries with some new approaches.

Approximal Caries

Bitewing radiography has a long history in dentistry. Currently, in everyday practice such radiographic examination has an important role in the dentist's armamentarium for the detection of approximal caries. It is possible to detect small approximal lesions amenable to preventive care. Given positioning mistakes of the cone and the curvature of the dental arches, however, only about half of the proximal surfaces of the permanent dentition are free of overlaps on bitewing radiographs. The corresponding figure for the primary dentition is approximately 80%.[44] Horizontal deviation in the direction of the beam may project enamel caries into dentin on the radiograph, possibly leading to a false-positive diagnosis. Therefore, radiolucencies in dentin must be associated with corresponding radiolucencies in enamel before the decision for invasive restorative therapy is made.[28] For these reasons bitewing radiographs should be taken only after careful clinical examination. This allows optimal orientation of the beam relative to areas with suspected caries in order to prevent overlaps.

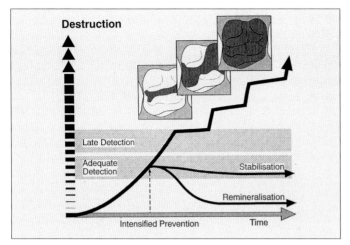

Fig 3-1 The carious process can start as soon as the teeth are erupted. In the early stages the changes are difficult or impossible to detect. Some of today's diagnostic methods are only able to detect the process at a stage at which a restoration is required (upper bar). Modern means of caries detection and monitoring should detect the carious process at a stage at which stabilization (arrestation) or even remineralization is still possible (lower bar).

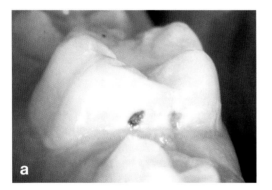 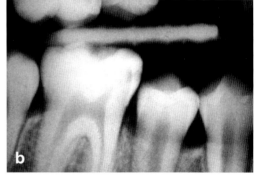

Figs 3-2a and 3-2b Cavitated approximal lesion *(a)* with corresponding bitewing radiograph *(b)*.

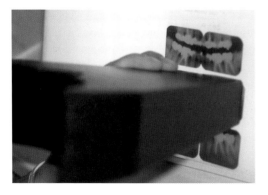

Fig 3-3 Radiographs should be read using a magnifying viewer.

Table 3-1 *In vitro* validity for the detection of dentinal caries on contacting approximal surfaces[31]

Method	Specificity	Sensitivity
Visual inspection	0.99	0.38
FOTI	0.97	0.67
Bitewing radiography	0.96	0.59

The specificity of radiographic diagnosis is 96% and the sensitivity 59% (Table 3-1).[31] A determining factor in the decision as to which therapeutic procedure to use is the condition of the approximal surface. If there is a surface discontinuity, ie, a cavitated surface, it will require restorative therapy together with general preventive measures. Various studies have dealt with the relationship between a given radiolucency in dental hard tissue and the status of the corresponding surface (Figs 3-2a and 3-2b). It has been shown that only about 10% of all approximal surfaces of permanent teeth with radiolucencies in enamel include clinically cavitated surfaces. However, the ratio increases to 100% if the radiolucency is visible in the inner half of dentin.[47] The status of the surface can only be assessed clinically when the teeth are temporarily separated. This method was therefore recommended as an aid to the diagnosis of posterior approximal caries.[35] It is important to note that the progression of a lesion through enamel may take years if oral hygiene, diet, salivary parameters, fluoride contacts, and other factors are favorable.[27,43] Judging the speed of penetration of caries is possible by comparing radiographs taken at different times. Such radiographs should, however, be taken, developed, and read (2x loupes, X-Produkter, Malmö, Sweden) under standardized conditions (Fig 3-3). The use of film holders is recommended to minimize overlaps.

Today, newer systems based on a charge-coupled device (CCD) or on storage phosphor plates are on the market. Both systems seem to be comparable in performance for the detection of approximal (and occlusal) caries.[38,55,56] In addition, these systems have the advantage of shorter exposure times compared with ultraspeed film in the range of 50% to 80%. The lower doses of radiation and the possibility of having instantaneous images that can be enhanced and stored electronically at low cost favor the increasing, widespread use of these systems.

Fiber-optical transillumination (FOTI) may be used as an additional auxiliary means for caries detection,[3,32,46] notably in the assessment of anterior teeth for which there is no appropriate radiographic assessment for caries. The sensitivity for approximal dentinal caries using a light source fitted with a special fiber-optic tip is 67% (Table 3-1).[31] This value is 8% higher, but no statistically different from the sensitivity achieved with bitewing radiographs. It should be noted that the potential of FOTI is only achieved after careful instruction in the method followed by thorough training, monitoring, and testing.[33] A study on 338 unrestored approximal surfaces in 53 students found FOTI to be the least reliable method examined for the identification of cavitated lesions.[10] Visual inspection after tooth separation may serve as a supplementary diagnostic tool to visual and radiographic examination.

Occlusal Caries

Historically, the detection of occlusal caries has been carried out with the use of a mirror, light, and explorer. The tactile sign of resistance while withdrawing the explorer has been considered diagnostic for caries, although dentists differ widely in their interpretation of this criterion.[29,54] The value of the explorer or probe in the detection of occlusal caries has recently been called into question by a number of investigators.[5,16,18,20,48,58] It has been conclusively demonstrated that conventional clinical methods result in remarkably low values for sensitivity when attempting to detect occlusal caries.[7,18,19,20,57] In the face of this evidence, it is difficult to defend the potential for iatrogenic damage of otherwise remineralizable lesions in fissures when using visual-tactile methods.[2] More modern alternative methods are available.

For occlusal surfaces, the specificity of a clinical examination exceeds 90%, ie,

sound surfaces are most often correctly recognized.[18,19,20,57] This is very important in the light of today's relatively small prevalence of occlusal caries. Surfaces that can be maintained unrestored for years with adequate preventive measures must not be treated prematurely by restorative dentistry. The sensitivity at the D_3 level (dentinal caries), ie, the ability to recognize with clinical examination methods diseased surfaces, varies between 12% and 82%.[18,19,20,57] The significant differences in the performance of the various "classical" clinical methods are related to different conditions of occlusal surfaces. Dentinal caries in teeth with a macroscopically intact occlusal surface is difficult to detect in everyday practice. Indeed, the lowest sensitivities have been found with teeth exhibiting macroscopically intact occlusal surfaces but revealing underlying dentinal caries histologically (Figs 3-4a, 3-4b, and 3-5a to 3-5d; Table 3-2). This phenomenon characterizes the so-called "hidden caries" found in between 10% and 50% of adolescents. Such caries is very difficult to diagnose correctly.[4,15,23,52,53] In such situations the use of an explorer does not improve caries detection. In the case of open lesions, the sensitivity increases to up to 82%. But even in these circumstances the use of a probe does not significantly improve the diagnostic capability. A detailed rating scheme could increase the performance[6] and thorough drying reveals opacity, which is a good indication of the carious process.[18] Instead of using mirror and probe, it is advised to use air-drying with a 3-in-1 syringe and a mirror alone. The intra-examiner reproducibility values are too low to allow monitoring of the carious process (Table 3-3).

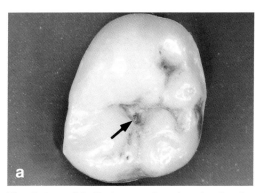 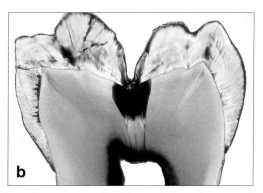

Figs 3-4a and 3-4b A noncavitated occlusal surface *(a)* and the corresponding histological section through the area marked by the arrow revealing the extent of the caries *(b)* (original magnification x 3.2).

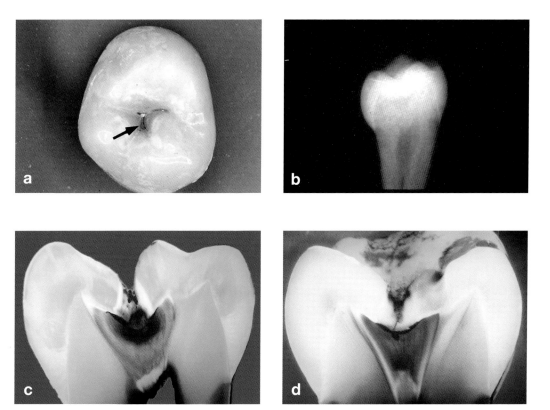

Figs 3-5a to 3-5d Occlusal surface *(a)*, radiograph *(b)*, and histological sections *(c and d)* showing the extension of caries (original magnification x 6.4).

Table 3-2 In vitro validity of different classical diagnostic methods employed by practicing dentists for occlusal surfaces at the D_3 level[18,19]

Methods	No caries (D_0) /enamel caries (D_1, D_2)
	Specificity
Visual inspection (n = 26 dentists)	0.93
Visual inspection combined with probing (n = 23)	0.93
Visual inspection with a magnifying glass (n = 26)	0.89
Bitewing radiography (BW) (n = 24)	0.83
Visual inspection combined with BW (n = 10)	0.87

Methods	Dentinal caries (D_3, D_4)	
	Sensitivity	
	No cavitation*	Cavitation
Visual inspection (n = 26 dentists)	0.12	0.62
Visual inspection combined with probing (n = 23)	0.14	0.82
Visual inspection with a magnifying glass (n = 26)	0.20	0.75
Bitewing radiography (BW) (n = 24)	0.45	0.79
Visual inspection combined with BW (n = 10)	0.49	0.90

*No cavitation = intact occlusal surface as judged by the naked eye.

Table 3-3 Interexaminer and intraexaminer reproducibility values of different classical diagnostic methods for occlusal surfaces at the D_3 level by practicing dentists[19,21]

Methods	Interexaminer reproducibility (Cohen's Kappa)		Intraexaminer reproducibility (Cohen's Kappa)	
	No cavitation	Cavitation	No cavitation	Cavitation
Visual inspection	0.18	0.61	0.49	0.51
Visual inspection combined with probing	0.24	0.45	–	–
Visual inspection with a magnifying glass	0.18	0.39	–	–
Bitewing radiography (BW)	0.45	0.84	0.55	0.67
Visual inspection combined with BW	0.46	0.85	–	–

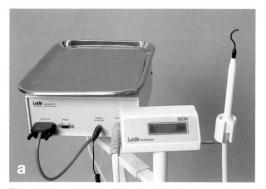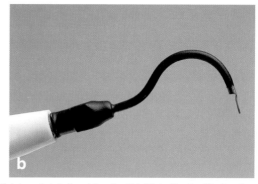

Figs 3-6a and 3-6b The electrical caries meter (ECM) *(a)* and details of the tip *(b)*. Note the facility for drying the occlusal surface.

It is not possible with bitewing radiography to detect reliably occlusal enamel lesions. The sensitivity of bitewing radiography for the detection of dentinal caries beneath a macroscopically intact surface (hidden caries) is 45%. The corresponding value for clinical inspection achieved by the same dental practitioners was below 15%[19] (Table 3-2). Hence, radiography can increase the low sensitivity of clinical diagnoses and can be useful in the detection of occlusal dentinal lesions.[11] Radiography is, however, associated with the unavoidable hazards of exposure to ionizing radiation. It is therefore strongly advised to review all available bitewing radiographs for occlusal dentinal lesions. It has been shown that radiographic appearance is of particular relevance to the level of infection of the dentin. When the tooth is radiographically sound, few bacteria can be recovered from dentin. In contrast, when a radiolucency is present in dentin, a large increase in recoverable bacteria may be found. It therefore may be concluded that if bacterial infection of demineralized dentin justifies operative intervention, the radiographic appearance of a dentinal lesion on bitewing radiographs is a good predictor of the need to intervene.[36] Lesions that are not detected radiographically may be treated using preventive measures.

The electrical resistance of a tooth is dependent on its condition.[37] Sound enamel and dentin lose their insulation properties with ongoing disintegration and replacement by a medium with better conductivity. This is the basis of the electric caries detector (Figs 3-6a and 3-6b). Electrical conductivity measurements are particularly suitable for the assessment of occlusal lesions with macroscopically intact surfaces. The electrical conductivity of a tooth changes with demineralization, even when the surface remains macroscopically intact. Several studies have demonstrated in vitro and in vivo the favorable performance of fixed frequency conductance measuring devices in the detection of occlusal dentinal caries.[14,21,36,37,50] A variable frequency method also appears to be promising for future development.[17] The disadvantage of the fixed frequency type of electrical detection system is the somewhat difficult measuring procedure. The sensitivities reported in various in vivo studies have been between 93% and 96%, which is significantly higher than with any traditional method. The respective specificities (71% to 77%) are typically smaller than with visual inspection.[21,50] These relatively small values for specificity indicate that 23% to 29% of sound teeth may be erroneously diagnosed as diseased and consequently at risk of being treated by invasive methods. Good reproducibility with this method is frustrated by factors including the fluid content of the lesion and the presence of porosity and organic material that may influence conductivity and thus the readings.

There are two widely used diagnostic light systems currently available. The one based on FOTI is especially suitable for approximal caries and the other, based on laser light, is best used for the detection of occlusal and smooth surface lesions. Among the fluorescence- and light scattering–based methods, there is presently only one system that is suitable for use in everyday practice. It is based on the detection of fluorescence radiation. Usually fluorescence is excited by (ultra)violet, blue, or green light producing fluorescence radiation with longer wavelengths that may be analyzed in the visible part of the spectrum. Spectral investigations on teeth with caries, however, revealed that a better contrast between sound and diseased regions can be achieved when fluorescence is excited in the red and detected in the near infrared region.[9] Under such conditions, fluorescence is much more intense within caries compared to sound dental tissues. This

allows optical probing into the tooth. Furthermore, the ratio between caries and sound tooth fluorescence intensity is high over the entire spectrum range of 700 to 800 nm indicating that fluorescent light can be used to discriminate between healthy and diseased tissue without the need for any spectral analysis.

On the basis of the above findings, a relatively simple instrument for caries detection has been developed (DIAGNOdent, KaVo, Biberach, Germany), containing a laser diode (655 nm, modulated, 1 mW peak power) as the excitation light source, and a photo diode combined with a long pass filter (transmission > 680 nm) as the detector. The excitation light is transmitted by an optical fiber to the tooth, and a bundle of nine fibers arranged concentrically around it serves for detection. The long pass filter absorbs the backscattered excitation and other short wavelength light and transmits the longer wavelength fluorescent radiation. To prevent the long wavelength ambient light passing through the filter, the laser diode is modulated and only light with the same modulation characteristic is registered. Thus the digital display shows quantitatively the detected fluorescence intensity (in units related to a calibration standard) according to real time and a maximum value (Fig 3-7a). A tapered fiber-optic tip has been designed for the detection of fissure caries (Fig 3-7b).

The assessment of a tooth with the laser fluorescence system is as follows: After calibration with a ceramic standard, the fluorescence of a sound area on the smooth surface of the tooth is measured to provide a baseline value. This value is then subtracted electronically from the fluorescence of the site to be assessed. To determine the extent of the caries, the

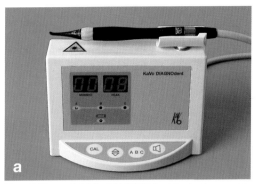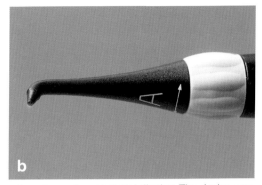

Figs 3-7a and 3-7b DIAGNOdent including real time and maximum (peak) digital display. The device consists of a probe, a fiber-optic lead, and a unit containing electronics and a laser diode *(a)*. Close-up view of the tapered tip *(b)*.

Table 3-4 In vitro validity for the detection of caries using laser fluorescence (DIAGNOdent) and electrical conductivity measurements (ECM) at the D_2 and D_3 level*[22]

	Specificity		Sensitivity		Likelihood ratio	
	D_2	D_3	D_2	D_3	D_2	D_3
Laser (moist teeth)	0.78	0.87	0.87	0.76	3.9	5.6
Laser (dried teeth)	0.72	0.79	0.83	0.84	3.0	4.0
ECM	0.64	0.78	·0.87	0.92	2.4	4.1

*Only teeth with a macroscopically intact occlusal surface were included.

instrument has to be worked around the site being assessed (Figs 3-8a to 3-8d and 3-9a to 3-9b). This ensures that the tip picks up fluorescence from the slopes of the fissure walls where caries is often initiated. A rising tone starting with a value of 10 helps the examiner to find the maximum fluorescence value for the site under assessment.

An overview of the in vitro performance at the D_2 and D_3 level of the laser system compared with electrical conductance measurements[22] is set out in Table 3-4. ECM and the DIAGNOdent were found to have comparable performance at the D_3 level. At the D_2 level, the detection of caries was more accurate with the laser. Performance values of ECM and DIAGNOdent at the D_1 level are not reported given that the two devices cannot differentiate between sound surfaces and early enamel lesions (D_1).[22]

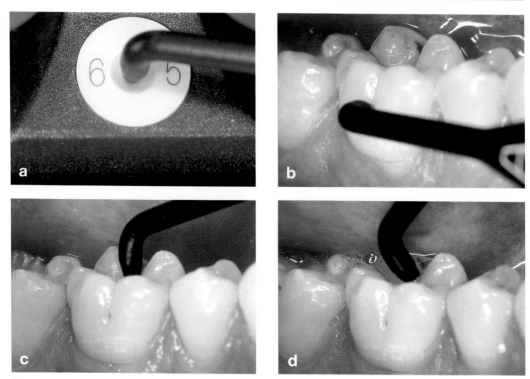

Figs 3-8a to 3-8d Once calibrated using a ceramic standard *(a)* and on a sound surface *(b)*, the tip of the laser device has to be carefully rotated around the vertical axis *(c and d)* until the maximum fluorescence value for the site being assessed is found. This ensures that the tip picks up the maximum fluorescence of the fissure walls in which the carious process starts.

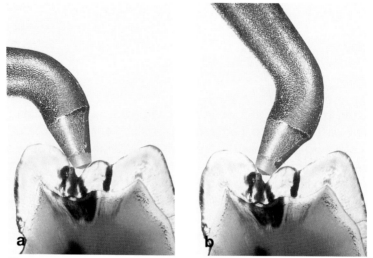

Figs 3-9a and 3-9b Histological section with the tip of the DIAGNOdent illustrating the importance of tilting of the tip to detect the carious process.

Table 3-5 Guidelines for the clinical use of DIAGNOdent in adult patients

Values	Guidelines
0 to 13	No active care is advised (NCA)
14 to 20	Preventive care is advised (PCA)
21 to 29 (approx)	Preventive or operative care is advised, depending on the patient's caries risk, the recall interval, etc (PCA or OCA)
Over 30 (approx)	Operative (and preventive) care is advised (OCA and PCA)

Generally, teeth to be assessed should be dried and cleaned to create optimal conditions for visual inspection. The laser system DIAGNOdent is, because of its high sensitivity values, especially useful for occlusal sites in which the visual diagnosis is equivocal. Experience with the device demonstrates that deposits, including plaque and calculus, in the fissure or on the tip, as well as staining and the presence of composites could give rise to a false positive reading. Thus, for this device, as well as for clinical detection, thorough cleaning is a prerequisite to the accurate diagnosis of caries. Screening of the whole fissure is only possible with careful tilting of the instrument.

The confirmed presence of caries with histological involvement of dentin should not necessitate operative intervention. The decision triggering restorative treatment is dependent upon a range of other variables, including the patient's case history and fluoride and dietary status, together with perceived caries activity and the status of the surface.[34] Triggers for operative intervention in daily practice are therefore at a DIAGNOdent value quoted in Table 3-5.

In order to receive information about cut-off values in vivo, six dental practitioners were asked to diagnose 332 teeth from 240 patients, (mean age, 19 years) either by visual inspection with magnification or with the aid of the DIAGNOdent. Prior to the study, the dentists had an audit meeting concerning caries detection. When a dentist decided to prepare a tooth, the extension of the caries was assessed with the assistance of a sharp probe. Using statistical methods, the best cut-off limits were determined and the guidelines set out in Table 3-5 developed for clinical use.[23]

Reproducibility was assessed by 11 other dentists in vitro.[23] These dentists were given initial instructions of 5 minutes duration prior to the assessment with no prior experience of the system. They were asked to initially assess the fluorescence of a sound smooth surface site (internal calibration of the tooth) and then of the site under study. Later in the same session each measurement was repeated. The quality of the intraexaminer and inter-examiner reproducibility was calculated using Cohen's Kappa statistic. The Kappa values were determined using the previously established cut-off levels for caries extending more than halfway through the enamel thickness (D_2) and for caries involving dentin. Cohen's Kappa for each of the 11 participating dentists was on average 0.90 (D_3 level) and 0.88 (D_2 level). Again, the reproducibility values achieved in an everyday practice setting were in the same order of magnitude.

Combined with the high caries detection performance of DIAGNOdent, the excellent reproducibility of this device indicates that the laser-based method may be suitable for the longitudinal monitoring of caries and, as a consequence, for assessing caries activity and the outcome of preventive interventions. Its potential application extends beyond locating dentinal lesions requiring operative intervention to facilitating the preventive-based management of dental caries.

It is suggested that a patient should always be examined clinically, first and foremost using a mirror and a 3-in-1 syringe without a probe. Drying makes decalcifications visible. If there is doubt as to the status of a particular site, further assessment should involve the use of the newer forms of diagnostic devices. This approach allows the dentist to combine the advantages of the greater specificity and speed of clinical examination with the greater sensitivity of the new devices. In no case should the detection of early caries be an indication for operative intervention. In addition, since the new devices appear to tolerate moisture on the teeth, they may find application in epidemiological surveys, although such uses require further research because specificity is still lower than for visual examination. In any case, it is important that the DIAGNOdent is tilted until the maximum peak value for a site is achieved.

Root Caries

In Switzerland, as in other countries, coronal caries has markedly decreased in recent decades, especially among adolescents.[45] This will enable many more individuals to keep their teeth into their old age. However, with gingival recession an increasing number of elderly people tend to have exposed root surfaces, bringing dentin and cementum into direct contact with the oral environment. Wallace et al[51] surveyed 603 patients older than 60 years and found 8% of exposed root surfaces to include caries or a filling. Fifty-five-year-old subjects had on average 14% of their root surfaces decayed or filled; this figure was 22% in 75-year-old patients.[8] A survey of 223 inhabitants of long-term care centers showed that 48% of the patients older than 70 years had at least one tooth affected by root surface caries (Lussi et al, unpublished data, 2000). Several investigations report root caries to be more frequent in men than in women.[1,49,51]

Dentin and cementum are more susceptible than enamel to both mechanical trauma and demineralization. The critical pH for the demineralization of root dentin appears to be about 6.7, while that of enamel is generally considered to be 5.5 under physiological concentrations of calcium and phosphate ions, and in the

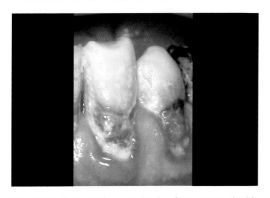

Fig 3-10 Root surface caries is often covered with plaque. This plaque must be removed to assess the surface.

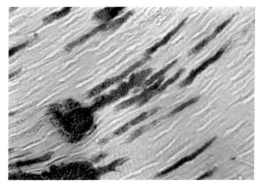

Fig 3-11 Invasion of microorganisms into the dentinal tubules with lateral spread of the bacteria.

range of 4.5 when fluoride is present in the surrounding environment.[13]

Caries on root surfaces, like coronal caries, is caused primarily by acids from the bacterial fermentation of sugars in dental plaque. Therefore, susceptible sites are mostly covered with plaque, stained yellow, brown, or black and may exhibit roughened surfaces. Since small lesions of caries are hardly discernible under extended bacterial plaque, mechanical cleaning of all root surfaces is, as it is for other surfaces, an important prerequisite to any clinical examination. Usually, no carious demineralization is to be expected directly subadjacent to dental calculus. Nevertheless, such deposits need to be removed in the process of completing a thorough examination (Fig 3-10).

Root caries is usually densely colored from yellowish-brown to dark brown or even black. It must be noted, however, that the color of a lesion does not correlate with its activity.[26,39] All colors may be associated with all degrees of caries activity. Signifi-

cantly higher levels of mutans streptococci and lactobacilli are present in soft rather than hard caries, in large rather than small lesions, and in lesions close to rather than remote from the gingival margin.[25] Mutans streptococci and lactobacilli seem to be the most reliable microbiologic indicators of the activity of a lesion. Surface hardness, as assessed with a sharp explorer, appears to be the most important parameter for the differentiation of root caries activity. Hard lesions appear to harbor significantly less cariogenic microorganisms such as mutans streptococci or lactobacilli than do leathery or soft lesions.[26] These findings correlate well with results from histologic investigations in which mineralizing processes and dead bacteria were found in hard lesions, whereas soft lesions, were invaded by microorganisms in the dentinal tubules (Fig 3-11) with lateral spread of the bacteria and loss of inorganic substance and organic matrix.[30,40–42] Soft, active lesions exhibit markedly lower pH-values than do inactive

Table 3-6 The validity of different methods presently used for the detection of noncavitated lesions of caries

Methods	Approximal surface	Smooth surface	Occlusal surface	Root surface
Visual (after drying)	−*	++	+	+
Visual and tactile	−	−	−	++
Light systems (FOTI, laser)	+†	+	++	+
Electrical conductance	−	+	++	+
Radiography	++	−	+	−

+, applicable; −, not applicable; ++, method of choice.
*Applicable after tooth separation.
†FOTI in posterior teeth only after supervised training.

sites.[12] Clinically, it may be concluded that, in contrast to occlusal sites, probing of root surfaces is of great value and that hard lesions may be judged "inactive" or "resting" whereas soft lesions must be considered "active" or "progressive." Leathery defects are somewhere in between, but should, as a precaution, be considered active rather than inactive.

Conclusions

In summary, it can be stated that a combination of several methods, depending on the surface being assessed, have to be used for optimal caries detection. An overview of the validity of different methods for detection of lesions of caries is set out in Table 3-6.

References

1. Beck JD, Hunt RJ, Hand JS, Field HM. Prevalence of root and coronal caries in a non-industrialized older population. J Am Dent Assoc 1985;111: 964–967.

2. Bergman G, Lindén LA. The action of the explorer on incipient caries. Sven Tandlak Tidskr 1969;62:629–634.

3. Choksi SK, Brady JM, Dang DH, Rao MS. Detecting approximal dental caries with transillumination: A clinical evaluation. J Am Dent Assoc 1994;125:1098–1102.

4. Creanor SL, Russell JI, Strang DM, Stephen KW, Burchell CK. The prevalence of clinically undetected occlusal dentine caries in Scottish adolescents. Br Dent J 1990;169:126–129.

5. Ekstrand K, Qvist V, Thylstrup A. Light microscope study of the effect of probing in occlusal surfaces. Caries Res 1987;21:368–374.

6. Ekstrand K, Ricketts DNS, Kidd EAM. Reproducibility and accuracy of three methods for assessment of demineralization depth on the occlusal surface: An in vitro examination. Caries Res 1997;31:224–231.

7. Ferreira Zandona AG, Analoui M, Beiswanger BB, et al. An in vitro comparison between laser fluorescence and visual examination for detection of demineralization in occlusal pits and fissures. Caries Res 1998; 32:210–218.

8. Fure S, Zickert J. Prevalence of root surface caries in 55-, 65-, and 75-year-old Swedish individuals. Community Dent Oral Epidemiol 1990;18: 100–105.

9. Hibst R. Optische Meßmethoden zur Kariesdiagnose. ZWR 1999;108:50–55.

10. Hintze H, Wenzel A, Danielsen B, Nyvad B. Reliability of visual examination, fibre-optic transillumination, and bite-wing radiography, and reproducibility of direct visual examination following tooth separation for the identification of cavitated carious lesions in contacting approximal surfaces. Caries Res 1998;32:204–209.

11. Hintze H, Wenzel A, Jones C. In vitro comparison of D- and E- speed film radiography, RVG, and visualix digital radiography for the detection of enamel approximal and dentinal occlusal caries lesions. Caries Res 1994;28:363–367.

12. Hojo S, Komatsu M, Okuda R, Takahashi N, Yamada T. Acid profiles and pH of carious dentine in active and arrested lesions. J Dent Res 1994; 73:1853–1857.

13. Hoppenbrouwers PMM, Driessens FCM, Borggreven JMPM. The mineral solubility of human tooth roots. Arch Oral Biol 1987;32:319–322.

14. Huysmans MC, Longbottom C, Hintze H, Verdonschot EH. Surface-specific electrical occlusal caries diagnosis: reproducibility, correlation with histological lesion depth, and tooth type dependence. Caries Res 1998;32:330–336.

15. Kidd EAM, Naylor MN, Wilson RF. Prevalence of clinically undetected and untreated molar occlusal dentine caries in adolescents on the Isle of Wight. Caries Res 1992;26:397–401.

16. Loesche WJ, Svanberg ML, Pape HR. Intraoral transmission of streptococcus mutans by a dental explorer. J Dent Res 1979;58;1765–1770.

17. Longbottom C, Huysmans MC, Pitts NB, Los P, Bruce PG. Detection of dental decay and its extent using AC impedance spectroscopy. Nat Med 1996;2:235–237.

18. Lussi A. Comparison of different methods for the diagnosis of fissure caries without cavitation. Caries Res 1993;27:409–416.

19. Lussi A. Impact of including or excluding cavitated lesions when evaluating methods for the diagnosis of occlusal caries. Caries Res 1996; 30:389–393.

20. Lussi A. Validity of diagnostic and treatment decisions of fissure caries. Caries Res 1991; 25:296–303.

21. Lussi A, Firestone A, Schoenberg V, Hotz P, Stich H. In vivo diagnosis of fissure caries using a new electrical resistance monitor. Caries Res 1995; 29:81–87.

22. Lussi A, Imwinkelried S, Pitts NB, Longbottom C, Reich E. Performance and reproducibility of a laser fluorescence system for detection of occlusal caries in vitro. Caries Res 1999;33: 261–266.

23. Lussi A, Megert B, Longbottom C, Braig F, Reich E, Francescut P. Clinical performance of a laser fluorescence device for detection of occlusal caries lesions. Eur J Oral Sci 2001; 109:1–6.

24. Lussi A, Menghini G, Steiner M, Marthaler TM. The impact of radiography and electrical conductivity measurements on the prevalence of occlusal caries in epidemiological surveys [abstract 124]. Caries Res 1997;31:322.

25. Lynch E. Relationships between clinical criteria and microflora of primary root caries. In: Stookey GK (ed). Early Detection of Dental Caries. Indianapolis: Indiana Univ School of Dentistry, 1996:195–242.

26. Lynch E, Breighton D. A comparison of primary root caries lesions classified according to colour. Caries Res 1994;28:233–239.

27. Marthaler TM, Steiner M, Bandi A. Werden verfärbte Molarenfissuren innerhalb von vier Jahren häufiger kariös als nichtverfärbte? Schweiz Monatsschr Zahnmed 1990;100:841–848.

28. Mileman PA, Mulder H, Van Der Weele LT. Factors influencing the likelihood of successful decisions to treat dentine caries from bitewing radiographs. Communtiy Dent Oral Epidemiol 1992; 20:175–180.

29. Newbrun E, Brudevold F, Mermagen H. A microradiographic evaluation of occlusal fissures and grooves. J Am Dent Assoc 1959;58:26–31.

30. Nyvad B, Fejerskov O. Active and inactive root surface caries: Structural entities? In: Thylstrup A, Leach SA, Qvist V (eds). Dentine and Dentine Reactions in the Oral Cavity: Proceedings of a Workshop 24–28 February 1987, Kage, Denmark. Oxford: IRI Press, 1987:165–180.

31. Peers A, Hill FJ, Mitropoulos CM, Holloway PJ. Validity and reproducibility of clinical examination, fiber-optic transillumination, and bitewing radiology for the diagnosis of small approximal carious lesions: An in vitro study. Caries Res 1993; 27:307–311.

32. Pieper K, Schurade B. Die Untersuchung mit der Kaltlicht-Diagnose Sonde. Eine Alternative zum Flügelbiss-Status? Dtsch Zahnarztl Z 1987;42:900–903.

33. Pine CM. Fiber-optic transillumination (FOTI) in caries diagnosis. In: Stookey GK (ed). Early Detection of Dental Caries. Indianapolis: Indiana Univ School of Dentistry, 1996:51–65.

34. Pitts NB. Diagnostic tools and measurements — Impact on appropriate care. Community Dent Oral Epidemiol 1997;25:24–35.

35. Pitts NB, Longbottom C. Temporary tooth separation with special reference to the diagnosis and preventive management of equivocal approximal carious lesions. Quintessence Int 1987; 18:563–573.

36. Ricketts DNJ, Kidd EAM, Beighton D. Operative and microbiological validation of visual, radiographic and electronic diagnosis of occlusal caries in non-cavitated teeth judged to be in need of operative care. Br Dent J 1995;179:214–220.

37. Rock WP, Kidd EAM. The electronic detection of demineralization in occlusal fissures. Br Dent J 1988;164:243–247.

38. Russell M, Pitts NB. Radiovisiographic diagnosis of dental caries: Initial comparison of basic mode videoprints with bitewing radiography. Caries Res 1993;27:65–70.

39. Schaeken MJM, Keltjens HMAM, Van der Hoeven JS. Effects of fluoride and chlorhexidine on the microflora of dental root surfaces and progression of root surface caries. J Dent Res 1991; 70:150–153.

40. Schüpbach P, Guggenheim B, Lutz F. Histopathology of root surface caries. J Dent Res 1990;69:1195–1204.

41. Schüpbach P, Guggenheim B, Lutz F. Human root caries: Histopathology of advanced lesions. Caries Res 1990;28:301–306.

42. Schüpbach P, Guggenheim B, Lutz F. Human root caries: Histopathology of arrested lesions. Caries Res 1992;26:153–164.

43. Schwartz M, Gröndahl HG, Pliskin J, Boffa J. A longitudinal analysis from bite-wing radiographs of the rate of progression of approximal carious lesions through human dental enamel. Arch Oral Biol 1984;29:529–536.

44. Stassinakis A, Grüninger A, Hugo B, Hotz P. Die Häufigkeit von Zahnüberlagerungen im Interdentalraum bei Bitewing-Röntgenbildern. Acta Med Dent Helv 1996;1:70–74.

45. Steiner M, Menghini G, Curilovic Z, Marthaler T. Kariesbefall der Schüler der Stadt Zürich im Zeitraum 1970-1993. Schweiz Monatsschr Zahnmed 1994;104:1210–1218.

46. Stephen KW, Russell JI, Creanor SL, Burchell CK. Comparison of fiber-optic transillumination with clinical and radiographic caries diagnosis. Community Dent Oral Epidemiol 1987;15:90–94.

47. Thylstrup A, Bille J, Qvist V. Radiographic and observed tissue changes in approximal carious lesions at the time of operative intervention. Caries Res 1986;20:75–84.

48. Van Dorp CSE, Exterkate AM, Ten Cate JM. The effect of dental probing on subsequent enamel demineralization. J Dent Child 1988; 55:343–347.

49. Vehkalahti M. Occurence of root caries and factors related to it. Proc Finn Dent Soc 1987; 83:835–899.

50. Verdonschot EH, Bronkhorst EM, Burgersdijk RCW, König KG, Schaeken MJM, Truin GJ. Performance of some diagnostic systems in examinations for small occlusal carious lesions. Caries Res 1992;26:59–64.

51. Wallace MC, Retief DH, Bradley EL. Prevalence of root caries in a population of older adults. Gerodontics 1988;4:84–89.

52. Weerheijm KL, Groen HJ, Bast AJJ, Kieft JA, Eijkman MAJ, Van Amerongen WE. Clinically undetected occlusal dentine caries: A radiographic comparison. Caries Res 1992;26: 305–309.

53. Weerheijm KL, Gruythuysen RJM, Van Amerongen WE. Prevalence of hidden caries. J Dent Child 1992;59:408–412.

54. Weerheijm KL, Van Amerongen WE, Eggink CO. The clinical diagnosis of occlusal caries: A problem. J Dent Child 1989;56:196–200.

55. Wenzel A. Digital radiography and caries diagnosis. Dentomaxillofac Radiol 1998;3:3–11.

56. Wenzel A, Borg E, Hintze H, Gröhndahl HG. Accuracy of caries diagnosis in digital images from charge coupled device and storage phosphor systems: An in vitro study. Dentomaxillofac Radiol 1995;24:250–254.

57. Wenzel A, Larsen MJ, Fejerskov O. Detection of occlusal caries without cavitation by visual inspection, film radiographs, xeroradiographs, and digitized radiographs. Caries Res 1991;25: 365–371.

58. Yassin OM. In vitro studies of the effect of a dental explorer on the formation of an artificial carious lesions. J Dent Child 1995;62:111–117.

59

Chapter 4

Assessment of Caries Risk in the Clinic— A Modern Approach

Douglas Bratthall, J. Ramanathan Stjernswärd, and Gunnel Hänsel Petersson

Introduction

This chapter deals with caries risk and how caries risk assessment may be performed for a patient. It is based on the view that the main etiological factors for dental caries are known and that these factors can be identified and often modified to the benefit of the patient.

A general discussion about the term *risk* is presented at the beginning of the chapter. This is followed by an explanation regarding the factors generally associated with caries risk. Finally, to illustrate and assess caries risk, a new concept, the Cariogram, is introduced.

Risk

The definition of risk is "the probability that some harmful event will occur." Consequently, caries risk is the probability that caries lesions will develop or progress. Assessment of caries risk is performed to predict if an individual will develop caries lesions during a specified period of time.

The assessment is based on a particular exposure status of etiological factors, supposed to remain stable during the period in question. Thus, *caries risk* relates to the likelihood of a person developing caries lesions for a subsequent period of time. The importance of properly predicting the occurrence of lesions is obvious; targeted preventive actions can be directed to those persons, or teeth, with a high risk of caries.

Factors to Be Considered in the Assessment of Caries Risk

Several attempts have been made to assess caries risk, but so far the "perfect" method is missing, which is not surprising considering the multifactorial etiology of dental caries. On the other hand, there are several factors and characteristics that often accompany the development of an increased number of caries lesions, which is the reason why an evaluation of such parameters is often helpful in caries risk assessment.

Figs 4-1a and 4-1b An illustration of the factors directly involved in biochemical events on the tooth surface.

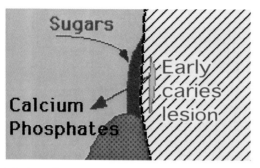

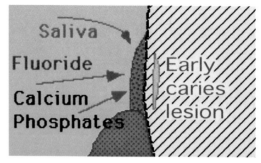

Fig 4-1a The figure illustrates in a simple way those factors that are directly involved in the biochemical events (on the tooth surface) resulting in caries lesions. The figure shows the dental plaque to which sugars or other fermentable carbohydrates are added. The acid formation results in calcium and phosphates being dissolved from the enamel.

Fig 4-1b This figure illustrates the remineralization stage. Acid formation has ceased and saliva buffers remaining acids. If fluoride is present, remineralization, where calcium and phosphates are redeposited into the enamel, is favored.

When considering the caries-causing factors, it is important to differentiate between factors that are directly involved in the biochemical events that occur on the tooth surface and result in caries lesions (Figs 4-1a and 4-1b), and factors or circumstances that are indirectly related to such events.

Biochemical Factors

These are factors that contribute to the development of the lesion to which the tooth surface is directly exposed. They are thus directly part of the causal chain (Table 4-1).

Each of the factors has to be considered in terms of dose and duration. For example, a large amount of plaque (high dose) only indicates high risk if present for a long period of time (long duration).

Strictly speaking, one could say that the only true risk factor is bacteria because the microorganisms "make" the acids that result in the demineralization. Fermentable carbohydrates constitute an essential factor. Fluorides and saliva are factors modifying the outcome of the bacterial actions. The favorable—or unfavorable—mix of these components determines whether caries lesions will develop over time.

Factors Contributing to Caries Risk and Prevalence

This group includes various factors that are not directly involved in "making" the caries lesion on the tooth surface, but may, in one way or another, be part of the causal chain (Table 4-2).

Table 4-1 Examples of factors to be considered in caries risk assessment

Direct factor	High caries risk	Low caries risk
Amount of plaque	Large amount of plaque on the teeth, indicating large numbers of bacteria that can produce acids, leading to low pH and demineralization	Few bacteria or absence of plaque, indicating good oral hygiene
Type of bacteria	Large proportion of "cariogenic" bacteria resulting in lower pH, sticky plaque, and prolonged acid production	Lower proportion of "cariogenic" bacteria
Type of diet	High in carbohydrates, in particular sucrose; "sticky" diet leading to low pH for longer periods	Low sugar content; non- "sticky" diet
Frequency of carbohydrate intake	High frequency of fermentable carbohydrate intakes resulting in low pH for longer periods of each day	Low frequency of fermentable carbohydrate intakes
Saliva secretion	Reduced saliva flow leading to prolonged sugar clearance time and to a reduced effect of other saliva protective systems	Optimal; helps to wash away sugars and acids
Saliva buffer capacity	Low buffer capacity resulting in low pH for prolonged periods	Optimal; relatively short time at low pH
Fluorides	Absent; reduced remineralization	Available; increased remineralization

Table 4-2 Examples of indirect factors to be considered in caries risk assessment

Indirect factor	High caries risk	Low caries risk
Socioeconomic circumstances	Unemployed, underprivileged, poor economy, poorly educated, not well-educated parents, and irregular dental check-ups leading to poor oral hygiene	Privileged, educated, employed, and regular dental check-ups resulting in good oral hygiene
General health	Serious disease or treatment of the disease affects salivary secretion, more cariogenic food intake; physical handicap may lead to poor oral hygiene	Good health and fitness associated with noncariogenic food intake and good oral hygiene
Epidemiological circumstances	Living in high DMF country/area, member of family with high DMF, high past caries experience, preexisting lesions and fillings in the mouth	Living in low DMF country, member of family with low DMF, low past caries experience, absence of preexisting lesions/fillings in the mouth
Clinical findings	Early signs of caries (white spots) in newly erupted teeth, exposed root surfaces, crowded teeth, deep fissures, natural retentive sites, and retentive sites caused by dental treatment	Absence of white spots in the teeth, no natural or treatment-induced retentive sites

These circumstances can result in more cariogenic food intake, in less than acceptable oral hygiene, saliva problems, and reduced fluoride support. However, it should be noted that they do not necessarily result in increased caries risk. For example, "poor economy" can, under certain conditions, promote caries if carbohydrate products are cheaper than protein-rich foods in that area. In another society, a poor economy may actually decrease caries risk because buying sweets would be considered a luxury.

Certain diseases, or their treatment, affect saliva secretion and can also result in more cariogenic food intake and in poor oral hygiene. In various ways, handicaps also can affect oral hygiene.

Epidemiological circumstances exist when a location or a family with high DMF can be characterized by frequent intakes of cariogenic food, high mutans streptococcal load, unacceptable oral hygiene, or low fluoride concentrations in the drinking water. High past caries experience indicates that individuals are susceptible to caries; moreover, the same factors that caused the past disease may still be in operation. The distribution of preexisting lesions and fillings reflects to some extent the cariogenic pressure that has been in operation. Fillings and cavities in anterior teeth in the mandible, for example, indicate a serious situation because these teeth are normally the last ones to be affected by caries.

Early signs of caries can reflect an ongoing carious process and are therefore not a real risk indicator because the risk stage has already passed. It is, however, a risk factor in the sense that the caries process may continue in the future. Newly erupted teeth and exposed root surfaces have relatively low resistance to caries. Crowded teeth and various retentive sites, including orthodontic appliances, indicate risk for increased plaque accumulation and reduced saliva flow over the involved tooth surfaces.

For each of the circumstances or indirect factors mentioned, the reason they may indicate increased caries risk is that they, in one way or another, reflect or contribute to the biochemical events on the tooth surface on which caries may develop.

Evaluation of Factors Influencing Caries Risk Assessment

Several studies have tried to evaluate how reliable the parameters described above are in the prediction of caries.[8,15,16] Some of these studies have related caries development to just one or two factors, while others have included a large set of factors. The studies have been both cross-sectional and longitudinal. Often, methods such as simple correlation, sensitivity/specificity, and positive/negative predictive values have been used to illustrate the results.[9,14] Such methods are suitable to test, for example, the accuracy of analytical methods, but are seldom useful for evaluating factors in a multifactorial disease. Consequently, nearly all previous attempts have given low or moderate values for predictive ability.

Risk and
Risk Assessment Models

Formal caries risk assessment has been described by Beck as a four-step process.[1] The first two steps involve identification of risk factors and the development of a multivariate assessment tool or model that uses the risk factors in a way that weighs them according to their level of statistical influence. The third step is the assessment process, which entails application of the caries risk model to individuals to identify their risk profiles. The fourth step is targeting the application of a disease-prevention regimen or treatment procedure that is matched to the risk profile of each individual.

According to Moss,[12] the first two steps of caries risk assessment have to date received the most attention. A wide variety of risk factors have been identified and a number of investigative teams have developed multivariate risk assessment models that can be used to assign risk profiles to individuals. These models have not, however, been as accurate as had been hoped and, as a consequence, have not enjoyed wide use in either public health or private practice settings.

In 1989, a risk assessment conference was held at the University of North Carolina.[13] The conclusions drawn included:

- Clinical variables were considered stronger predictors than nonclinical variables.
- Past caries experience was viewed as the most significant predictor; other important variables were accepted, including socioeconomic status, fluoride exposure, tooth morphology, and microbial agents.

- Regression models using multiple factors and longitudinal data were considered to be the preferred analysis.

In 1998, Powell[15] published a review article for the purpose of summarizing and evaluating prediction models. Conclusions from this review included:

- Clinical variables, especially past caries experience, were confirmed as the most significant predictor of future caries development.
- The status of the most recently erupted/exposed surface was the most successful measure of past caries experience.
- Bacterial levels were included in the most accurate prediction models.
- Sociodemographic variables were most important to caries prediction models for young children and older adults.

Thus, several sources encourage the inclusion of "past caries experience" in risk assessment models. A high past caries experience indicates that the person has previously had active caries. This condition may remain prevalent in the patient. If newly erupted tooth surfaces show signs of caries, this indicates that the person has active caries. However, in another situation, the activity may be a sign of past activity. For example, a 50-year-old person may have had active caries as a teenager. Having changed behavior, he may no longer have active caries. The high past caries experience is therefore not a good parameter to predict future caries in such cases. If successful measures are introduced to reduce caries activity, past caries experience loses its value as a predictive instrument.

Dental caries is a disease that can be prevented, treated, and controlled. The practicing dentist, however, still needs a tool that will be of assistance in assessing and predicting caries risk in patients. A working model for caries risk assessment is therefore required for use in everyday practice.

Cariogram

The Cariogram is a computer program that serves as a new risk assessment model. This program assesses and graphically illustrates the caries risk for a patient, expressed as the "chance to avoid new caries" in the coming year. The Cariogram can also demonstrate how and to what extent the various caries-causing factors may affect this "chance."

The original Cariogram was first presented in 1996. It was developed as part of a project aimed at describing the factors of importance for the caries decline in recent times in industrialized countries.[7] It appeared that there was a need to find a simple way to relate this caries decline to various strategies, such as reduced sucrose intake, improved oral hygiene, and promotion of the proper use of fluorides. The Cariogram has similarities with the circles of Keyes,[11] but differs in that it provides for the possibility to single out individual risk or resistant factors. Based on the original Cariogram concept, an interactive version for caries risk assessment was developed.[5] The original purpose of the program was educational in that it illustrates a possible risk evaluation. It does not diminish the responsibility of the dentist, but it may help in making correct decisions.

The aims of the Cariogram are to:

- Illustrate the chance to avoid caries
- Illustrate the interaction of caries-related factors
- Express caries risk graphically
- Recommend targeted preventive actions
- Motivate patients in the clinical setting
- Provide an educational program

Five Sectors of the Cariogram

The Cariogram is a pie-circle diagram, as seen on the computer screen. The diagram is divided into five sectors in the following colors: green, dark blue, red, light blue, and yellow, indicating the different groups of factors related to dental caries. An explanation of each sector is set out in Fig 4-2.

Implications of "Chance to Avoid Caries"

The "chance to avoid caries" (green sector) and caries risk are explanations of the same process, but are expressed inversely. When the chance is high, the caries risk is small and vice versa, as follows:

Caries risk	Chance to avoid caries	Cariogram
High risk	Low chance	Small green sector
Low risk	High chance	Large green sector

The Cariogram works as follows: The patient is examined and data are collected for some factors of direct relevance to

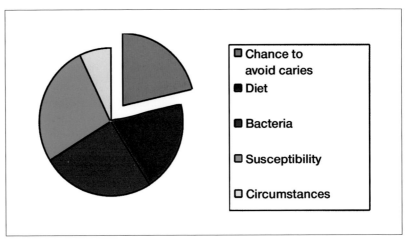

Fig 4-2 The Cariogram for caries risk assessment. The dark blue sector "Diet" is based on a combination of diet contents and diet frequency. The red sector "Bacteria" is based on a combination of amount of plaque and mutans streptococci. The light blue sector "Susceptibility" is based on a combination of fluoride therapies, saliva secretion, and saliva buffer capacity. The yellow sector "Circumstances" is based on a combination of caries experience and related diseases. The green sector shows an estimate of the "chance to avoid caries."

caries, namely bacteria-, diet-, and susceptibility-related factors. The various factors are given a score according to a predetermined scale, and entered into the computer program. According to a weighted formula, the program presents a pie diagram in which "bacteria" appears as a red sector, "diet" as a dark blue sector, and "susceptibility" as a light blue sector. In addition, "circumstances" are presented as a yellow sector. The four sectors are mapped out and what is left—the chance to avoid caries—appears as a green sector (Fig 4-2). Details of the factors that are included and the data needed to give scores for the Cariogram are presented in Table 4-3.

Accuracy of the Cariogram

In an article entitled "Caries Risk Assessment: A Comparison Between the Computer Program "Cariogram," Dental Students and Dental Instructors,"[10] the Cariogram program was applied to a set of patients. The outcome of the risk evaluation was compared with assessments made by dental students and faculty.

A questionnaire was given to the participants, containing descriptions of five patients with detailed information on nine factors generally associated with caries. The participants were asked to rank the patients according to their "chance to avoid dental caries" during the coming year.

The results indicated that 86% of the respondents ranked the patients for caries risk either identically to, or with only one deviation from, the program. No difference was seen between students and teachers.

It was concluded that the opinion of caries risk according to the Cariogram was in agreement with that of the majority of the respondents. In addition, the use of the

Table 4-3 Caries-related factors and the data needed to create a Cariogram*

Factor	Comment	Information/data required
Caries experience	Past caries experience, including cavities, fillings, and missing teeth due to caries. Several new caries lesions definitely appearing during preceding year should give a high score even if number of fillings is low	DMFT, DMFS, new caries experience in the past year
Related diseases	General disease or conditions associated with dental caries.	Medical history, medications
Diet, contents	Estimation of the cariogenicity of the food, in particular sugar content	Diet history, lactobacillus test count
Diet, frequency	Estimation of number of meals and snacks per day, mean for "normal" days	Questionnaire results, 24-hour recall, or dietary recall (3 days)
Plaque amount	Estimation of oral hygiene, for example according to Silness-Löe Plaque Index (PI). Crowded teeth leading to difficulties in removing plaque interproximally should be taken into account	Plaque index
Mutans streptococci	Estimation of levels of mutans streptococci (*Streptococcus mutans, Streptococcus sobrinus*) in saliva, for example using a mutans streptococci test	Mutans streptococci test
Fluoride program	Estimation of to what extent fiuoride is available in the oral cavity over the coming period of time	Fluoride exposure, patient's views
Saliva secretion	Estimation of amount of saliva, for example using paraffin-stimulated secretion and expressing results as mL/min of saliva	Stimulated saliva test, secretion rate
Saliva buffer capacity	Estimation of capacity of saliva to buffer acids, for example using the Dentobuff test	Dentobuff test

*For each factor, the examiner has to gather information by interviewing and examining the patient, including some saliva tests. The information is then given a score on a scale ranging from 0 to 3 (0 to 2 for some factors), according to predetermined criteria. The score "0" is the most favorable value and the maximum score of "3" (or "2") indicates a high, unfavorable risk value. Further information, together with a detailed description and explanation as to how to use the Cariogram, is available.[2-6]

Figs 4-3 to 4-5 Examples of Cariogram estimation of caries risk. Values have been entered in the boxes to the right, according to predetermined scales.

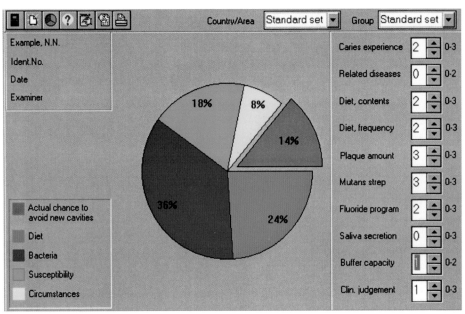

Fig 4-3 Data for a patient with high caries risk (small green sector).

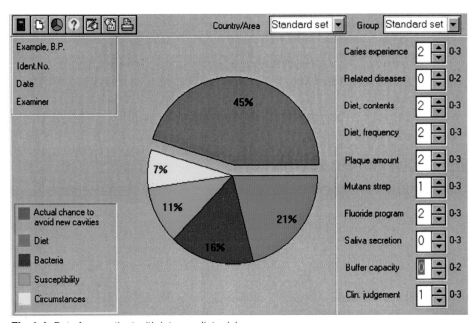

Fig 4-4 Data for a patient with intermediate risk.

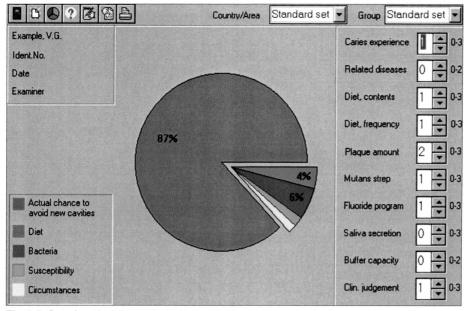

Fig 4-5 Data for a low-risk patient.

program encouraged discussions about the relative impact of the various etiological factors of caries. It is believed that the Cariogram can serve to complement the teaching of caries risk. Several new studies are now underway to further evaluate the program.

The Cariogram can assess caries risk for a patient and be used to illustrate simply how various caries-related factors can interact (Figs 4-3 to 4-5). This computer program model is useful in various clinical situations in which there is a need to discuss the importance of the various etiological factors of caries. In its interactive version, it is possible to use the program to demonstrate how the caries risk may change as a result of various cor-

rective actions. The program is also an educational interactive program for the computer, developed to extend the understanding of the multifactorial complexity of dental caries. It acts as a guide when estimating the individual caries risk, but it does not replace personal, professional judgement of caries risk. The Cariogram is a tool to motivate the patient and may serve to complement clinical decision making when selecting preventive strategies for the patient.

References

1. Beck JD. Identification of risk factors. In: Bader JD (ed). Risk Assessment in Dentistry. Chapel Hill: Dept. of Dental Ecology, Univ of North Carolina School of Dentistry, 1990:8–13.

2. Bratthall D, Hänsel-Petersson G, Stjernswärd JR. Cariogram manual [in Japanese]. Tokyo: Oral Care, 1999.

3. Bratthall D, Hänsel-Petersson G, Stjernswärd JR. Cariogram manual [in Portuguese]. São Paulo: BCE Corporation, 1998.

4. Bratthall D, Hänsel-Petersson G, Stjernswärd JR. Cariogramhandboken. Stockholm: Förlagshuset Gothia AB, 1997.

5. Bratthall D, Hänsel-Petersson G, Stjernswärd JR. Kariogramm Anleitung. Vaduz, Liechtenstein: International Health Care Foundation, 1999.

6. Bratthall D, Hänsel-Petersson G, Stjernswärd JR, Bian JY. Cariogram manual [in Chinese]. Beijing: National Committee for Oral Health, 1999.

7. Bratthall D, Hänsel-Petersson G, Sundberg H. Reasons for the caries decline: What do the experts believe? Eur J Oral Sci 1996;104(4, part 2):16–422.

8. Demers M, Brodeur J-M, Simard PL, Mouton C, Veilleux G, Frechette S. Caries predictors suitable for mass-screenings in children: A literature review. Community Dent Health 1990;7:11–21.

9. Douglass CW. Risk assessment in dentistry. J Dent Educ 1998;62:756–761.

10. Hänsel-Petersson G, Carlsson P, Bratthall D. Caries risk assessment: A comparison between the computer program "Cariogram", dental students and dental instructors. Eur J Dent Educ 1998; 2:184–190.

11. Keyes PH. Recent advances in dental caries research. Int Dent J 1962;12:443–464.

12. Moss ME, Zero DT. An overview of caries risk assessment, and its potential utility. J Dent Educ 1995;59:932–940.

13. Newbrun E, Leverett D. Risk assessment dental caries working group summary statement. In: Bader JD (ed). Risk Assessment in Dentistry. Chapel Hill: Dept. of Dental Ecology, Univ of North Carolina School of Dentistry, 1990:304.

14. Pitts NB. Risk assessment and caries prediction. J Dent Educ 1998;62:762–770.

15. Powell LV. Caries prediction: A review of the literature. Community Dent Oral Epidemiol 1998;26: 361–71.

16. Powell LV. Caries risk assessment: Relevance to the practitioner. J Am Dent Assoc 1998;129: 349–53.

Part 2

Preservation of Tooth Tissues

Chapter 5

Decision Making in Restorative Dentistry

Emiel H. Verdonschot and Alphons J.M. Plasschaert

Introduction

General dental practitioners make numerous diagnostic and treatment decisions on a daily basis. For the most part, these decisions are made in an implicit, intuitive way and there is evidence that dental practitioners do not share a common decision-making process.[11] For many dentists, decision making has become a routine, rather than a problem-solving process based on scientific principles. In problem solving, generally two strategies can be employed. First, algorithms exactly define the relation between the variables involved and the solution to the problem. Examples are Ohm's law, univocally relating the electrical current and resistance to the voltage, and "if...then" procedures such as, "If it rains, then I will take the bus." An algorithmic problem-solving strategy generates only one solution. Second, a heuristic problem-solving strategy aims at increasing the probability of finding one or more valuable solutions to a problem. It does not prescribe the problem-solving process, nor will it always lead to the same outcome.

This aspect of heuristic problem solving is a major factor in the interobserver variability reported by many investigations on diagnostic and treatment decisions made by dentists.[2-4,16]

Dental problems in general, and restoration-related problems in particular, require a heuristic problem-solving approach.[14] However, existing literature includes indications that general dental practitioners have a tendency to solve restorative problems in an algorithmic way. For example, dentists decide whether to replace restorations in situations where secondary caries has been noted at the margins of amalgam restorations. However, the number of restorations replaced by dental practitioners greatly exceeds the reported prevalence of secondary caries.[6,9] Hence, numerous false-positive restorative treatment decisions are still being made, based on false-positive diagnoses of secondary caries, causing substantial overtreatment. Besides discomfort to the patients, overtreatment causes an unnecessary increase in the cost of dental health care and a decrease in the survival time of restorations.

This, in turn, will inevitably result in earlier tooth loss. Many incorrect decisions to replace restorations can be ascribed to marginal fracture, a phenomenon intimately related to amalgam restorations and their age. When dentists apply a diagnostic test for secondary caries (such as visual-tactile inspection) they may interpret marginal fracture as being secondary caries, and because secondary caries is considered a progressive disease, the decision is made to replace the restoration. Expressed in an algorithmic way, this problem-solving process could be represented by: "If there is marginal fracture, then there is secondary caries; if there is secondary caries, then the restoration should be replaced."

Alternatively, a heuristic problem-solving approach would first question the outcome of the diagnostic test and its relation to disease: "Is there truly marginal fracture and, if so, what is the probability that this is associated with secondary caries?" Secondly, given the probability of a marginal fracture being related to secondary caries, the available treatment alternatives would be weighed against each other. Valid solutions to the problem are "wait and watch," "apply sealant," "repair restoration," and "replace restoration." All treatment alternatives possess different longevity and cost characteristics, making each decision a challenge, and the outcome in terms of chosen treatment rather unpredictable. However, the outcome in terms of health gain or "quality adjusted years," ie, the contribution of the selected treatment to the quality of life experienced by the patient, will become measurable by application of decision analysis to diagnostic procedures and restorative treatment planning.[1]

Probabilities and Utilities

Decision analysis is a tool in the hands of the dentist that facilitates the provision of treatment-related information to patients, including the proposed treatment alternatives and the cost of treatment. Patients will be able to weigh the proposed treatment options, discuss the advantages and disadvantages with the dentist, and make choices. For the dentist, the advantage is that treatment discussed with a patient and delivered on a decision-analysis basis secures the quality of care desired by patients, health care insurance companies, and health care authorities. In the tract between observation and treatment, two main types of decisions have to be made by the dental clinician. A diagnostic decision is required to ascertain the precise nature of the problem, and a treatment decision is subsequently needed to select the most appropriate treatment alternative. The relation between the two types of decisions is obvious as incorrect diagnoses will most likely have an adverse effect on subsequent treatment decisions.[5,13]

Decision analysis is ruled by probabilities and utilities. In diagnosing small occlusal caries lesions, the prevalence of the disease is important. If the prevalence of small occlusal caries lesions in a population is 0.2, then this indicates that 2 out of 10 patients within this population have one or more small occlusal caries lesions. On a patient level, a prevalence of 0.2 means that 20% of the occlusal surfaces have small occlusal caries lesions. Epidemiological surveys may reveal this prevalence,[8,15] which is therefore considered an a priori probability, indicating that the practitioner could use this knowledge to improve the quality of diagnostic decision

Table 5-1 Contingency table of a practitioner's radiographic diagnosis of occlusal caries in 100 extracted teeth relative to the true state of disease, as observed from tooth sections

		Observations from sectioned teeth (True state of disease)	
		Caries present	Caries absent
Radiographic diagnosis (estimated state of disease)	Caries present	12 (true-positive)	16 (false-positive)
	Caries absent	8 (false-negative)	64 (true-negative)

making. Other useful a priori probabilities are related to the ability of the practitioner to correctly detect initial occlusal caries lesions, and to correctly identify those surfaces that do not have caries lesions. These probabilities are referred to as the sensitivity and the specificity of the diagnostic test applied by the practitioner. The sensitivity of a diagnostic test is the proportion of correct positive diagnoses, and the specificity is the proportion of correct negative diagnoses. Let us assume that the diagnostic test consists of bitewing radiography. If a shadow is discerned beneath the occlusal dentino-enamel junction, the test outcome is positive, ie, the disease (caries) is present. If no shadow can be observed, the test outcome is negative. Suppose we take 100 extracted premolar and molar teeth with no obvious caries lesions, mount them in blocks simulating a patient's posterior dentition, and take bitewing radiographs. A practitioner is asked to examine the radiographs and to state whether or not occlusal caries is present in

each tooth. The teeth are subsequently cut into thin sections, and from the sections it is verified if occlusal caries is present. This observation is used as the "gold standard" observation—the true state of disease to which the diagnosis is compared. The comparison between radiographic diagnosis and gold standard observations for the practitioner is contained in a contingency table (Table 5-1). From Table 5-1 the following a priori probabilities, pertaining to this specific practitioner's diagnostic performance, can be calculated:

Prevalence of occlusal caries:
$$\frac{(12+8)}{(12+8+16+64)} = 0.20$$
Sensitivity of bitewing examination:
$$\frac{12}{(12+8)} = 0.60$$
Specificity of bitewing examination:
$$\frac{64}{(16+64)} = 0.80$$

The above probabilities play a role in the performance of the practitioner in diagnosing caries lesions from bitewing radiographs. A majority of the diagnoses (true-positives plus true-negatives) is correct and provide a solid base for treatment decision making. However, a certain proportion of diagnostic decisions will be incorrect (false-positives plus false-negatives) and, as a result, incorrect treatment decisions are likely to be made. For ease of explanation it is assumed that only two treatment alternatives, ie, no treatment and restorative treatment, are available. Based on a false-positive diagnosis, an occlusal surface will be restored although this surface is in fact caries-free. Conversely, a false-negative diagnosis causes a carious surface to be left unrestored although in fact a restoration should have been placed. Patients value both types of incorrect treatments differently.[7] In general, they are less concerned about having caries lesions that remain unrestored than receiving restorations in sound teeth. The value that patients attribute to treatment outcomes are called utilities. Utilities are scaled from 0, indicating a minimum value attached to a treatment outcome, to 100, which represents the maximum value. In the present case, utility values of 100 can be assigned to the treatment decisions based on true-positive and true-negative treatment outcomes. To estimate the utilities of both incorrect treatment outcomes, it is imperative to know the patient's or the public's opinion in this respect. For the case presented, the utilities for false-positive and false-negative treatment outcome are fixed at 5 and 20, respectively.

Decision Analysis in Diagnostics

The objective of the current decision analysis is to estimate the value of bitewing radiography as a diagnostic test for small occlusal caries lesions. The value of applying bitewing radiography can be determined relative to a situation in which bitewing radiography is not applied and no restorative treatment will be conducted. In these circumstances, the relation between observation, diagnosis, treatment decisions, and treatment utility can be represented as in Fig 5-1. Other diagnostic tests can be applied but were not included in the analysis of the case.

In Fig 5-1, a population of 100 patients with an occlusal caries prevalence of 0.20 is the subject of the decision analysis. Hence, 20 patients have occlusal caries. When bitewing radiography is applied with a sensitivity of 0.60, 12 patients ($0.60\times$ 20) with occlusal caries lesions are correctly identified (true-positives), and 8 patients ($20-12$) with caries lesions receive a false-negative diagnosis. In the population, 80 patients have no occlusal caries lesions. The specificity of bitewing radiography is 0.80, causing 64 patients (0.8×80) to be correctly classified as having no occlusal caries (true-negatives), whereas 16 patients ($80-64$) receive a false-positive diagnosis. Thus, the probability of the diagnostic test outcome of bitewing radiography being positive is 0.28 ([12+16]/100). The probability of a negative diagnostic test outcome is 0.72 ([8+64]/100). These probabilities are included in Fig 5-1. If the test outcome is positive, restorative treatment is provided. Twelve patients with a positive test outcome (43%, P = 0.43) legitimately receive,

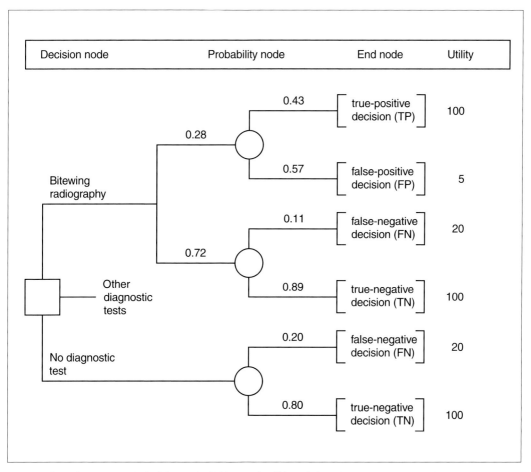

Fig 5-1 Decision tree model of the probabilities and utilities of decision outcomes to calculate the estimated utility of bitewing radiographs in occlusal caries diagnosis.

restorative treatment and 16 patients (57%, P = 0.57) receive unnecessary restorative treatment. Likewise, 11% (P = 0.11) of the negative test outcomes are false, and 89% (P = 0.89) are correct. The overall utility of bitewing radiography can be calculated by multiplication of probabilities and utilities:

$$(0.28 \times 0.43 \times 100) + (0.28 \times 0.57 \times 5) + (0.72 \times 0.11 \times 20) + (0.72 \times 0.89 \times 100) = 75$$

The overall utility of no bitewing radiography is 84 ([0.2 × 20] + [0.8 × 100]). The result of this decision analysis is that the utility of bitewing radiography is less than that of not using a diagnostic test for occlusal caries at all. Therefore, this practitioner should not use bitewing radiography for the detection of small occlusal caries lesions.

Decision Analysis in Restorative Dentistry

One of the assumptions in the preceding analysis of the diagnostic problem was that only one treatment alternative, ie, restorative therapy, would be available. In fact, given a small occlusal caries lesion, many treatment options are available. If the lesion is arrested and demineralization is compensated by remineralization, the provision of no treatment could be considered. If the lesion is small and restricted to the enamel, or if it has progressed just beyond the dentinoenamel junction with no cavitation, and doubt exists as to whether remineralization will compensate for mineral loss, preventive interventions such as fluoride varnish, chlorhexidine varnish, or sealant application may be considered. If the outer layers of the dentin are demineralized, a preventive resin restoration may be placed. When the deeper layers of the dentin are decayed, a restoration of composite resin, glass ionomer, compomer, or amalgam is probably indicated. The problem of choosing the correct treatment is limited to eight treatment alternatives. If we assume that the practitioner has sufficient knowledge and skills to apply all of the above treatment alternatives, he or she may select the option that yields the highest utility for the patient. A patient may have a strong preference for a durable solution leading to a relatively high utility for amalgam as the restorative material. A high utility for composite resin restorations exists if the patient prefers esthetic restorations, whereas sealants may receive a high utility if a patient wishes to postpone restorative treatment. The utility values can be obtained through sensitivity analysis, in which the patient expresses preference for one treatment alternative relative to other alternatives. The utility of the preferred treatment alternative, for example a restoration, is compared to a no-restoration option that will result in total caries arrest with probability P, and one that will result in toothache caused by pulpitis with probability 1 − P. The latter option is clearly associated with zero utility, whereas an untreated, arrested caries lesion is associated with a utility of 100. The model of this sensitivity analysis is depicted in Fig 5-2. The sensitivity analysis starts with the selection of a value for P, such as 0.40, for the "caries arrest" option. The "pulpitis" option will then occur with a probability of 0.60. The patient is asked what he prefers: a restoration or a 40% chance of caries arrest combined with a 60% chance of getting pulpitis. Clearly, the patient will prefer the no treatment/caries arrest option; however, the associated probability of pulpitis is too high. Therefore, the patient will most likely choose the restorative treatment. The value of P is subsequently increased until the patient has no preference for a restoration. This may, for example, be attained at P = 0.90, when the probability of pulpitis is 0.10. The expected utility of restorative treatment is then equal to the sum of the utilities of both no treatment options, thus (0.90 × 100) + (0.10 × 0) = 90. The utility of preventive treatment can be determined similarly.

The model contained in Fig 5-3 can be employed to estimate the utility of amalgam and composite restorations with respect to esthetics and durability. Both treatment options are initially offered for the same amount of money, eg, $100, and the patient (or a population) is asked which treatment modality is preferred. If a preference for composite resin as a restorative

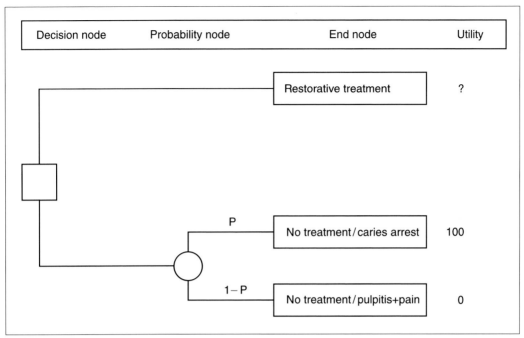

Fig 5-2 Decision model used in a sensitivity analysis to estimate the utility of restorative treatment.

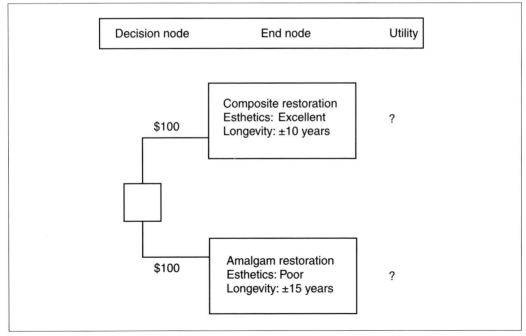

Fig 5-3 Decision model used in a sensitivity analysis to estimate the utility of amalgam and composite restorations.

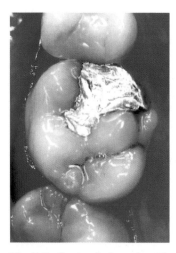

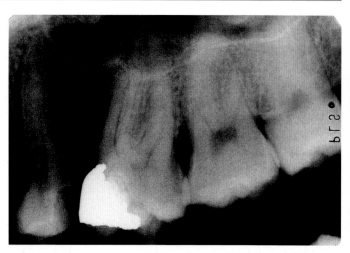

Fig 5-4 Occlusal view of a 10-year-old mesio-occlusal amalgam restoration in the left maxillary first molar of a 30-year-old woman.

Fig 5-5 Radiograph of the left maxillary first molar from Fig 5-4 showing a mesial overhang and the presence of a cement lining near the pulp.

material exists, the price of an amalgam restoration is decreased (or that of a composite resin increased) until their is no preference for either modalities. Suppose this equilibrium is reached at a price of $25 for an amalgam restoration compared to $100 for a composite restoration. The amounts can be rescaled to obtain estimated utilities of 25 and 100 for amalgam and composite restorations respectively. This type of analysis enables the practitioner to weigh the advantages of two treatment alternatives against each other. Similar analyses may be conducted to estimate the utility of glass-ionomer and compomer restorations.

Given the various utilities for restorative treatment options and the probabilities of disease progression, a decision analysis of a specific case will be considered. The case involves a 30-year-old female patient with good oral hygiene. About 10 years previously her dentist placed a mesio-occlusal amalgam restoration in the left maxillary first molar (Fig 5-4). On examination the gingivae did not bleed on probing and the pocket depth around the tooth did not exceed 3 mm. A pocket of 5 mm was found mesial to the left maxillary second molar. The outcome of an electrical pulp test indicated that the tooth was vital. A periapical radiograph revealed a large mesial overhang on the restoration and angular bone resorption mesial to the left maxillary second molar, but no periapical radiolucency (Fig 5-5). The question is, should the practitioner replace this restoration? If so, what restorative material should be used?

The analysis of this case starts with an investigation of the causal relationships between the observations. Apparently, the existing amalgam restoration did not cause the associated periodontal problems. The radiopaque area beneath the amalgam restoration is probably a lining of cement, which indicates that the preparation was close to the pulp. This did not, however, cause endodontic or periapical problems. The observed periodontal pocket and angular bone defect are related to the mesial site of the left maxillary second molar and are clearly independent of the amalgam restoration in the adjacent first molar. The overhang on the amalgam restoration could have had an effect on periodontal health, but did not lead to pocket formation or angular bone resorption during the previous 10 years. Clinically it appears that two cusps are undermined and weakened by the amalgam restoration, and that the left maxillary second premolar contains a disto-occlusal tooth-colored restoration. The radiograph indicates that the radiopacity of this restorative material is very low. In comparison to the left maxillary second premolar, second molar, and third molar, the pulp space of the left maxillary first molar is reduced, possibly because of reparative dentinal formation.

Based on the causal relationships, three variables could possibly influence the decision to replace the existing amalgam restoration: (1) the probability of pulpitis, a periapical periodontitis, or periodontal disease related to the amalgam overhang, (2) the probability of restoration failure because of bulk fracture, marginal fracture, or cusp fracture, and (3) the probability of tooth loss due to the restoration or restorative procedures. In this analysis, reparable shortcomings of the restoration were classified as failed features.

The decision to replace the amalgam restoration should be based on the prognosis of the tooth and the probability of possible failures. From the literature, data can be obtained regarding the durability of existing and newly placed restorations of amalgam and composite. These data can be used to estimate the probability that the present restoration (in case of no treatment) or the various treatment options (if treatment were conducted) will fail within a 9-year time span. Suitable estimates of the probabilities of "restoration failure," "periodontal and endodontic problems," and "tooth loss" were obtained from the recent literature.[10,12] Plasmans et al reported on the 8.5-year survival of extensive amalgam restorations and Van Dijken et al on the 3-year survival of extensive posterior composite restorations. The probabilities of failure reported in the latter publication were multiplied by 3 to obtain 9-year failure probability estimates. The utilities for this analysis were thought to be applicable to an average patient.

In a decision tree, the possible treatment decisions, ie, "no treatment," "restorative treatment," and "removal of cervical overhang," are related to the estimated probabilities and utilities of treatment outcomes (Fig 5-6). The probability of treatment outcome was estimated for the "replace with amalgam" and "replace with composite" options, and were adjusted for the other treatment options, ie, "no treatment," and "removal of cervical overhang," given the probabilities of the amalgam replacement. A maximum utility was assigned whenever no change to the existing or new situation occurred, and a zero utility was assigned to the occurrence

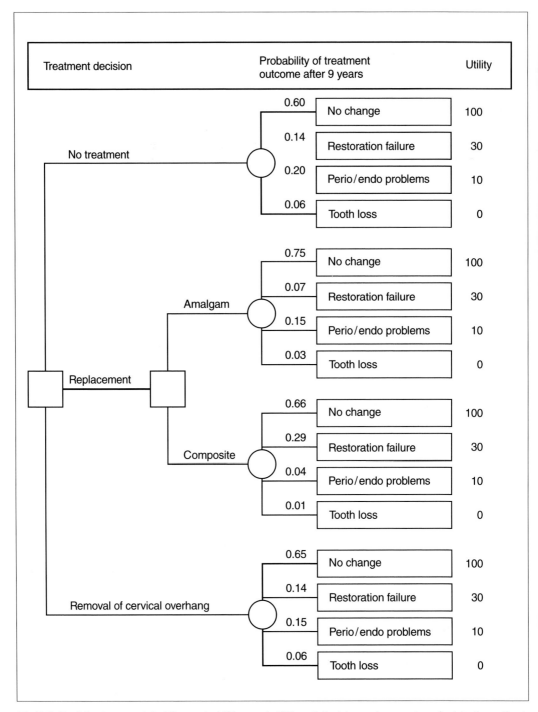

Fig 5-6 Decision tree model of the probabilities and utilities of decision outcomes to calculate the estimated utility of "no treatment," "restoration replacement," and "removal of cervical overhang" for the case presented in Figs 5-4 and 5-5.

of tooth loss. Given both scale limits, restoration failure and periodontal and endodontic problems were associated with utility values of 30 and 10, respectively. The decision analysis results in the following utilities for the four treatment options:

No treatment:
$(0.60 \times 100) + (0.14 \times 30) + (0.20 \times 10) + (0.06 \times 0) = 66.2$

Replacement of restoration with amalgam:
$(0.75 \times 100) + (0.07 \times 30) + (0.15 \times 10) + (0.03 \times 0) = 78.6$

Replacement of restoration with composite:
$(0.66 \times 100) + (0.29 \times 30) + (0.04 \times 10) + (0.01 \times 0) = 75.1$

Removal of cervical overhang:
$(0.65 \times 100) + (0.14 \times 30) + (0.15 \times 10) + (0.06 \times 0) = 70.7$

Based on this decision analysis, the practitioner should choose the treatment alternative with the highest yield of utility for this patient, ie, replacement of the existing amalgam restoration with a new amalgam restoration.

Discussion

Decision analysis is a tool, not a philosophy. It serves the purpose of improving the performance of a practitioner in diagnostic and treatment decision making, by weighing the probabilities and utilities of the treatment outcomes. The described procedures to obtain utility values for treatment outcomes and probabilities are given as examples and are not generally applicable. The clinician should bear in mind that decision analysis can be applied to individual patient's treatment plans. It challenges the practitioner to design a decision tree and to reflect on the values of probabilities and utilities. In doing this, the practitioner will develop a problem-solving strategy based on scientific reasoning and on data published in the scientific literature. The dental practitioner utilizing decision analysis in this way will be practicing evidence-based dentistry.

In this chapter, a decision analysis of a case of amalgam replacement has been presented. The survival and failure probabilities for the restoration were derived from the literature. The selection of these probabilities and the construction of the decision tree may be open to various criticisms. However, it was the authors' intention to provide an example pertaining to an individual case, not for a range of cases. The outcome is applicable to the "average" patient. The outcome of the analysis would not be applicable to the patient who assigns low utilities to amalgam as a material or its esthetics. Nor would it be applicable to those dentists who lack experience in applying large posterior composite resin restorations. One might also dispute the choice of a 10-year survival report to estimate the survival of amalgam restorations, and of a 3-year study to estimate the probabilities of failure and tooth loss when an existing amalgam restoration is replaced by a composite restoration. In the analysis, it was decided not to select a long-term study on posterior composite survival because, contrary to amalgam, composite restorations have been modified and improved upon considerably over the past 10 years. The selection of a 9-year survival study on composites would relate to outdated materials and procedures and, as a consequence, result in an underestimation of the survival of current composites.

To date, reports on the application of decision analyses are predominantly descriptions of diagnostic and treatment-planning problems in respect to individual patients. It is realistic, however, to apply decision analyses on diagnostic and therapeutic problems to a larger population, based on the probability of disease within the population and the utility values for the population. It is possible, for example, to determine the prevalence of secondary caries associated with amalgam restorations in a country or region, and to collect data on the utilities of treatment options including preventive interventions and replacement by various types of restorations for the population. The information obtained can be used in a decision analysis resulting in general recommendations or clinical guidelines. These will aid the practitioner in making decisions regarding restoration replacement, but could also serve the purpose of enhancing knowledge and treatment planning skills in undergraduate and continuing education. It would be an important step toward evidence-based dentistry.

References

1. Anusavice KJ. Decision analysis in restorative dentistry. J Dent Educ 1992;56:812–822.

2. Bader JD, Shugars DA. Variation in dentists' clinical decisions. J Public Health Dent 1995; 55:181–188.

3. Elderton RJ, Nuttall NM. Variation among dentists in planning treatment. Br Dent J 1983;154: 201–206.

4. Espelid I, Tveit AB, Fjelltveit A. Variations among dentists in radiographic detection of occlusal caries. Caries Res 1994;28:169–175.

5. Fyffe HE, Kay EJ. Assessment of dental health state utilities. Community Dent Oral Epidemiol 1992;20:269–273.

6. Hewlett ER, Atchison KA, White SC, Flack V. Radiographic secondary caries prevalence in teeth with clinically defective restorations. J Dent Res 1993;72:1604–1608.

7. Kay EJ, Blinkhorn AS. A qualitive investigation of factors governing dentists' treatment philosophies. Br Dent J 1996;180:171–176.

8. Lussi A. Impact of including or excluding cavitated lesions when evaluating methods for the diagnosis of occlusal caries. Caries Res 1996;30: 389–393.

9. Panaite MA, Verdonschot EH, Plasschaert AJM. Impact of patient and practice variables on re-restoration decisions [abstract 1400]. J Dent Res 1999;78(special issue):280.

10. Plasmans PJJM, Creugers NHJ, Mulder J. Long-term survival of extensive amalgam restorations. J Dent Res 1998;77:453–460.

11. Plasschaert AJM, Verdonschot EH, Wilson NHF, Blinkhorn AS. Decision making in restorative dentistry: Intuition or knowledge based? Br Dent J 1995;178:320–321.

12. Van Dijken JWV, Kieri C, Carlén M. Longevity of extensive Class II open-sandwich restorations with a resin-modified glass-ionomer cement. J Dent Res 1999;78:1319–1325.

13. Verdonschot EH, Angmar-Mänsson B, ten Bosch JJ, et al. Developments in caries diagnosis and their relationship to treatment decisions and quality of care. Caries Res 1999; 33:32–40.

14. Verdonschot EH, Plasmans JJM. Operative procedures prior to reconstructive therapy. Quintessence Int 1988;19:469–475.

15. Weerheijm KL. Prevalence of hidden caries. J Dent Child 1992;59:408–412.

16. Wenzel A, Verdonschot EH, Truin GJ, König KG. Accuracy of visual inspection, Fiber-Optic transillumination, and various radiographic image modalities for the detection of occlusal caries in extracted non-cavitated teeth. J Dent Res 1992;71:1934–1937.

Chapter 6

Initial Management: To Drill or Not to Drill?

Fabio Toffenetti

Introduction

The preceding chapters have shown that operative dentistry must no longer be considered to be limited to restorative techniques and materials science concepts; preventive and therapeutic criteria are now important considerations in the field. The treatment plan for each patient must be based on caries risk assessment,[30] radiographic examinations, and precise classification of the patient into a specific treatment need category. Only then is it possible to choose the most appropriate restorative treatment for teeth with established lesions, ranging from opening and restoring initial lesions of caries to waiting for evidence of the effects of remineralizing therapy, supported by measures preventing the extension of caries to the neighboring teeth. New materials and techniques are available today for the treatment of initial caries lesions that have irreversibly progressed into dentin. The purpose of these materials and techniques is to make the treatment as minimally invasive as possible, avoiding, wherever possible, the use of rotary instruments.

The alternative approaches to the management of initial caries lesions involving dentin include:

- Sealing the lesions without tooth preparation
- Mechanical preparation and the placement of a so-called preventive resin restoration (PRR)—the combination of a small restoration with fissure sealing
- The use of air abrasion for the preparation of pits and fissures to be restored with a PRR
- Chemical preparation and a PRR
- Manual instrumentation and the use of atraumatic restorative treatment (ART) techniques.

These new treatment methods avoid the need for extension to achieve prevention, greatly reducing the need for rotary instrumentation and the time taken for cavity preparation. The use of adhesive techniques can be effective even in the absence of a conventional approach to cavity preparation.

Figs 6-1 and 6-2 A therapeutic approach based on medical concepts helped manage the active caries and periodontal disease in the mouth of this patient. The successful outcome has been maintained for almost 15 years.

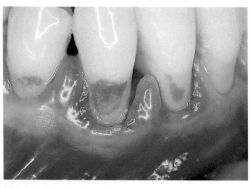

Fig 6-1 Illustration of active caries and periodontal disease on presentation.

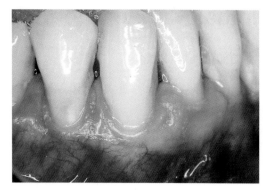

Fig 6-2 The long-term successful outcome.

Beyond new materials and techniques, the changes in the general philosophy of caries management have greatly transformed the nature of operative dentistry. The treatment of caries based on the chemomicrobial theory of pathogenesis, as proposed by Miller in 1890[40] and other pathogenetic theories discussed by Black in 1908,[6] have been superseded. Successful treatment now may not be assumed unless caries is managed as an infectious disease as described in 1991 by Anderson.[1] In this chapter, caries is described in terms of an infectious disease and a method of treatment based more on the medical therapy of infection than on the surgical removal of lesions is proposed (Figs 6-1 and 6-2). From this viewpoint, the only rationale for cleaning and sealing open lesions is to eliminate reservoirs of pathogenic microorganisms.

Many authors state that this approach to treatment is not yet accepted in clinical practice. McCoy[38] underlines the need for undergraduate students to learn medical criteria for the treatment of caries and for the dentist to secure adequate reimbursement for this type of therapy, which is not yet recognized by insurance companies. Osborne[46] suggests changes to preclinical education, whereby the students are taught to consider caries as an infective disease, considering risk assessment, prevention, and nonsurgical management, before planning traditional surgical management in the clinical situation.

Mandel[37] points out that the traditional management of caries in most dental practices presently constitutes overtreatment, with insufficient attention being given to possible preventive approaches. Irregularities in the availability of services and access to caregivers for a substantial segment of the population results, in contrast, in a great deal of undertreatment.

To sum up the preventive philosophy one may quote the maxim, "if in doubt prevent, wait, and reassess," as a substitute to the old concept, "if in doubt fill," which has been taught in good faith for decades.[24] The aim of treatment is to eradicate disease, restore function, and prevent the onset of future disease. If the etiological factors are not identified and managed, the lesions will sooner or later reappear in other sites or at the margins of restorations. Secondary caries typically manifests as a new primary lesion adjacent to an existing restoration.[41] In other words, secondary caries is a result of a failure to treat the causative factors of the caries process. More than 50% of cases of replacement of restorations are still attributed to secondary caries, indicating how little is understood about the treatment of the underlying cause of caries.

Initial Treatment: Diagnosis and Treatment Decisions

In operative dentistry, as in all other fields of medicine and dentistry, a precise, early diagnosis followed by preventive, interceptive, or other necessary treatment is paramount to the success of therapy. In operative dentistry, diagnosis is based on visual inspection, judicious light-pressure use of a blunt probe, traditional and increasingly digital radiographic examinations, and the use of recent diagnostic tools such as fiber-optic transillumination, electrical conductance measurements, and laser quantitative fluorescence. The details of these diagnostic techniques have been described in preceding chapters.

As has been reported, a clinical examination conducted by a calibrated, well-trained operator, together with good quality bitewing radiographs, allows for a sufficiently precise diagnosis of pathological conditions of the teeth. The risk of caries can be ascertained and the patient can be classified into a specific treatment category. Single lesions can be rated according to their severity and the best method of treatment identified.

In order to make immediate decisions regarding initial treatment, it is important to know if the patient is to be classified as: (1) no care advised (NCA) and, therefore, dentally fit; (2) preventive care advised (PCA), apparently healthy but at risk of caries and, therefore, to be treated with preventive measures, or as a patient with initial lesions that can be remineralized with prophylactic methods; or (3) operative care advised (OCA), when the lesions are not reversible and must be treated by means of operative intervention.[49] Borderline cases are difficult to classify and treat. If in doubt, it is wise to plan intense preventive treatment and to apply the newest remineralization techniques with the option to modify the treatment on recall.

During the initial examination it is possible to ascertain the presence of caries lesions, classify them according to their severity and activity, and establish a treatment plan.[10] However, initial examination findings can lead to underestimation of the prevalence of initial lesions and to inadequate restorative decisions (Figs 6-3 and 6-4), particularly in relation to approximal surfaces.[52] Multiple examinations can increase the number of carious surfaces correctly diagnosed, but can also increase the number of sound surfaces

Figs 6-3 and 6-4 "Hidden caries." It is now relatively common to observe dentinal caries under apparently healthy enamel. This seems to be related to the acid resistance of fluoride-exposed enamel. When in doubt, a small diagnostic cavity may be opened using atraumatic techniques such as air abrasion.

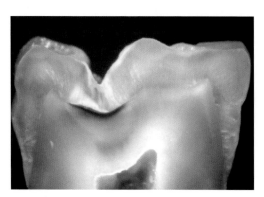

Fig 6-3 Ground section of hidden caries.

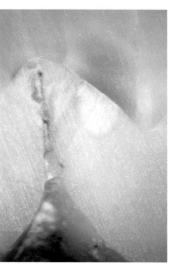

Fig 6-4 Because of the orientation of the enamel prisms, caries has developed in the dentin lateral to the occlusal fissure.

incorrectly diagnosed as carious and subsequently restored.[22] The use of bitewing radiographs is still considered essential to approximal caries diagnosis, with the necessary exposure to ionizing radiation being justified by the high diagnostic yield. Bitewing examination is also useful in monitoring early approximal lesions treated according to the medical approach.[51] Intraoral digital radiography, when compared with conventional film-based radiography, affords a reduction in the overall dose of radiation given to the patient and presents no significant problems with respect to the reliability of diagnosis.[43] The use of other modern diagnostic tools may improve sensitivity and permit the possibility of diagnosing

very early initial lesions, but with a reduced specificity, and the possibility of false positive results.[29,36,58] The highest diagnostic success rate is obtained by the combined use of the different tools.[35]

Bitewing radiography has proven high reliability, allowing the clinician to identify lesions in approximal surfaces and to classify the identified lesions according to their depth, development, and progression. The studies of Groendal and coworkers first proposed the classification of approximal caries lesions,[19] which was subsequently modified by Pitts[50] to provide the current scoring system. This standardized system is useful for diagnosis and monitoring, epidemiology purposes, and in the calibration of examiners.

0= radiographically sound surface
1= lesion in the outer half of enamel
2= lesion in the inner half of enamel
3= lesion in the outer half of dentin
4= lesion in the inner half of dentin

Subclinical lesions of a value less than 1 can be identified by the most modern diagnostic tools. For value 2 and more extensive lesions, clinical examination is sufficient. It is presently believed that preventive therapy according to the medical model may result in the remineralization of initial lesions of value 2, and possibly early value 3 lesions. For value 3 and more extensive lesions, the treatment of choice is operative intervention. At this stage, a cavity has formed and preparation followed by a restoration is therefore necessary to avoid plaque trap formation.[23]

Initial Treatment: Cavity Preparation

The new concepts of treatment, according to etiological principles, have therefore affected both the theory and clinical practice of dentistry. The indications for cavity preparation are that preventive measures would be insufficient, remineralization has not occurred, or it is necessary to remove the infected (and some of the affected) dentin in order to interrupt continuing cavitation and thereby avoid the forming of bacterial plaque nests.[42] Cavity preparation should be performed in accordance with guidelines for the conservation of sound tooth structures and while taking advantage of the possibilities offered by new instruments and techniques. Fluoride-releasing restorative materials and ad-

hesive restorative techniques should be used in the provision of restorations.

Adhesive dentistry allows conservation of sound tooth structures. Extension for prevention has been replaced by fissure sealing. Undermined, sound enamel may be preserved and strengthened by the use of adhesive materials; geometric, retentive preparations can be avoided and decalcified enamel may be preserved if glass-ionomer materials are used.

The widespread use of magnification aids during cavity preparation and the consequent use of small-diameter preparation instruments have greatly contributed in recent years to more controlled and conservative tooth preparation procedures.

With these considerations in mind, Mount and Hume have proposed a new classification for cavities[42] based on the site and size of the lesion. The three sites considered are:

• Site 1: Pits, fissures, and enamel defects on the occlusal surfaces of posterior teeth and smooth surfaces on anterior teeth
• Site 2: Approximal enamel immediately below contact areas with adjacent teeth
• Site 3: The cervical one-third of the crown, or the exposed root

The four sizes are:

• Size 1: Minimal involvement of dentin.
• Size 2: Moderate involvement of dentin. The tooth is strong enough to support the restoration.
• Size 3: Beyond moderate involvement of dentin. The restoration is designed to provide support to the tooth.
• Size 4: Extensive caries and bulk loss of tooth structure.

93

The location and severity of lesions can be indicated using two digits, making record keeping easier both in clinical practice and epidemiologic surveys. For instance, a 1.3 cavity is an occlusal cavity with loss of tooth structure requiring a strengthening restoration, and a 3.1 cavity is an initial cervical lesion. The form of the prepared cavity should be dictated by the size of the caries lesion. Extension into sound enamel must only extend to tissue capable of remineralization.

When to Prepare a Cavity

The question as to when to prepare a cavity is not posed when a lesion has caused frank cavitation and when the patient is in pain. In such cases, cavity preparation and the placement of a restoration is essential for two fundamental reasons: to relieve the patient's symptoms and to restore tooth form and function to eliminate bacterial plaque traps that may maintain the infection. In the presence of numerous open cavities and active disease in patients at high risk for caries, the preliminary phase of therapy should be excavation of all the cavities followed by temporary restoration with cariostatic materials such as zinc oxide–eugenol cements and glass-ionomer materials.

When the patient presents with small initial lesions, the size and nature of the lesions should be determined in order to decide whether the patient should be treated with prophylactic measures only (PCA) or with both preventive and operative procedures (OCA). The basis of treatment of a patient with caries is, in all cases, the application of all known preventive methods[4]: dietary assessment and counseling, professional tooth cleaning and instruction in oral hygiene techniques, and the prescription of chlorhexidine mouthrinses followed by fluoride applications[55] in the form of dentifrices, rinses, fluoridated salt, and fluoride varnishes.[9,47] The preventive armamentarium has proven its effectiveness and reliability over time but remains undervalued and underutilized by the profession.[2]

Once a carefully targeted treatment has been planned based on data collected on caries risk, lesion activity, and the site, size, number, and distribution of lesions, decisions remain to be made regarding the different restorative options available. It is possible to select from among many different restorative approaches, both traditional and innovative, to restore tooth form and function and, more importantly, to form a seal between restoration and the remaining tooth structure.

Modern technology, underpinned by biologic studies and materials science research, has provided new instruments and methods that make the treatment of initial lesions less invasive, less painful, less expensive, more conservative, and more affordable. Clinical research has also helped to identify the indications for many of these methods. Other methods still await scientific validation and cost-benefit analysis.

Ultraconservative Sealed Restorations

The research group lead by Mertz-Fairhurst undertook significant studies on fissure-sealing techniques, and in recent years

Figs 6-5 to 6-7 Stained fissures can be sealed without tooth preparation. A transparent sealer may help diagnose failures or recurring caries. There is ample evidence that early primary caries may be arrested by such a procedure.

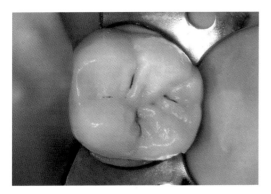

Fig 6-5 Stained fissure in the occlusal surface of a mandibular molar in a young patient.

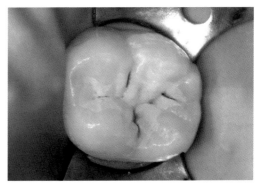

Fig 6-6 Acid etching of the occlusal pits and fissures.

Fig 6-7 Sealing with a transparent resin may assist in the early detection of any subsequent occlusal caries.

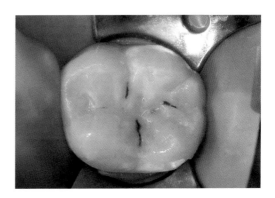

investigated the behavior of small caries lesions left untreated under occlusal sealants. During the 1970s, several clinical and microbiologic studies demonstrated that initial caries can be sealed without negative effects.[18,20] Clinical and microbiologic research has subsequently shown that sealed initial lesions become arrested with complete absence of symptoms.[39] A comparison between this simple method and traditional and sealed amalgam restorations has been undertaken. Occlusal sealants, in contrast to restorations of amalgam, asymptomatically arrested lesion progression without loss of form and function of sound tooth tissues. A pilot study on the densitometric computer-assisted analysis of radiographic images of sealed teeth containing initial lesions has demonstrated the ability to objectively detect changes in the radiographic density of sealed lesions.[7] It would therefore appear that it is not to the disadvantage of the patient that initial occlusal lesions are sealed, assuming periodic clinical and radiologic monitoring (Figs 6-5 to 6-7).

Figs 6-8 to 6-12 Modern adhesive dentistry based on the use of resin systems allows more conservative approaches to the preparation of teeth with the preservation of sound tissues subadjacent to the caries.

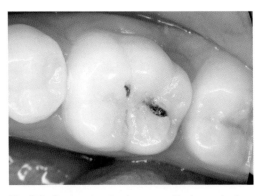

Fig 6-8 Occlusal caries in a mandibular molar in a young patient.

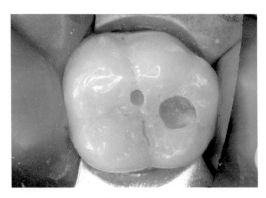

Fig 6-9 Conservative cavity preparation dictated only by the location and extent of the caries.

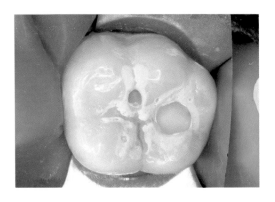

Fig 6-10 After preparation and etching, remnants of a preexisting fissure sealer are evident on the occlusal surface. In order to reduce the polymerization shrinkage stress of the resin-based restorative material, a layer of glass-ionomer cement, resin-modified glass ionomer, or flowable composite resin is placed on the occlusal floor of the cavities.

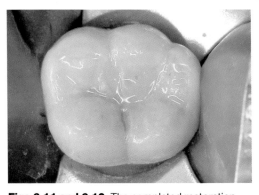

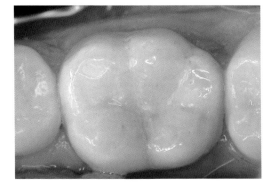

Figs 6-11 and 6-12 The completed restoration.

Preventive Resin Restorations

A very conservative, but somewhat more traditional technique for the management of small- to medium-sized caries lesions in the pits and fissures of posterior teeth was proposed by Simonsen in 1977.[56] The concept is to restore the small lesions with the minimum possible sacrifice of sound tissues, while preventing further caries in the surrounding sound structures (Figs 6-8 to 6-12).

Limited access to the caries is achieved using a small diamond bur. The carious dentin is excavated using a small round bur operating at low speed. Because an adhesive restoration of composite resin will follow, it is not necessary to prepare beyond the lesion. When caries is limited to enamel, there is no need to prepare into dentin, as is necessary for a restoration of amalgam. Very often small preventive resin restorations (PRRs) can be performed without anesthesia. It is, however, advisable to place such restorations under rubber dam. After etching both the cavity and the surrounding fissures, the cavity can be restored with a flowable composite that may also act as a fissure sealant. Larger cavities are better filled with a wear-resistant composite, followed by a fissure sealant to seal the adjacent fissures.

Initial studies[56,57] and more recent clinical trials have shown PRRs to be reliable and clinically effective.[26,60] At present, the PRR is state-of-the-art in the treatment of initial occlusal caries. Different methods of tooth preparation for PRRs are being studied with the advantage of the restorative procedure being less traumatic to the patient and minimally invasive to the tooth. PRRs can be placed in teeth prepared using, for example, air abrasion or chemical caries removal techniques.

Initial approximal caries lesions can be managed through the marginal ridge and then restored with an adhesive composite restoration and fissure sealant in much the same way as a PRR.[27] Other conservative approaches in such situations include the so-called tunnel restoration[21] and the lateral slot (buccal or lingual) restoration. The aim of such approaches is to preserve the integrity of the marginal ridge.

Air Abrasion

Adhesive dentistry based on resin adhesive systems has greatly reduced the need to prepare sound tooth structures for resistance and retention. Current recommendations are to obtain only access to the lesion in order to complete excavation of the carious dentin. The use of a caries indicator dye is advocated as a routine procedure, followed by the careful excavation of carious tissue using small round burs operating at low speed. The restoration of the cavities may then proceed using a resin-based adhesive and restorative system.

A further development towards minimally invasive, atraumatic treatment of small lesions is provided by air abrasion units. Air abrasion equipment has been produced and tested since 1950. However, in the 1950s the resin-based adhesive restorative materials that currently complement air abrasion preparation were not available. As a consequence, high-speed rotary systems were selected for development, allowing a faster and more accurate geometric preparation of cavities for principally silver amalgam and cast gold restorations. Today, air abrasion preparation, coupled with resin-based adhesive systems, is considered an effective and safe alternative to the use of rotary instrumentation and traditional restoratives in managing small initial lesions.[33] The air abrasion units produced by many different manufacturers are powered by compressed air at the pressure of 7 to 11 atm (40 to 140 psi) and use abrasive aluminum oxide powders of 20- to 50-pm particle size.

Studies have shown that air abrasion units can effectively cut enamel, dentin, and restorative materials when defective or failed restorations of amalgam or composite are to be replaced.[61] The use of air abrasion units also appears to be safe as far as the tooth vitality is concerned.[34] Some studies suggest, following initial access preparation, the use of specific abrasive powders to make the excavation of carious tissue safe and more precise, with the aim of rendering the whole procedure more conservative and less traumatic.[25] However, while air abrasion is very effective in cutting sound dental structures, it is less effective in achieving caries removal.

The placement of an adhesive restoration following air abrasion preparation is to be performed with great care because air abrasion is not a substitute for acid etching.[53] Air abrasion alone results in reduced bond strength to enamel and dentin as compared with acid etching of the enamel and dentinal cavity walls.[44,54] Contrary to what was initially believed, acid etching of the cavity walls should always be performed after air abrasion preparation.

To summarize the qualities of air abrasion, it may be stated that air abrasion has advantages in the preparation of initial occlusal and cervical lesions and in the management of approximal lesions provided careful protection of the adjacent tooth surface.[8]

Disadvantages of air abrasion include its inability to remove caries and provide precise preparations for prosthodontics. Abrasive overspray is not considered dangerous, although it may sometimes disturb patients with chronic respiratory disorders and is messy in the office environment. Air abrasion units are still very expensive and time is required to gain clinical skills and proficiency with the technique.

Rubber dam, protective face masks, high-velocity suction units with good flow rate, a filter system to prevent abrasive degradation of metal pumps and clogging of suction lines, disposable abrasion-resistant mouth mirrors, and 2x magnifying aids with face-shield protection are important in the appropriate use of air abrasion.

Chemical Caries Removal

Given the aim of making the treatment of caries less traumatic, chemical methods of caries dissolution were developed in the 1970s.[32] The Caridex system was based on the combined use of an organic acid solution and sodium hypochloride.

Following the modern trend of minimally invasive operative dentistry, new methods of caries dissolution, based on the combined use of amino acids and a weak solution of sodium hypochloride, are now available on the market.[11] Studies on alternative enzyme solutions are reported in the literature, indicating a growing interest in minimally invasive operative procedures.[5] The use of chemical caries removal is also advocated in situations with poor access, especially in cases in which caries is to be removed but traditional instrumentation is ineffective.[45]

The recommended clinical procedure for the chemical management of caries consists of repeated applications of the chemical solutions over the caries. The caries is gently removed with specially designed hand instruments. The use of a caries indicator dye helps to identify where sound, uninfected dentin remains.[31] Multicenter studies demonstrate that this method is effective and safe for the preservation of the sound, surrounding structures.[12] The application time is longer than the time needed for rotary preparation, but as a compensation, no injection nor the use of rotary instrumentation is usually necessary. Careful case selection is advisable because not every case is suitable for this approach. The reported indications are root caries, coronal caries with open access or where access can be easily gained, recurrent caries under restorations or at the margins of crowns, and excavation of deep caries approaching the pulp.

Studies have repeatedly shown that adhesion to dentin underlying caries is usually less effective than it is to sound dentin. The chemical treatment of caries does not further lower bond strength values,[13] allowing effective adhesive restorations to be placed.

Atraumatic Restorative Treatment

Atraumatic restorative treatment (ART), as studied at Groeningen University and pre-sented to the World Health Organization in 1994,[14] was developed for developing countries in which caries often leads to extraction.[16] In Africa, more than 90% of dentinal lesions go untreated.[17] One of the major obstacles to the traditional treatment of such lesions is the need for expensive electrically powered technological equipment and technique-sensitive materials. ART, in contrast, is based on the use of simple manual instrumentation for lesion access and caries removal. Drying with compressed air is replaced by the use of cotton pellets. No anesthesia is usually needed and the technique can be taught to nonmedical staff. One of the greatest advantages of the technique is that it makes it possible to reach and treat people who would otherwise never receive any oral care (Figs 6-13 to 6-15).

The ART method uses a small number of hand instruments that can be readily carried around by operators. ART is performed by a seated operator on a horizontally positioned patient (a table can be readily adapted to the task). Occlusal lesions are generally treated with the access and caries excavation being performed manually. After they are cleaned with water and cotton pellets, ART cavities are treated and conditioned with the liquid of the glass-ionomer cement used for the restoration. The cement is then mixed, inserted in slight excess into the cavity, and protected with petroleum jelly. Digital pressure with a gloved finger allows for both better adaptation of the material to the cavity and sealing of the adjacent fissures. Excesses are removed with a sharp instrument before complete setting of the glass-ionomer material.

One of the justifications for the method is the belief that glass-ionomer cement

Figs 6-13 to 6-15 ART is a pragmatic approach to the management of occlusal caries (courtesy of Dr Taco Pilot, Groeningen University).

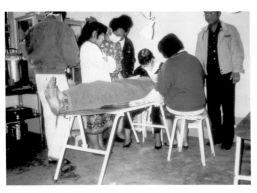

Fig 6-13 ART restoration is indicated in communities lacking modern amenities, including electricity, running water, and compressed air.

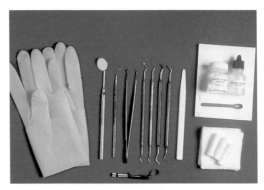

Fig 6-14 With a minimum of equipment, it is possible to successfully treat medium-sized occlusal caries lesions.

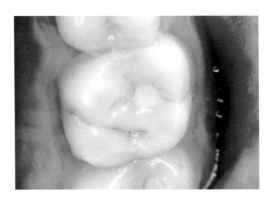

Fig 6-15 A completed ART restoration.

releases fluoride ions capable of preventing secondary caries and arresting residual caries under simple restorations. Studies have not yet confirmed this view.[59]

An instruction manual in many languages and instruction courses for field operators are available. Notwithstanding some negative criticism,[3] ART is being promoted as a caries treatment for communities in particular need of dental care. As an emergency treatment, it can be useful in the care of handicapped and house-bound elderly patients.

The available data on the first field trials in rural areas of Thailand indicate that after 3 years the survival rate of ART restorations (88% at 3 years) was close to that for amalgam restorations performed under the same conditions. No statistical differences were found between ART restorations in children and adults or between those applied by dentists and dental nurses.[48] More recent field trials with evaluations of the restorations at 3 years indicate that with improved materials enhanced results are obtained.[15]

Summary and Conclusions

New methods for the early diagnosis of caries lesions are increasing the frequency of identification of initial lesions capable of healing through remineralization. Given effective preventive programs, the surgical management of caries can be postponed until there is progressive involvement of dentin.

The simultaneous development of atraumatic, minimally invasive methods of cavity preparation and adhesive restorative techniques has contributed greatly to the conservative management of caries. The outdated concept of extension for prevention has been reversed to promote prevention of extension.

The benefits of recent developments in the management of caries can be seen in the reduced need for restorations and in the increased preservation of sound tooth structures—a distinguishing feature of modern operative dentistry for both initial lesions and the retreatment of preexisting lesions. The use of rotary instrumentation at high, medium, and low speeds may be reduced in conventional preparations as a consequence of adhesive techniques. Alternative instrumentation and methods allow increasingly conservative approaches to the management of initial caries lesions.

References

1. Anderson MH, Molvar MP, Powell LV. Treating dental caries as an infectious disease. Oper Dent 1991:16;21–28.

2. Anusavice KJ. Chlorhexidine, fluoride varnish, and xylitol chewing gum: Underutilized preventive therapies? Gen Dent 1998;46:34–38.

3. Anusavice KJ. Does ART have a place in preservative dentistry? Community Dent Oral Epidemiol 1999;27:442–448.

4. Anusavice KJ. Treatment regimens in preventive and restorative dentistry. J Am Dent Assoc 1995;126:727–743.

5. Beltz RE, Herrman EC, Nordbo H. Pronase digestion of carious dentin. Caries Res 1999; 33:468–472.

6. Black GV. A Work on Operative Dentistry. Vol 1: The pathology of the hard tissues of the teeth. Chicago, Medico-Dental Publishing, 1908.

7. Briley JB, Dove SB, Mertz-Fairhurst EJ, Hermesh CB. Computer-assisted densitometric image analysis (CADIA) of previously sealed carious teeth: A pilot study. Oper Dent 1997; 22:105–114.

8. CRA Newsletter. Status report, air abrasion for caries removal. 1997(Dec):2–3.

9. De Bruyn H, Arends J. Fluoride varnishes–A review. J Biol Buccale 1987; 15: 71–82.

10. Ekstrand KR, Ricketts DN, Kidd EA, Qvist V, Schou S. Detection, diagnosing, monitoring, and logical treatment of caries in relation to lesion activity and severity: An in vivo examination with histological validation. Caries Res 1998; 32:247–254.

11. Ericson D. The efficacy of a new gel for chemomechanical caries removal [abstract 360]. J Dent Res 1998;77:1252.

12. Ericson D, Zimmerman M, Raber H, Gotrick B, Bornstein R, Thorell J. Clinical evaluation of efficacy and safety of a new method for chemomechanical removal of caries: A multi-centre study. Caries Res 1999;33:171–177.

13. Frankenberger R, Oberschachstieg H, Krämer N, Petschelt A. Bond strength to dentin after mechanical and chemical removal of simulated caries [abstract 1015]. J Dent Res 1999; 78(special issue):232.

14. Frenken J, Makoni F. A treatment technique for tooth decay in deprived communities. World Health 1994;47:15–17.

15. Frenken J, Holmgren CJ. How effective is ART in the management of dental caries? Community Dent Oral Epidemiol 1999; 27:423.

16. Frenken J, Phantumvanit P, Pilot T, Songpaisan Y, van Amerongen E. Manual for the Atraumatic Restorative Treatment approach to control dental caries. Groeningen: WHO Collaborating Center for Oral Health Services Research, 1997.

17. Frenken J, Pilot T, Songpaisan Y, Phantumvanit P. Atraumatica restorative treatment (ART): Rationale, technique and development. J Public Health Dent 1996:56;135–140.

18. Going RE, Loesche WJ, Grainer DA, Syed SA. The viability of microorganisms in carious lesions five years after covering with a fissure sealant. J Am Dent Assoc 1978;97:455–462.

19. Groendal HG, Hollender L, Malmcrona E, Sundquist B. Dental caries and restorations in teenagers. 1. Index and score system for radiographic studies of approximal surfaces. Swed Dent J 1977;1:45–50.

20. Handelman SL, Buonocore MG, Schoute PC. Progress report on the effect of a fissure sealant on bacteria in dental caries. J Am Dent Assoc 1973; 87:1189–1191.

21. Hasselroth L. Tunnel restorations: A three-and-a-half-year follow-up study of class I and II tunnel restorations in permanent and primary teeth. Swed Dent J 1993;17:173–182.

22. Heaven TJ, Firestone AR, Weems RA. The effect of multiple examinations of approximal caries and the restoration of approximal surfaces. Oral Surg Oral Med Oral Pathol Oral Radiol Endod 1999; 87:386–391.

23. Hennequin M, Lasfargues JJ. La demarche diagnostique en cariologie. Real Clin 1999;10: 515–5405.

24. Hoersted-Bindslev P, Mjor IA (eds). Modern Concepts in Operative Dentistry. Copenhagen: Munksgaard, 1988.

25. Horiguchi S, Yamada T, Inokoshi S, Tagami J. Selective caries removal with air abrasion. Oper Dent 1998;23:236–243.

26. Houpt M, Fukus A, Eidelman E. The preventive resin (composite resin/sealant) restoration: Nine-year results. Quintessence Int 1994;25: 155–159.

27. Hunt PR. Micro-conservative restorations for approximal carious lesions. J Am Dent Assoc 1990; 120:37–40.

28. Huysmans MC, Longbottom C, Hinze H, Verdonschot EH. Surface-specific electrical caries diagnosis: Reproducibility, correlation with histological lesion depth, and tooth type dependence. Caries Res 1998;32:330.

29. Huysmans MC, Longbottom Ch, Pitts NB. Electrical methods in occlusal caries diagnosis: An in vitro comparison with visual inspection and bite-wing radiography. Caries Res 1998; 32:324–329.

30. Johnson N (ed). Risk Markers for Oral Diseases. Cambridge: Cambridge Univ Press, 1991.

31. Kidd EA, Joyston-Bechal S, Beighton D. The use of a caries detector dye during cavity preparation: A microbiological assessment. Br Dent J 1993;174:245–248.

32. Kronman J, Goldman M, Habib CM, Mengel L. Electron microscopic evaluation of collagen structure induced by N-chloroglycerine (GK 101). J Dent Res 1977;56:1539–1545.

33. Kutsch VK. Microdentistry: A new standard of care. J Mass Dent Soc 1999;47:35–39.

34. Laurell K, Carpenter W, Daugherty D, Beck M. Histopathologic effects of kinetic cavity preparation for the removal of enamel and dentin. Oral Surg Oral Med Oral Pathol Oral Radiol Endod 1995;80:214–225.

35. Lussi A, Firestone A, Schoenberg V, Hotz P, Stich H. In vivo diagnosis of fissure caries using a new electrical resistance monitor. Caries Res 1995;29:81–87.

36. Lussi A, Imwinkelried S, Pitts N, Longbottom C, Reich E. Performance and reproducibility of a laser fluorescence system for detection of occlusal caries in vitro. Caries Res 1999; 33:261–266.

37. Mandel I. Dentistry at the millennium: Overtreatment and undertreatment. Dental Abstr 1999; 44:250–254.

38. McCoy, RB. Caries risk treatment—Where are you? [editorial]. Oper Dent 1997;22:241.

39. Mertz-Fairhurst EJ, Ergle JW. Cariostatic and ultraconservative sealed Class-I restorations: Ten-year results [abstract 1892]. J Dent Res 1995;74:248.

40. Miller WE. The Micro-organisms of the Human Mouth. Philadelphia: SSC White, 1890.

41. Mjor IA, Toffenetti F. Secondary caries: A literature review with case reports. Quintessence Int 2000;31:165–179.

42. Mount GJ, Hume WR. Preservation and Restoration of Tooth Structure. London: Mosby, 1998.

43. Naitoh M, Yuasa H, Toyama M, et al. Observer agreement in the detection of proximal caries with direct digital intraoral radiography. Oral Surg Oral Med Oral Pathol Oral Radiol Endod 1998;85:107–112.

44. Nikaido T, Katumi M, Burrow MF, Inokoshi S, Yamada T, Takatsu T. Bond strength of resin to enamel and dentin treated with low-pressure air abrasion. Oper Dent 1996;21:218–224.

45. Nordbo H, Brown G, Tjan AH. Chemical treatment of cavity walls following manual excavation of carious dentin. Am J Dent 1996;9:67–71.

46. Osborne JW. Operative dentistry for the new millennium: A problem-specific approach to operative dentistry. Oper Dent 2000;25:59–61.

47. Petersson LG. Fluoride mouthrinses and fluoride varnishes. Caries Res 1993;27(suppl 1): 35–42.

48. Phantumvanit P, Songpaisan Y, Pilot T, Frenken J. Atraumatic restorative treatment (ART): A three-year community field trial in Thailand—Survival of one-surface restorations in permanent dentition. J Public Health Dent 1996;56:141–145.

49. Pitts NB. Patient caries status in the context of practical, evidence-based management of the initial caries lesion. J Dent Educ 1997;61: 861–865.

50. Pitts NB. Score system for behaviour of radiologically diagnosed aproximal carious lesions. Community Dent Oral Epidemiol 1985;3: 268–272.

51. Pitts NB. The use of bite-wing radiographs in the management of dental caries: Scientific and practical considerations. Dentomaxillofac Radiol 1996;25:5–16.

52. Poorterman JH, Aartman IH, Kalsbeek H. Underestimation of the prevalence of approximal caries and inadequate restorations in a clinical epidemiological study. Community Dent Oral Epidemiol 1999;27:331–337.

53. Rinaudo PJ, Cochran MA, Moore BK. The effect of air abrasion on shear bond strength to dentin with dental adhesives. Oper Dent 1997;22:254–259.

54. Roeder LB, Berry EA, You C, Powers JM. Bond strength of composite to air-abraded enamel and dentin. Oper Dent 1995;20:186–190.

55. Schaeken MJ, Keltjiens HM, Van Der Hoeven JS. Effects of fluoride and chlorhexidine on the microflora of dental root surfaces and progression of root-surface caries. J Dent Res 1991;70:150–153.

56. Simonsen RJ. Preventive resin restorations: Three-year results. J Am Dent Assoc 1980;100: 535–539.

57. Simonsen RJ, Stallard RE. Sealant-restorations utilizing a diluted filled resin: One year results. Quintessence Int 1977;8:77–84.

58. Stookey GK, Jackson RD, Zandona AG, Analoui M. Dental caries diagnosis. Dent Clin North Am 1999;43:665–677.

59. Van Amerongen WE. Dental caries under glass ionomer restorations. J Public Health Dent 1996;56:150–154.

60. Walker J, Floyd K, Jakobsen J, Pinkham JR. The effectiveness of preventive resin restorations in pediatric patients. ASDC J Dent Child 1996;63:338–340.

61. Wright GZ, Hatibovic-Kofman S, Millenaar DW, Braverman I. The safety and efficacy of treatment with air abrasion technology. Int J Paediatr Dent 1999;9:133–134.

Chapter 7

Replacement or Repair of Dental Restorations

Nairn H. F. Wilson, James C. Setcos, and Paul Brunton

Introduction

Traditional dental teaching has perpetuated the view that those restorations that do not satisfy strict quality requirements should be replaced. This outdated mechanistic approach, which typically involves the removal of the entire restoration, including any bases and liners, stems from the erroneous thinking that all marginal and interfacial defects, irrespective of their nature, location, or extent, are associated with the free flow of oral fluids in the tooth-restoration interface. Such thinking also tends to extend to the view that microleakage, as demonstrated under laboratory conditions, occurs clinically and will inevitably lead to secondary caries and pulp pathology with associated clinical symptoms. In the process of pursuing such a "drill and fill" approach to operative dentistry, hindsight has revealed that countless serviceable restorations, notably in the mouths of low caries–risk patients, must have been unnecessarily replaced.[4]

This cyclic repeated restoration is accompanied by the associated loss of tooth tissue by progressive cavity enlargement[8] and repeated insults to the pulp, as well as misuse of patient's time, resources, and tolerance of interventive dental care. It is all too easy to be critical, however, when looking retrospectively, in particular, when it has been the exception rather than the rule for patients to have low caries risk. Furthermore, when clinicians have a population of patients with high caries risk and are hard-pressed to deliver the greatest good to the greatest number, it is acknowledged, as recently evidenced by work on the atraumatic restorative treatment (ART) technique, that a pragmatic rather than an idealistic approach to the delivery of care has many merits.[5]

Notwithstanding the expanding options for dental care, it remains the case that where there is clear evidence of frank failure of a restoration, there are few, if any, alternatives to making arrangements to provide a replacement restoration

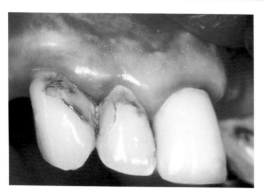

Fig 7-1 Stained and deficient composites in the right maxillary lateral incisor and canine.

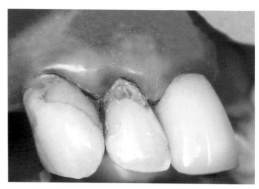

Fig 7-2 After attempted refinishing, composites still show unacceptable marginal discrepancies.

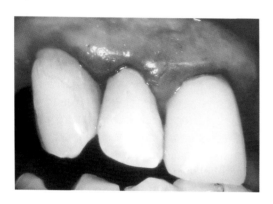

Fig 7-3 Replacement composites immediately following placement.

(Figs 7-1 to 7-3). In such circumstances, the challenge is to minimize the consequences of the intervention while maximizing the quality of the outcome, having identified and, wherever possible, managed the underlying cause of the failure.

Operative dentistry, as currently taught in dental schools around the world, will continue to constitute the major component of everyday clinical practice. Modern-day dentistry must, in addition to meeting patients' ever-increasing expec-

tations, cope with the legacy of pre-existing restorations provided according to traditional principles. Regrettably, many patients remain at risk for recurrent disease, and it is therefore inevitable that, for the foreseeable future, over 50% of all restorative dentistry may continue to be the replacement of restorations.[1] Notwithstanding such considerations, it is suggested that teachers, researchers, and practitioners work together to shift the thought process from "diagnose and treat" to "predict and prevent." An important element of such new thinking relates to the maintenance and repair, rather than the replacement, of deteriorating yet serviceable restorations in patients who maintain a good standard of oral health. These patients have a favorable oral environment in which minimal interventive care should be considered.[7] Central to such thinking is the acceptance that the repair of restorations is not substandard "cheapskate" care. In contrast, such care, given clinical indication and the application of appropriate techniques, should increasingly be viewed as the most appropriate and contemporary form of care in a patient-centered approach to the lifelong provision of high quality restorative dentistry.

The repair of a restoration may include an element of refurbishment, a procedure that should normally preempt and delay repair or replacement. Refurbishment procedures typically involve the refinishing of a restoration, with or without recontouring. Refurbishment may be limited to the margins of a restoration or involve all of the exposed surfaces (Figs 7-4 to 7-8). Following the use of finishing procedures using existing finishing systems, the effects of which can alone greatly influence the clinician's decision making, the application of a surface coating (resurfacing) would appear to offer certain advantages. Loss of anatomic form (wear) in posterior composites (especially earlier generations of composites) may be seen after several years of clinical service (Fig 7-9). For composite restorations with wear but no other defects, the procedure of "resurfacing" by bonding a layer of new composite to replace the lost material has been reported.[2] Although much of the surface glaze and other thin coating applied over the surface of a restoration may be lost within a few days of application, there can be advantages gained by filling in microscopic marginal defects and cracks in the composite or margin enamel, thereby achieving decreased rates of wear.[3]

In discussing the criteria and techniques to underpin the proposed shift to the increasing use of repair procedures as part of the wider concept of preservative dentistry, it is acknowledged that, to date, the clinical evidence to support the efficacy of repairs is largely anecdotal. Robust clinical data, which can not be derived by a summation of clinical anecdote, is essential. As in many aspects of present-day operative dentistry, the need for new groundbreaking research is substantial. The global expenditure on operative dentistry, although never quantified objectively, is considered to be immense, yet the investment in researching and validating new procedures is, by all accounts, trivial.

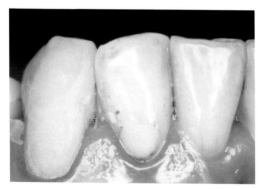

Fig 7-4 Staining associated with otherwise satisfactory composite in the right mandibular lateral incisor.

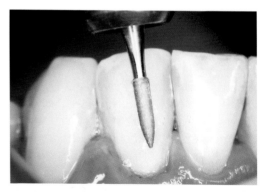

Fig 7-5 Fine-particle diamond finishing bur used to remove stain and smooth the composite surface.

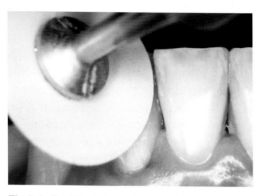

Fig 7-6 Flexible disk used to polish the composite surface.

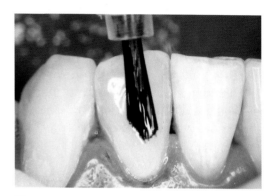

Fig 7-7 Application of unfilled resin as a surface "glaze."

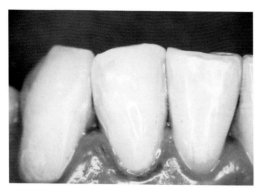

Fig 7-8 Refinished restoration after light activation of resin applied to the surface.

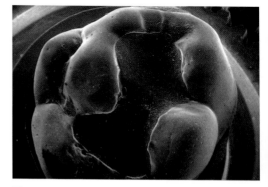

Fig 7-9 Cast of molar tooth restored with a posterior composite, showing marginal discrepancy due to loss of composite material after several years of clinical service.

Criteria for Refurbishment and Repair

Criteria for the refurbishment and repair of restorations may be considered to fall into one of two categories: patient-centered and tooth-specific criteria. As with all other decision-making criteria, however, there is considerable overlap and linkage amongst the criteria, which, as a consequence, should be applied collectively rather than individually. In such decision making, the views and wishes of the patient must be taken into account if the treatment to be provided is to be truly patient-centered and specific. Such reinforcing of the relationship between clinical and patient requirements is considered to have many significant advantages beyond improved communication and a mutual understanding of the desired outcome of treatment.

Patient-Centered Criteria

In general, refurbishment and repair procedures should be limited to patients who are regular attenders, maintain a good standard of oral health, and are dentally motivated. Exceptions to such criteria may include patients with special needs, including elderly patients with conditions that complicate and limit oral hygiene, cooperation, and tolerance of dental procedures. In this respect, patients who have been provided with sophisticated forms of advanced restorative dentistry and have lost manual dexterity and mobility pose a particular problem.

Further patient-centered criteria relate to the patient's understanding and accept-ance of refurbishment and repair procedures as having advantages over replacement therapies. Research in the field of refurbishment and repair versus replacement is much needed. It is possible that in accepting the refurbishment and repair approach, patients may be committing themselves to ongoing care involving a succession of minor interventions with occasional major replacement procedures when and if frank failure, such as bulk fracture, occurs. This is in contrast to more traditional treatment, which involves fewer interventions, but more replacement procedures than would otherwise be necessary. Some evidence of patients' acceptance of an ongoing program of minor interventions in preference to the traditional approach to restorative care is provided by the emerging trend to favor the relatively frequent application of materials requiring minor intervention in the management of noncarious cervical lesions. Admittedly, esthetic considerations greatly influence patients' thinking when restorations will be included in the smile, but increasingly there are opportunities to be noninterventive, yet satisfy the esthetic expectations of the patient.

Tooth-Specific Criteria

Having ascertained that patient-centered criteria are satisfied, individual restored tooth units remain to be assessed regarding the appropriateness of applying repair and associated refurbishment procedures. Research is needed to define and validate tooth-specific criteria. Meanwhile, it is suggested that a new lesion of caries immediately adjacent to an existing restoration

109

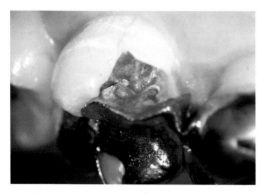

Fig 7-10 Cuspal fracture adjacent to a cast gold inlay.

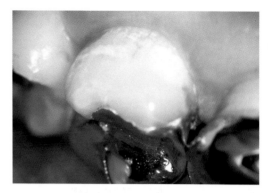

Fig 7-11 Bonded composite effecting cuspal repair.

and/or the deterioration of the existing restoration(s) should be limited, but at the same time sufficient to warrant intervention if a repair is to be justified. In practical terms, this would require new caries to be active and to involve dentin and, in the case of an existing restoration, for there to be a progressive defect that threatens the viability of the restored tooth unit before intervention could be justified. Esthetic deterioration with or without the presence of a lesion, even if inactive and limited to enamel but compromising to the patient's dental attractiveness, could be considered to justify a repair and associated refurbishment. As in modern-day management of primary caries, the decision regarding the nature of the necessary intervention should in many cases be deferred pending the outcome of preventive management. This also applies to the findings of an exploratory procedure to investigate, for example, the extent to which marginal staining may have penetrated in a pulpal direction, giving rise to worrisome interfacial staining. To effectively undertake such assessments,

the use of magnification is considered important.[10] Clinicians unfamiliar with the use of magnifying aids should, however, be mindful of the possibility of being excessively interventive in their assessments given that relatively few existing restorations are found to have ideal characteristics when examined with the aid of loupes, let alone an operating microscope.

As with patient-centered criteria, tooth-specific criteria may be overridden by confounding factors, the most notable of which may be the risk of failure to restore the tooth if a replacement restoration were planned. For example, an ambitious repair of a large intracoronal compound restoration in the molar tooth of an elderly patient may offer better prospects of success than a replacement that, despite all care and attention, may lead to no other option than the provision of an unwanted crown. A cuspal fracture may be readily repaired[6] (Figs 7-10 and 7-11). Special considerations may also apply when, for example, considering the restorative options for a restored abutment tooth in a complex prosthesis. These considerations share a great deal of commonality with the considerations relating to the options for restoring endodontic access cavities in fixed partial dentures.

Repair Techniques

Techniques for effective repairs remain to be fully investigated given the inherent problems of linking new and clinically aged materials to form a mechanically robust restored tooth unit. The technique varies with the material of the restoration being repaired, the material selected to complete the repair, and the functional requirements of the repair. Notwithstanding such considerations, certain principles apply to all repairs.

Cavity Preparation

The principles of cavity preparation for repairs are considered to include:

1. Access
2. Lesion management
3. Bonding (retention) form and finishing

Access
Access is required for effective instrumentation in the preparation and subsequent procedures integral to the placement of the repair. Poor access may result in failure to manage the lesion and in less-than-ideal adaptation, as well as porosity and voids in the repair as seen in certain restorations placed in minimal extension preparations. In creating access, careful consideration must be given to creating space for a repair of functional thickness and the avoidance of placing new margins and the junction between the repair and the existing restoration directly under an occlusal contact. For proximal surfaces, special instrumentation is needed to remove restoration overhangs and refinish the surface (Figs 7-12 to 7-14).

Lesion management
Lesion management in repair procedures differs from that in routine cavity preparation in that the clinician may be left with considerable uncertainties as to whether the entire lesion has been accessed, let alone managed. Where uncertainties are encountered, the clinician must weigh the disadvantages of a replacement restoration rather than a repair against the risk of having failed to access and manage the entire lesion being treated. Clearly, if diseased tissue is found to extend up to or even under the exposed section of the existing restoration, access should be extended. However, because arrangements should be made to bond and seal the repair to both the exposed section of the existing restoration and the new cavity walls and margins, the decision may be made to leave some residual softened dentin and thereby minimize the risk of pulpal involvement.

Bonding (retention) form and finishing
In addition to the resistance and retention form that typically exists within a preparation for a repair, it is considered prudent to maximize the bonding form through appropriate finishing of the walls and margins of the preparation. Roughening of the cut surface and margins of the existing restoration is contraindicated given that,

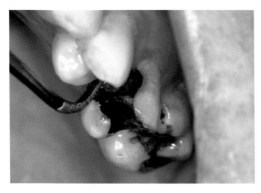

Fig 7-12 Removal of an amalgam overhang using a safe-sided diamond tip in a sonic handpiece.

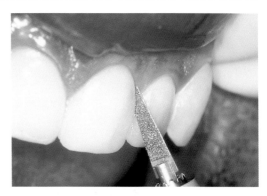

Fig 7-13 Ledge removal and smoothing along the proximal margin of a veneer using a safe-sided diamond tip in a reciprocating handpiece.

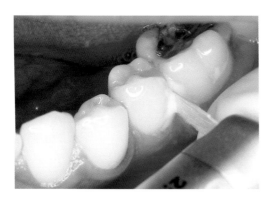

Fig 7-14 Interproximal polishing of a restoration using polishing paste together with a wooden tip in a reciprocating handpiece.

irrespective of the materials involved, the outcome is typically air inclusions and evidence of less-than-ideal adaptation at the interface between the repair and the remaining portion of the existing restoration.

Management of Exposed Dentin

In most cases, the preparation for a repair is relatively shallow and operatively exposed dentin may be appropriately managed by etching and bonding. In deep preparations, there may be merits in placing a base of, for example, a glass-ionomer cement, in a manner similar to that employed in procedures to replace restorations.

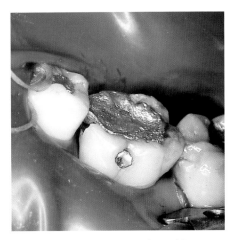

Fig 7-15 Amalgam restoration with a reparable marginal defect.

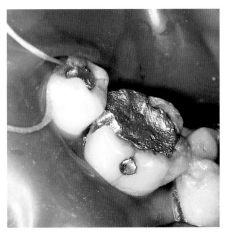

Fig 7-16 Repair preparation completed using a diamond tip in a sonic handpiece.

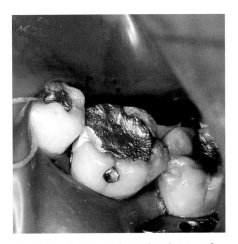

Fig 7-17 Completed repair prior to refurbishment of the restoration.

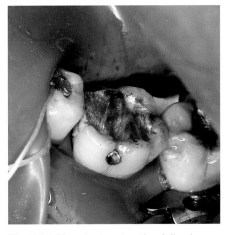

Fig 7-18 Repaired restoration following refurbishment and polishing.

Placement of the Repair

The precise procedure to be followed is dependent on the material of the restoration to be repaired and the material selected to complete the repair. Experience indicates that whatever the circumstances of the repair, an adhesive approach should be considered even in the case of an amalgam repair to an existing amalgam restoration, as may occur in the management of ditching without associated caries[9] (Figs 7-15 to 7-18). In all cases, the directions for the use of the selected materials must be

113

meticulously followed, with great care being taken to achieve good adaptation of the repair material to, in particular, the margins of the preparation. Appropriate finishing should be extended to include all the restored surfaces, not just the repair.

Postoperative Monitoring

Given the lack of objective data on the performance of repairs to restorations in clinical service, there is a good case for recommending special care in the monitoring of repairs. A particular concern is the failure to identify an interfacial gap between repair and restoration and, as a consequence, leakage that may be clinically significant but masked when, in particular, the restorations and repair are metallic. Such concerns may be alleviated by the use of magnification to visually inspect the repair and associated restoration at each review and by the routine use of compressed air and thermal and electrical pulp tests to complement a detailed visual inspection.

Considerations for the Future

It is understood that many clinicians already view the repair of restorations as an established part of their everyday practice. Data on the techniques found to be most successful and on the clinical performance of repairs, notably in terms of the extension of the longevity of repaired restorations, would be an invaluable addition to data that must be collected from randomized controlled trials. Such trials, out of necessity for ethical approval, must be preceded by a fully comprehensive review of the relevant literature and possibly certain simulation investigations followed by any necessary pilot studies. Concurrently, the profession at large should apply existing knowledge and understanding, tempered by intuition to develop proposals for new approaches, instrumentation, techniques, and devices to facilitate the provision of repairs. Thereafter, meaningful pragmatic (field) studies and cost-benefit analyses may be planned to determine the lasting value of repairs as opposed to replacement restorations. Whatever the outcome of this program of research, it may be confidently predicted that repairs, in a similar manner to preservative restorative techniques, are equally, if not more, demanding compared with traditional techniques.

References

1. Burke FJT, Cheung SW, Mjör IA, Wilson NHF. Reasons for the placement and replacement of restorations in vocational training practices. Prim Dent Care 1999;6:17–20.

2. Crumpler DC, Bayne SC, Sockwell S, Brunson D, Roberson TM. Bonding to resurfaced posterior composites. Dent Mater 1989;5:417–424.

3. Dickinson GL, Leinfelder KF. Assessing the long-term effect of a surface penetrating sealant. J Am Dent Assoc 1993;124:68–72.

4. Elderton RJ. Clinical studies concerning re-restoration of teeth. Adv Dent Res 1990;4:4–9.

5. Frencken JE, Makoni F, Sithole WD. ART restorations and glass ionomer sealants in Zimbabwe: Survival after 3 years. Community Dent Oral Epidemiol 1998;26:372–381.

6. McDaniel RJ, Davis RD, Murchison DF, Cohen RB. Causes of failure among cuspal-coverage amalgam restorations: a clinical survey. J Am Dent Assoc 2000;131:173–177.

7. Mjör IA. Repair versus replacement of failed restorations. Int Dent J 1993;43:466–472.

8. Mjör IA, Reep RL, Kubilis PS, Mondragon BE. Change in size of replaced amalgam restorations: a methodological study. Oper Dent 1998;23: 272–277.

9. Paterson FM, Paterson RC, Watts A, Blinkhorn AS. Initial stages in the development of valid criteria for the replacement of amalgam restorations. J Dent 1995;23:137–143.

10. Whitehead SA, Wilson NHF. Restorative decision-making behaviour with magnification. Quintessence Int 1992;23:667–671.

115

Chapter 8

Biologic Aspects: Adverse and Beneficial Effects of Restorative Materials

W. Rory Hume

Introduction

In most cases, tooth restoration is in the best interest of patients. It is indisputably better than leaving progressive caries untreated, and is in most cases better than treating the disease by extracting teeth. The incidence of adverse systemic effects of restorative materials in patients is at present extremely low (Fig 8-1). In the case of dental amalgam, there is a long-standing controversy about whole-body safety. There are also more recent concerns related to chemicals released into the body from resin-based materials .

The health risks for dentists and other dental workers from dental restorative materials are also not great, providing that appropriate precautions are taken.

The great majority of adverse responses to dental restoratives are in the tissues immediately adjacent to the area restored, most commonly the dental pulp and, if the pulp dies and the pulp space becomes infected, the periapical tissues. Pulp sensitivity or pulp death after restoration place-

ment are, unfortunately, relatively common. There is good evidence that these problems are related to the nature of the restorative materials used.

Some restorative materials release chemicals that have direct and local therapeutic effects. These include zinc oxide–eugenol (ZOE), some materials which contain antibiotics and corticosteroids, and glass-ionomer cements, which contain fluoride, calcium, and phosphate.

The aim of this chapter is to provide information that will help dentists and patients to evaluate the balance between benefits and risk and, in the case of pulpal responses, to help dentists make choices that help to avoid adverse effects and manage them if they have already occurred.

An understanding of several factors can provide a common, sound basis for both understanding and avoiding adverse effects and for using materials therapeutically. These factors include: the dynamics of release of chemicals from restorative materials into the local environment and into the body as a whole, the concen-

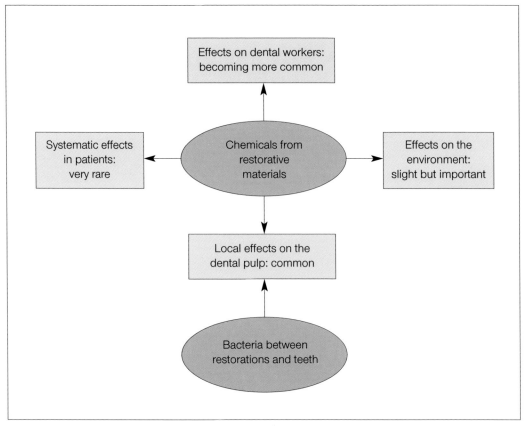

Fig 8-1 The principal risks of adverse effects related to restorative materials.

trations of such chemicals that develop in the tissues, the biologic effects of the chemicals at the concentrations achieved, and the time for which they are present before they leave the body.

This chapter comprises three sections:

1. Concerns about systemic health effects related to the use of dental amalgam
2. Possible adverse systemic effects of resin-based materials
3. Pulpal responses to restorative materials, both adverse and beneficial

Dental Amalgam

Dental amalgam is made by mixing an alloy of several metals, most commonly silver, tin, and copper, with mercury. Although each of the metals has the potential to cause adverse effects at high concentrations, attention has historically been focused on mercury, principally because mercury and some mercury compounds are potential toxins at relatively low concentrations.

The simplest way to explain the risks posed by mercury to people who work in

MERCURY

- LIQUID to VAPOR—neurotoxic risk to dental workers

- INORGANIC compounds—safest form, eg, dental amalgams

- ORGANIC compounds—risk to the environment from dental waste

Fig 8-2 The three forms of mercury and the nature of related risks in dentistry.

dental offices, patients, and the environment is to briefly describe the toxicology of the three basic types of mercury and the risks they pose. More detailed descriptions of the toxicology of mercury have been published.[7,22,41]

From a toxicologic viewpoint, there are three forms of mercury: elemental mercury, inorganic compounds of mercury, and organic compounds of mercury (Fig 8-2). Each is quite different from the others.

Elemental Mercury

Elemental mercury is, at the temperature of the biosphere, either a liquid or a vapor. Un-ionized elemental mercury is highly lipid soluble. When mercury vapor is inhaled, it is rapidly taken up across the alveoli into the blood and it remains un-ionized for several minutes thereafter. During this time it is distributed throughout the body tissues. Because it is highly lipid soluble at this time, elemental mercury passes readily across capillary walls into the brain. These capillaries, the "blood-brain barrier," are permeable to chemicals that are lipid soluble, but are relatively impermeable to

chemicals that are not lipid soluble. After a few minutes, the un-ionized mercury becomes ionized, Hg^{++}. In most of the body this is not a problem, because in the general circulation Hg^{++} can diffuse back into the blood and is cleared by the kidneys into the urine. But Hg^{++} cannot get out of the brain as easily because of the unique nature of the blood-brain barrier.

If the mercury vapor level is low, then the slow rate of clearance from the brain can match the slow rate of uptake. All humans inhale small amounts of mercury vapor all of the time because mercury is part of the biosphere, but at low levels it does not accumulate in the brain. However, if the vapor intake is high, then the slow rate of clearance cannot match the rate of uptake and the levels of mercury in the brain tissue therefore increase. When the levels of tissue mercury become sufficiently high, some basic enzymes in the glycolytic pathway are inhibited and brain cell function is changed. The first symptoms are usually tremors and fatigue. With increasing levels tremors get worse, then basic neural functions become impaired, leading to insanity and then death.[41,67]

Dentists and dental workers, like people who work in other industries that use liquid mercury, are at risk from mercury vapor. It is important to keep the level of mercury vapor in the dental work environment as low as possible by practicing what is termed "mercury hygiene."[44]

The surfaces of dental amalgam restorations release very low levels of mercury vapor when abraded,[21,43,63,65,66] but the level appears to be so low as to pose no risk to patients.[12,13,59] Measurement of brain mercury levels in 101 autopsy subjects with known dental amalgam status and dental amalgam history showed no association between these factors.[61]

Inorganic Compounds

Inorganic compounds of mercury are the safest forms. If swallowed, they are absorbed relatively poorly into the body as ionized mercury, which is readily excreted via the kidneys. Some ionized mercury is taken up from swallowed particles of amalgam, for example, but the rate of uptake is slow and the excretion via the kidneys is good. Similarly, swallowed liquid mercury droplets form a surface coat of mercuric chloride through reaction with HCl in the stomach. Mercuric chloride is poorly absorbed from the gut. The mercury droplets reach the feces essentially intact and are excreted.

Organic Compounds

The third form of mercury from a toxicologic viewpoint is organic compounds. Some of these are highly toxic and dangerous. The prime and very relevant example is methyly mercury, which in moderate doses can cause severe neurological damage and death. Mercury from industrial waste can be converted by anaerobic bacteria in river or sea mud to methyly mercury, which can enter the food chain via fish and damage human health.[42] Fortunately, there is no evidence that the bacteria in the human mouth can convert mercury from dental amalgam into organic compounds of mercury. However, this potential chain of events is important from the point of view of industrial pollution risk from dentistry. The dental industry is one of the sources of mercury in wastewater. The dental profession is under sustained pressure in many parts of the world to minimize the environmental risk of mercury.

It is important to know when discussing the risks of mercury with patients that mercury is a component of the normal human diet. Anything that is grown in the earth, anything that eats things that grow in the earth, or anything that comes from the sea has mercury in it. The normal daily human diet contains approximately 21 μg of inorganic mercury and 3.8 μg of organic mercury. The maximum theoretical amount of additional mercury intake from the wearing down of amalgam fillings in a heavily restored mouth has been calculated at 1.3 μg per day. The normal blood mercury level in humans is in the 3- to 5-ng/mL range. Amalgam removal studies show that the uptake into the body from amalgam in a heavily restored mouth can add less than 1 ng/mL to the blood mercury level. We know that the toxic level of mercury in blood is approximately 30 ng/mL. It is also highly relevant that there is no evidence of any difference in morbidity or mortality between people who have never had amalgam fillings, those who have amalgam fillings, and those who have had amalgam fillings removed.[8,11,59]

Rarely, local allergic reactions occur on the mucosa adjacent to amalgam restorations. This can be a true allergy to mercury, or it might be an allergic response to silver or tin. The allergy is usually a whitened patch with a surrounding reddened area; its appearance is identical to lichen planus.

There undoubtedly will be continuing pressure on the dental profession to find alternatives to dental amalgam. The reasons for this are not related to any direct risk to patients' health, but rather to the indirect risks that amalgam used in dentistry poses through industrial pollution.

Resin-Based Materials

Several chemicals are known to be released from resin-based dental materials. There is no evidence of systemic toxicity for either patients or dental workers from any of these chemicals, although as will be described below they can pose local (pulpal) toxic risks to patients. The known risk of these chemicals is allergy, principally to dental workers, and the suggested risk to patients is estrogenicity.

Most composite resins are made up of filler particles, usually glass or silica, and a matrix, which is primarily a mixture of bisphenol A glycidyl methacrylate (Bis-GMA) and triethyleneglycol dimethacrylate (TEGDMA).[60] Bis-GMA is a large molecule and is very viscous at room temperature. To be usable as a dental material, it has to have some ability to flow and it is therefore mixed with a much more fluid resin monomer, TEGDMA. For stiff, packable composites the TEGDMA pro-

portion is about 15%, while for flowable composites, bonding resins, or fissure sealants the TEGDMA proportion is much higher, in the 50% to 60% range.

When Bis-GMA–TEGDMA mixtures are cured, the conversion, or polymerization, of Bis-GMA is relatively complete, but the polymerization of TEGDMA is much less so.[16,17] Many studies have shown that substantial amounts of TEGDMA diffuse out of the cured composites, bonding resins, or fissure sealants.[23–27,30,35] Approximately 30 μg of TEGDMA is released into the biophase from a routine, composite resin filling during the first 3 days after it is placed into a tooth (Fig 8-3).[26]

Another resin monomer, hydroxyethyl methacrylate (HEMA) is used as the principal constituent of all successful dentin-bonding primers.[39] HEMA works as a primer in contact with dentin because it is relatively hydrophilic. Bis-GMA and TEGDMA are hydrophobic, so they have very little chance on their own of adhering to dentin. After HEMA has cured, TEGDMA–Bis-GMA mixtures wet it and the sequence can therefore adhere to dentin moderately well.[49]

HEMA polymerizes quite poorly, particularly at the surface of dentin, which is a complex mixture of collagen, apatite, and water. After bonding resin is placed and cured on dentin, approximately 20 μg of HEMA per restored tooth diffuses into the biophase.[24,35]

Composite resin restorative materials therefore release moderate amounts of TEGDMA and, if bonding resins are used, HEMA into the body. It is also important to note that both TEGDMA and HEMA can diffuse out of resin-based filling materials, through gloves, and into the skin of dentists and dental assistants.[48]

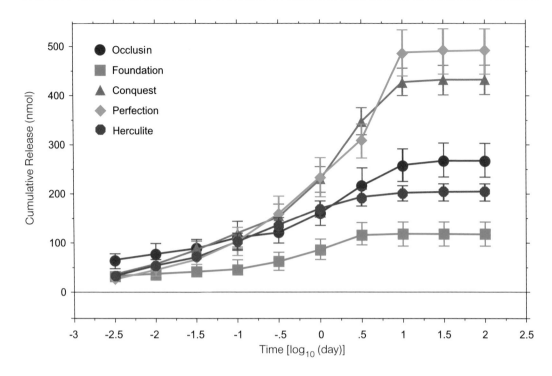

Fig 8-3 Direct cumulative release of TEGDMA (means and standard deviations shown) in nanomoles from five commercially available composite resins. The time point shown is the end-point of the collection period. The $\log_{10}$ time scale shown is 4.32, 14.4, 43.2, 144, and 432 minutes and 1, 3, 10, 30, and 100 days. The total amounts of TEGDMA released from the various resins were in the range 100 to 500 nmol (30 to 150 µg).

We now have some information about what happens to TEGDMA when it enters the body.[57] It is distributed quite widely throughout all tissues, apparently metabolized in the liver, and excreted over about a 3-day period. The dynamics of distribution and excretion appear to be similar whether it is swallowed or absorbed through the skin. Fortunately, the TEGDMA concentrations that are achieved in various tissues in the body following administration of doses well above those that are known to be released from composite resin restorations are well below the

known levels for toxicity.[58] So there appears to be very little risk of any whole-body toxic effects from TEGDMA, for either patients or dental workers.[57] The distribution and clearance dynamics for HEMA appear to be similar (Reichl and Hume, unpublished data, 2000).

However, HEMA, in particular, is known to be a potent allergen.[38] There are many case reports of people who work with HEMA in dentistry and in the printing industry becoming sensitive to it.[9,38,39,40,46]

Allergic responses to HEMA or TEGDMA in patients seem, to date, to be

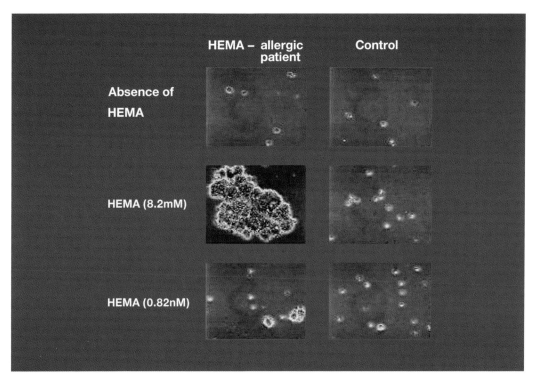

Fig 8-4 Lymphocytes in culture from a HEMA-allergic dentist in the absence and presence of HEMA, compared with lymphocytes from a nonallergic human control. The cell clumping (blast formation) is a strong indication of immune activation (Jewett and Hume, unpublished data, 2000).

quite rare.[29,51] In one case report, a patient had severe respiratory distress after receiving fissure sealants and the symptoms were not relieved until after the sealants were removed.[29] However, allergic responses are becoming more common in dentists and dental assistants (Fig 8-4). For example, 30 cases of allergic responses to resin-containing materials in Finnish dental workers were reported during the 2-year period from 1993 through 1994 (Forsten L, personal communication, 1995). The most common symptom is fingertip dermatitis, sometimes so severe that people cannot work. Other whole-body allergic symptoms,

such as bronchoconstriction and skin rashes elsewhere occur less commonly.

The other possible adverse effects related to composite resins revolve around the potential estrogenicity of bisphenol-A. All present data indicate that it is very unlikely that this is in any way important to patient health or safety. However, since there have been concerns expressed about this matter both in the scientific literature[19,52,62] and in the lay press,[56] the matter is worth describing in some detail.

Olea et al[52] proposed that bisphenol-A might be released from dental resin-based materials because it is a precursor of Bis-

GMA. Their concern was that bisphenol-A, which is estrogenic in its actions on cells at moderate concentrations, could have effects on children such as accelerating puberty in girls and reducing sperm counts in boys. They tested the saliva of patients who had received one brand of fissure sealant available in Spain and composite resin fillings for the presence of bisphenol-A. They reported detecting substantial amounts of bisphenol-A in the saliva of these patients.

Two groups attempted to duplicate these results and could not do so.[30,50] In both studies, a broad range of fissure sealants commercially available in the US was examined for any evidence of release or leaching of bisphenol-A into water. Each group used high-performance liquid chromatography, the same technology that Olea et al had used. Neither group was able to detect any released bisphenol-A. Both groups[30,50] showed that the major released component from the fissure sealants was TEGDMA. TEGDMA has no known estrogenic properties. It was strongly suggested[30] that Olea et al, who had not reported finding TEGDMA in their samples, had made an analytic error and had misidentified TEGDMA as bisphenol-A. The other possible interpretation was that the one fissure sealant that Olea et al had tested was contaminated with bisphenol-A. Bisphenol-A is added to Bis-GMA for use in electronic circuit boards, and this form of Bis-GMA could possibly have been used in the manufacture of the sealant that Olea et al tested.

More recently, Fung et al[19] looked again at the possibility of bisphenol-A release from fissure sealants into the saliva of human volunteers, using an improved detection technology, an ultraviolet fluores-cent system linked to high-pressure liquid chromatography (HPLC). The system had a sensitivity limit of five parts per billion, which was substantially more sensitive than the methods used previously. They confirmed that the major chemical released from fissure sealants was TEGDMA, but they also found trace amounts of bisphenol-A, just above the five parts per billion level, in the saliva of some of the subjects who had received the sealants. They could not detect bisphenol-A in the saliva after more than 3 hours had passed since the placement of the sealants. They also found no evidence of bisphenol-A in the blood of the volunteers.

The concentrations of bisphenol-A demonstrated[19] in saliva for the 3 hours during which it was detectable were in the nanomolar range. Bisphenol-A in the nanomolar concentration range was shown to stimulate the proliferation of estrogen-sensitive human breast cancer cells.[52] However, in a more recent study[3] it was shown that in the same range of concentrations, the chemical did not have a proliferative effect on human gingival epithelial cells. Markedly higher concentrations of bisphenol-A were required to damage cells.[3]

Despite the extremely low apparent probability of adverse local or systemic effects from bisphenol-A, there are likely to be more studies in the coming years on these matters.[62] At present all data indicate strongly that there is no biologic risk from bisphenol-A released from fissure sealants or other resin-based restorations. According to G. Christiansen, "There is more estrogenicity in a mother's kiss than there is in a fissure sealant" (personal communication, 2000).

Pulpal Responses to Restorative Materials

Ever since fillings, as we understand them, were first described,[14] there have been reports of patients having pulpal pain in the days and weeks after restoration placement, and pulp death in the weeks, months, or years thereafter.

Fauchard[14,15] proposed that the pressure of condensation of metal fillings onto the dentin caused the problem. He believed that placing a base, a plastic material that was flowed onto the dentin and then set, before condensing the metal filling reduced the pressure and therefore reduced the risk of pulpal damage. His theory of why the problems occurred was very probably not correct, but bases worked and they still do.

Between 1850 and 1950 it was generally accepted that metal restorations damaged the pulp by conducting heat into or out of the tooth as patients ate hot or cold foods.[4] Dentists used bases to decrease this thermal conductivity.

In the 1920s, when tooth-colored filling materials (silicate cement and direct filling acrylic resin) first became available, dentists discovered that if a base was not used, there were major problems with pulp sensitivity and pulp death.[47] This presented a logical difficulty, because both materials were themselves very good insulators. The profession needed another explanation for why the materials caused such problems, and that explanation was that they released toxic chemicals that could damage the pulp. The idea at that time was that a base material, such as zinc phosphate cement or, later, calcium hydroxide cement, would protect the pulp against chemicals released from the silicate cement or the acrylic resin.

In the 1970s and 1980s a new hypothesis was proposed, namely that microleakage between fillings and tooth structure allowed bacteria to grow beneath the fillings and that products of bacterial metabolism caused chronic pulpal inflammation, leading to pulpal death. There is strong experimental evidence supporting this hypothesis.[5,6,10,45] The concept explains why bases have always worked to reduce the incidence of late pulpal death. It also led to the practice of "total etch, total seal," which is a very appealing and worthwhile idea.[20] Unfortunately, a total seal is difficult to achieve with resin-based systems, particularly with large composite resin restorations, because resins shrink as they cure. It is rational to use a glass-ionomer cement base beneath large composite resin restorations to compensate for this tendency to leak.[36]

It is important to note that while the bacterial microleakage hypothesis provides a logical explanation for chronic inflammation, and therefore pulpal death months or years after restoration, it does not provide an explanation for short-term, acute inflammation or for pulpal death soon after tooth restoration. We can expect pulpal cell damage, and therefore acute inflammation, in response to the trauma of cavity preparation. There is also abundant and direct evidence that chemicals released from some filling materials can diffuse through dentin and into the pulp in sufficient concentration to damage pulpal cells.[33,35,36] It is worthwhile to summarize what is known about this.

Many restorative materials have toxic components and are themselves toxic if they are placed directly into tissue culture.[35] This includes such things as zinc oxide–eugenol, any of the acid-base

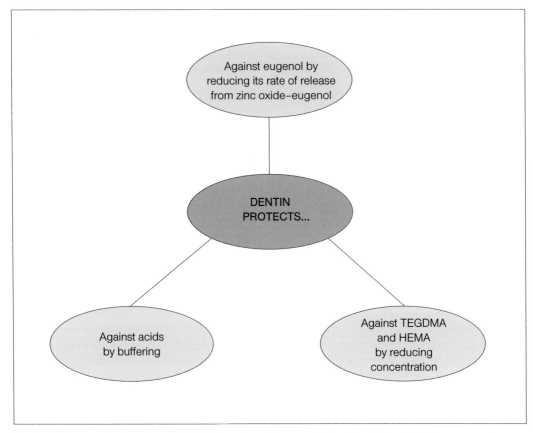

Fig 8-5 Three mechanisms by which dentin reduces the potential toxicity of chemicals from restorative materials.

reaction materials such as zinc phosphate cement, silicate cement, or glass-ionomer cement, and all of the resin-based materials, whether primers, bonding resins, or composite resin filling materials.[31,35,36]

Fortunately, dentin protects against this toxicity in most cases (Fig 8-5).[31,35] Dentin substantially reduces the rate of release of eugenol from zinc oxide–eugenol, reducing the resultant concentration in the pulp from one that would be toxic to one that is in the therapeutic range as a local anesthetic and anti-inflammatory.[32,34] Zinc oxide–eugenol is toxic to bacteria in dentin immediately adjacent to the zinc oxide–eugenol, which is part of the reason why it is so useful in dentistry. However, zinc oxide–eugenol is also toxic if it is placed directly onto the exposed pulp or onto other soft tissue. In this way, dentin converts a potentially toxic material into one that is therapeutic.[34] Dentin buffers strong acid extremely well,[68] so acids or acid materials can be placed onto intact dentin without risk to the pulp. This means that materials such as zinc phosphate cement can be used and, if necessary, dentin can be acid-treated without placing

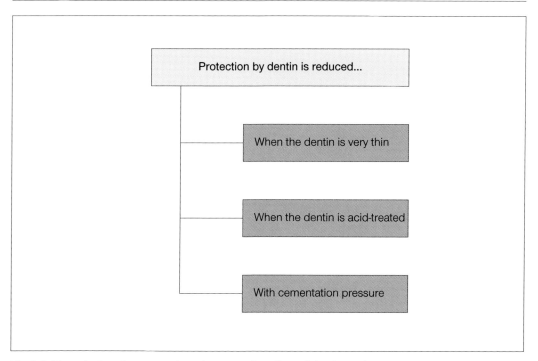

Fig 8-6 Three factors that can reduce the protective effect of dentin against the toxicity of chemicals from restorative materials.

the pulp at risk. Dentin also reduces to some degree the concentration of TEGDMA and HEMA released from restorative resin systems.[24,25] However, with very thin dentin, and dentin that has been acid-treated so that the smear layer is removed, the concentrations of TEGDMA and HEMA can be high enough to cause substantial amounts of damage to the cells in the pulp (Fig 8-6).[18,53,55]

The protective effect of dentin requires that the restorative material stay on one side of dentin while the pulp is on the other. It is possible, during the cementation of a closely fitting crown or inlay onto acid-treated dentin, to force low-viscosity cements through the dentinal tubules into the pulp space.[2] When this happens, quite severe, immediate pulp damage or death can occur due to the loss of dentin's protective effect (Fig 8-6).

It is worthwhile to review briefly three examples of chemical release from restorative materials that have beneficial or therapeutic effects. As was explained above, when zinc oxide–eugenol is placed onto dentin, it releases eugenol in amounts that develop antibacterial concentrations within the dentin but subtoxic concentrations within the adjacent pulp.[32,34] The levels of eugenol in the pulp tissue are sufficient to reduce inflammation and pain, through actions as a nonsteroidal anti-inflammatory and as a local anesthetic.[34]

127

The concentrations in the two tissues are maintained within an order or magnitude for several weeks. The release of both a corticosteroid and an antibiotic from the material Ledermix (Wyeth Lederle, Glostrup, Denmark) has been studied in detail.[1,37] The initial rates of release are relatively high and persist for only a few days. The material can therefore be expected to suppress pulpal or periapical inflammation for 1 or 2 days, but to have little other effect. There is strong direct evidence that glass-ionomer cements release fluoride into the local aqueous environment, and good clinical evidence that this release reduces the risk of caries adjacent to glass-ionomer cement restorations.[28,54,64] There is preliminary evidence that glass-ionomer cement may also contribute to the remineralization of adjacent dentin through release of calcium and phosphate (Ngo H and Mount GJ, personal communication, 1999).

Summary

Fortunately, systemic risks from restorative materials are rare, although concerns about both dental amalgam and resin-based materials are very likely to continue. Local effects on the pulp can be minimized through understanding two basic concepts: first, the desirability of developing an antibacterial seal; and second, using available materials in ways that minimize chemical risks to the tissue. Both zinc oxide–eugenol and steroid-antibiotic mixtures can have positive, therapeutic effects on the pulp. Glass-ionomer cement releases fluoride in sufficient concentrations to reduce the risk of secondary caries.

References

1. Abbott PV, Hume WR, Heithersay GS. The release and diffusion through human coronal dentine in vitro of triamcinolone and demeclocycline from Ledermix paste. Endod Dent Traumatol 1989;5:92–97.

2. Al-Fawaz A, Gerzina TM, Hume WR. Movement of resin cement components through acid-treated dentin during crown cementation in vitro. J Endod 1993;19:219–223.

3. Babich H, Tipton DA. In vitro cytotoxicity of bisphenol A to human gingival epithelial S-G cells. In Vitro Mol Toxicol 1999;12:233–244.

4. Black GV. A Work on Operative Dentistry in Two Volumes. Vol 1: The pathology of the hard tissues of the teeth. Chicago: Medico-Dental, 1908.

5. Brännström M. Dentin and Pulp in Restorative Dentistry. London: Wolfe Medical, 1987.

6. Brännström M, Nordenvall J. Bacterial penetration, pulpal reaction and inner surface of concise enamel bond. Composite fillings in etched and unetched cavities. J Dent Res 1978;57:3–8.

7. Bryant RW. Dental amalgams. In: Mount GJ, Hume WR (eds). Preservation and Restoration of Tooth Structure. London: Mosby, 1998: 113–114.

8. Choi BC. Risk assessment in dentistry: Health risks of dental amalgam revisited. J Can Dent Assoc 1996;62:328–332.

9. Clemmensen S. Sensitizing potential of 2-hydroxyethylmethacrylate. Contact Dermatitis 1985:12;203–208.

10. Cox CF, Keall CL, Keall HJ, Ostro E, Bergenholz G. Biocompatibility of surface-sealed dental materials against exposed pulps. J Prosthet Dent 1987;57:1–8.

11. Department of Health and Human Services' Committee to Coordinate Environmental Health and Related Management. Dental amalgam: A scientific review and recommended public health service strategy for research, education and regulation. Washington, DC: Department of Health and Human Services, 1993.

12. Eley BM. Dental amalgam: A review of safety. London: British Dental Association, 1993.

13. Eley BM, Cox SW. The release, absorption and possible health affects of mercury from dental amalgam: A review of recent findings. Br Dent J 1993;175:355–362.

14. Fauchard P. Le Chirurgen Dentiste. Paris: Pierre-Jean Mariette, 1728.

15. Fauchard P. Le Chirurgen Dentiste [Traité des Dents], ed 2. Paris: Pierre-Jean Mariette, 1746.

16. Ferracane JL, Condon JR. Rate of elution of leachable components from composite. Dent Mater 1990;6:262–287.

17. Ferracane JL, Greener HE. Fourier transform infrared analysis and degree of polymerization in unfilled resins-methods comparison. J Dent Res 1984;63:1093–1095.

18. Fuks AB, Cleaton-Jones P. Pulp response to a composite resin inserted in deep cavities with and without surface seal. J Prosthet Dent 1990; 63:129–134.

19. Fung EYK, Ewoldsen NO, St. Germain HA Jr, et al. Pharmacokinetics of bisphenol A released from a dental sealant. J Am Dent Assoc 2000; 131:51–58.

20. Fusayama T. A Simple Pain-free Adhesive Restorative System by Minimal Reduction and Total Etching. Tokyo: Ishiyaku Euroamerica, 1993:6, 74.

21. Gay DD, Cox RD, Reinhardt JW. Chewing releases mercury from fillings [letter]. Lancet 1979;1:985–986.

22. Gerstner HB, Huff JE. Clinical toxicology of mercury. J Toxicol Environ Health 1977;2:491–526.

23. Gerzina TM. The in vitro bioavaliability of components of some dental restorative resins [thesis]. Sydney: Univ of Sydney, 1995.

24. Gerzina TM, Hume WR. Diffusion of monomers from bonding resin-resin composite combinations through dentine in vitro. J Dent 1996; 24:125–128.

25. Gerzina TM, Hume WR. Effect of dentine on release of TEGDMA from resin composite in vitro. J Oral Rehabil 1994;21:463–468.

26. Gerzina TM, Hume WR. Effect of hydrostatic pressure on the diffusion of monomers through dentin in vitro. J Dent Res 1995;74:369–373.

27. Geurtsen W. Substances released from dental resin composites and glass ionomer cements. Eur J Oral Sci 1998;106:687–695.

28. Gilmour ASM, Edmunds DH, Newcome RG. Prevalence and depth of artificial caries-like lesions adjacent to cavities restored with a glass ionomer or a dentin-bonded composite material. J Dent Res 1997;76:1854–1861.

29. Hallström U. Adverse reaction to a fissure sealant: Report of a case. ASDC J Dent Child 1993;60:143–146.

30. Hamid A, Hume WR. A study of component release from resin pit and fissure sealants in vitro. Dent Mater 1997;12:98–102.

31. Hume WR. A new technique for screening chemical toxicity to the pulp of dental restorative materials and procedures. J Dent Res 1985:64:1322–1325.

32. Hume WR. An analysis of the release and the diffusion through dentin of eugenol from zinc oxide-eugenol mixtures. J Dent Res 1984;63:881–884.

33. Hume WR. Pulp protection during and after tooth restoration. In: Mount GJ, Hume WR (eds). Preservation and Restoration of Tooth Structure. London: Mosby, 1998;203–210.

34. Hume WR. The pharmacology and toxicology of zinc oxide-eugenol. J Am Dent Assoc 1986;113:789–791.

35. Hume WR, Gerzina TM. Bioavailability of components of resin-based materials which are applied to teeth. Crit Rev Oral Biol Med 1996;7:172–179.

36. Hume WR, Massey W. Disease dynamics of the dental pulp. In: Mount GJ, Hume WR (eds). Preservation and Restoration of Tooth Structure. London: Mosby, 1998:37–44.

37. Hume WR, Testa AE. Release of 3H-triamcinolone from a steroid-antibiotic mixture. J Endod 1980;7:509–514.

38. Kanerva L, Estlander T, Jolanki R, Tarvainen K. Dermatitis from acrylates in dental personnel. In: Menne T, Maibach HI (eds). Hand Eczema Book. Boca Raton, FL: CRC Press, 1994:231–254.

39. Kanerva L, Turjanmaa K, Estlander T, Jolanki R. Occupational allergic contact dermatitis from 2-hydroxyethly methacrylate (2-HEMA) in a new dentin adhesive. Am J Contact Dermat 1991;2:24–30.

40. Katsuno K, Manabe A, Itoh K, et al. A delayed hypersensitivity reaction to dentine primer in the guinea-pig. J Dent 1995;23:295–300.

41. Klaassen CD. Heavy metals and heavy-metal antagonists. In: Hardman JG, Limbird LE, Molinoff PB, Ruddon RW, Goodman GA (eds). Goodman and Gilman's. The Pharmacological Basis of Therapeutics. New York: McGraw-Hill, 1998:1649–1671.

42. Kurland LT, Faro SN, Siedler H. Minamata Disease. World Neurol 1960;1:370–390.

43. Mackert JR Jr. Factors affecting estimation of dental amalgam mercury exposure from measurements of mercury vapor levels in intraoral and expired air. J Dent Res 1987;66:1775–1780.

44. Martin FE. Hazards to the operator and staff. In: Mount GJ, Hume WR (eds). Preservation and Restoration of Tooth Structure. London: Mosby, 1998:253–258.

45. Massey WL, Romberg D, Hunter N, Hume WR. The association of dentinal microflora with tissue changes in human carious pulpitis. Oral Microbiol Immunol 1993;8:30–35.

46. Mathias CGT, Caldwell TM, Maibach HI. Contact dermatitis and gastrointestinal symptoms from hydroxyethylmethacrylate. Br J Dermatol 1987;100:447–449.

47. McGehee WHO. A Textbook of Operative Dentistry. Philadelphia: P. Blakiston's Son & Co, 1930.

48. Munksgaard EC. Permeability of protective gloves to (di)methacrylates in resinous dental materials. Scand J Dent Res 1992:100;189–192.

49. Nakabayashi N, Takarada K. Effect of HEMA on bonding to dentine. Dent Mater 1992;8:125–132.

50. Nathanson D, Lertpitayakun P, Lamkin MS, Edalatpour M, Chou LL. In vitro elution of leachable components from dental sealants. J Am Dent Assoc 1997;128:1517–1523.

51. Nathanson D, Lockhart P. Delayed extra oral hypersensitivity to dental composite material. Oral Surg 1979;47:329–333.

52. Olea N, Pulgar R, Perez P, et al. Estrogenicity of resin-based composites and sealants used in dentistry. Environ Health Perspect 1996;104:298–305.

53. Qvist V. Resin restorations: Leakage, bacteria, pulp. Endod Dent Traumatol 1993;9:127–152.

54. Qvist V, Laurberg L, Pulson A, Teglkers PT. Longevity and cariostatic effects of everyday conventional glass ionomer and amalgam restorations in primary teeth: three year results. J Dent Res 1997;76:1387–1396.

55. Qvist V, Staltze K, Qvist J. Human pulp reactions to resin restorations performed with different acid-etch restorative procedures. Acta Odontol Scand 1989;47:253–267.

56. Raloff J. Estrogenic agents leach from dental sealant. Sci News 1996;149:214.

57. Reichl FX, Durner J, Kunzelmann KH, et al. Clearance of dental composite component TEGDMA in Guinea pigs. J Dent Res 2000;79:190.

58. Reichl FX, Durner J, Mückter H, et al. Effect of dental materials on gluconeogenesis in rat kidney tubules. Arch Toxicol 1999;73:381–386.

59. Richardson GM. Assessment of mercury exposure and risks from dental amalgam: Final report. Ottawa: Medical Devices Bureau, Environmental Health Directorate, Health Canada, 1995.

60. Ruyter I E, Sjøvik I J. Composition of dental resin and composite materials. Acta Odont Scand 1981;39:133–146.

61. Saxe SR, Wekstein MW, Kryscio RJ, et al. Alzheimer's Disease, Dental Amalgam and Mercury. J Am Dent Assoc 1999;130:191–199.

62. Soderholm K-J, Mariotti A. BIS-GMA-based resins in dentistry: Are they safe? J Am Dent Assoc 1999;130:201–209.

63. Svare CW, Peterson LC, Reinhardt JW. The effect of dental amalgams on mercury levels in expired air. J Dent Res 1981;60:1668–1671.

64. Tantbirojin D, Douglas WH, Versluis A. Inhibitive effect of a resin-modified glass ionomer cement on remote enamel artificial caries Caries Res 1997; 31:275–280.

65. Vimy MJ, Lorscheider FL. Intraoral air mercury released from dental amalgam. J Dent Res 1985;64:1069–1071.

66. Vimy MJ, Lorscheider FL. Serial measurements of intraoral air mercury: Estimation of daily dose from dental amalgam. J Dent Res 1985;64:1072–1075.

67. Vroom FQ, Greer M. Mercury vapor intoxication. Brain 1972;95:305–318.

68. Wang J-d, Hume WR. Diffusion of hydrogen and hydroxyl ion from various sources through dentine. Int Endod J 1988;21:17–26.

Part 3

Restoration of Tooth Tissues

Chapter 9

Adhesion

Paul Lambrechts, Bart Van Meerbeek, Jorge Perdigão, and Guido Vanherle

Introduction

The more practitioners understand the clinical and substrate variables that may influence the formation of an effective hybrid layer, the greater the likelihood that clinicians will succeed in creating durable resin-dentin bonds. The ultimate goal in enamel-dentin bonding is the hybridization of demineralized tooth structure and the adhesion of restorative materials to tooth tissues. Gwinnett[6] compared resin-dentin bonding to "links in a chain in which the assemblage of the links is only as strong as the weakest link. It is generally agreed that the weak link in the resin bonded assembly to enamel and dentin lies at the tissue/resin interface. This connection is fashioned by the clinician. Therefore, an understanding of how this link is created and factors influencing its performance are basic to predicting the clinical effectiveness of bonded restorations." Therefore, the "dos and don'ts" of the process should be carefully considered.

Substrate Variables

Enamel

It is important to consider carefully the quality of the enamel and prism orientation. The inorganic, hydroxyapatite content of enamel varies from 86% by weight for immature enamel to 98% for mature enamel, and is concentrated in the crystallites of the enamel prisms. The outer surface comprises prismless or aprismatic enamel. Therefore, it is advisable to prepare, or at least roughen, the enamel surfaces during operative procedures to expose prism rods in a perpendicular, longitudinal, or tangential orientation.

The quality and angulation of a bevel plays a crucial role in achieving the best possible exposure of the enamel prisms. The development of the SonicSys system (KaVo, Biberach, Germany), with its torpedo, hemispheric, and space-shuttle shaped tips, greatly facilitates correct enamel bevel angulation in all types of cavities. It contributes tremendously to the realization of the new philosophy of "downsizing the restoration."

Acid etching with phosphoric acid (35%) removes about 10 μm of the top surface of enamel, exposing the prism cores (4 μm remaining diameter) to a depth of 10 to 20 μm. The surface-free energy doubles to 72 dyne/cm. One also has to be aware of the three potential enamel etching patterns: Type I in which the prism cores are dissolved; Type II in which the prism peripheries are dissolved; and Type III in which no clear prism structures are recognized. Clinically, however, the operator has no control over the type of prism core dissolution. The final etching effect depends on enamel instrumentation; the chemical composition, fluoride content, and prismatic or aprismatic nature of the enamel; and the type of tooth being restored (permanent or primary).[28]

The way in which the etchant is activated (active rubbing and/or repeated top-up) together with the type of etchant (gel or liquid) determines the efficiency of enamel acid etching. Use of the correct etching time (minimum of 15 s) and the complete removal of the etchant and dissolved calcium phosphates during rinsing (10 to 20 s) are essential steps. After drying, it is crucial to maintain a clean etched surface with no moisture or saliva contamination. Therefore, isolation under rubber dam is to be preferred over isolation with cotton rolls.[28]

The resin-enamel bond strength is mainly the result of the cumulative cross-sectional area of the taglike resin extensions (macrotags and microtags) that infiltrate the etched enamel surface. Resin-bonded enamel contains microtags of resin as small as 0.05 μm in diameter. Lengthening the tag does not increase the cumulative cross-sectional area of the tags

or, as a result, the enamel-resin bond strength. After effective curing of the bonding resin, the infiltrated resin will have enveloped apatitic crystallites in the etched enamel, increasing the bond strength and making the crystallites more resistant to cariogenic, endogenic, and exogenic acids.

It is important to be aware of the conditioning effect of weak mineral etchants, mild organic acids, and self-etching primers. Various demineralizing acidic agents have been tested for the simultaneous conditioning of enamel and dentin. The type, concentration, and application time of the etchant are selected to obtain an appropriate enamel etch pattern without causing extreme demineralization of dentin. Nitric acid (2.5%), citric acid (10%), maleic acid (10%), pyruvic acid (10%), polyacrylic acid (20%), and oxalic acid (1.5 to 3.5%) have been suggested. However, when concentrating on dentinal conditioning, one has to be careful not to neglect optimal enamel etching. Bond strength tests and findings in repect of long-term clinical performance indicate that weak mineral etchants and mild organic acids are not as efficient in the conditioning of enamel as traditional phosphoric acid etchants.[28]

Self-etching primers such as Clearfil Liner Bond 2 (Kuraray, Osaka, Japan) etch through the dentinal smear layer and about 1 μm into the underlying dentin, resulting in good bond strength to dentin. The degree of enamel etching is, however, minimal and depends on whether or not the enamel has been prepared.[1,24] The use of self-etching primers saves time clinically because such agents are simply dried with air and do not require separate acid-etching and water-rinsing steps prior to drying. They also offer the important advantage of the avoidance of the exactitudes of wet and dry bonding procedures. No long-term clinical data are yet available on the clinical effectiveness of the enamel bonding achieved with self-etching primers.

Dentin

Before commencing dentin bonding procedures, it is wise to first characterize the type of dentin. Is the dentin sensitive with open tubules or is it altered by physiologic or reactive sclerosis, caries, abrasion, or erosion? Dentin is subjected to continuous physiologic and pathologic changes affecting its microstructure, composition, and permeability. The number of tubules is 45,000/mm^2 at the pulpal side; 35,000/mm^2 1 mm from the pulp; 23,000/mm^2 2 mm from the pulp; and 19,000/mm^2 subjacent to the amelodentinal junction. Much more information is required on the mechanical properties of both normal and abnormal forms of dentin.

Caries-affected tubular dentin is generally sclerotic and almost impermeable. Acid etching of caries-affected dentin does not significantly increase the permeability of the tubular dentin.[21] However, as soon as the cavity is extended beyond caries-affected dentin into normal, relatively permeable dentin, total etching will increase the permeability. Sclerotic dentin is hypermineralized both within and around the tubules. The tubules are filled with acid-resistant calcium phosphate whitlockite crystals, which, as a consequence of their acid resistance, are only minimally demineralized by acidic conditioners. Resin tag formation in sclerotic dentin is more variable and includes short, blunt, funnel-shaped tags containing a core of mineral crystals. Because there is plenty of mineral at the tubular and intertubular level in sclerotic dentin, glass-ionomer adhesives should be used to take advantage of the chemical bonding potential. It remains to be determined which component (chemical or micromechanical) dominates in bonding performance.

Improvements in the hybridization of dentin and in the creation of hybridized resin tags have resulted in major reductions in microleakage. This prevents bacterial invasion and pulpal irritation.

Removal of the Smear Layer

Typically, tooth surfaces that have been prepared with cutting instruments are irregularly covered with a smear layer 0.5 to 2.0 μm thick, covering the underlying substrate. It is burnished onto the underlying surface and cannot be removed by scrubbing or rinsing. Smear plugs fill the openings to the tubules. Furthermore, the smear layer and plugs are usually contaminated with bacteria, saliva, blood cells, and denatured collagen. As Winkler stated, "To remove or not to remove the smear layer? That's the question" (personal communication, 2000).

The smear layer was preserved in bonding with early generation systems because it was thought to serve as a barrier that protected the pulp from noxious stimuli and reduced the outward flow of tubular fluid. However, the smear layer is an unstable substrate for bonding. If high bond strengths and good seal are to be achieved, dentin must be suitably conditioned to remove or modify the smear layer and to permit diffusion of monomers into the subjacent demineralized collagen matrix.[27]

Smear layers under restorative materials may gradually dissolve over time by hydrolysis and allow bacterial penetration. Chronic pulpal reactions are largely caused by the irritating effects of bacteria that invade restoration interfaces by microleakage and subsequently reach the pulp.

It is therefore advisable to demineralize and remove the smear layer from the dentinal surface with acids that at the same time also demineralize the underlying dentin, exposing a fresh collagenous matrix. Van Meerbeek et al[28] devised a classification based on the clinical approach to the management of the smear layer and the subsequent sequence of steps to achieve bonding.

Effect of Tubular Fluid Flow

During clinical cavity preparation, conditioning, and bonding, few clinicians realize how much intratubular fluid shifts across dentin. The quantities of fluid are not apparent macroscopically and evaporate at a high rate. Most acidic conditioners are hypertonic, causing outward tubular fluid flow, and possibly discomfort to the patient. Therefore, isotonically formulated acidic conditioners may be found to be biologically superior.[17]

To maximize the rate of diffusion into dentin, primers and adhesive monomers are highly concentrated in their solvent systems. These concentrated solutions can osmotically induce outward fluid movement through the tubules and cause transient pain. This can be avoided if the practitioner manages dentin as a dynamic continuum of the pulp. Tubular fluid flow, although problematic, is not incompatible with intratubular monomer diffusion and resin tag formation.

Wet or Overwet Surfaces

Gwinnett et al[7] and Kanca[11] recommend that after conditioning and rinsing, the bonding primer should be applied to wet dentin. The dentin should be kept wet to maintain the 15- to 20-nm spaces between the collagen fibers and to prevent collagen collapse. The moist surfaces are then primed with hydrophilic monomers that are dissolved in a water-miscible solvent. These monomers can diffuse into the subsurface of dentin, polymerize in situ, and permit the coupling of resin composites through a bonding agent to form hybridized dentin. However, if each collagen fiber is to be completely enveloped by resin during bonding, the water must be displaced from the collagen matrix. If too much water is present, the adhesive resins may not be able to compete successfully with the water on the collagen fiber surface, thereby leaving voids.[10] Also, intratubular globules of primer and blisterlike water droplet structures covered with adhesive resin may result from the application of acetone-based primers to dentin that is overwet. The resin-infiltrated layer must be free of any porosity or defects that can act as stress raisers under function or permit the hydrolysis of collagen fibers. The major problem with wet bonding and acetone-based primers is technique sensitivity. It is difficult to estimate how moist is moist. Acetone is often combined in primers intended for wet-bonding approaches to displace water. Adhesive resins are very soluble in acetone, which evaporates very rapidly from dentinal surfaces. The volatility of the solvent can be a great disadvantage because it can evaporate from containers, changing the concentration and also the efficacy of the bonding agent. During wet-bonding procedures, it is speculated that when monomers in acetone are first applied to moist conditioned dentin, they mix with the residual water, causing the resin monomer to come out of solution before it is able to diffuse into the collagen matrix. This process may physically block further monomer penetration. However, with each consecutive coating of primer, the acetone in the primer may redissolve the monomer and permit it to diffuse further into the demineralized dentin.[17]

Every dentist is able to recognize and evaluate the frosty white appearance of etched enamel. In contrast, it is much more difficult to determine when the moist surfaces in a complex cavity are overwet. Moist bonding is not easily defined clinically and may lead to less-than-ideal bonds if the dentin is excessively wet. Wet bonding is very technique sensitive with only a small window of opportunity.[26]

Water-based primers, such as Scotchbond Multipurpose (3M, St. Paul, MN), are also recommended for wet bonding. A mixture of water, HEMA, and a copolymer is applied and the surface is then air dried to evaporate as much water as possible. Because there is a difference in volatility of the solvent versus the solute, the water concentration drops by evaporation during air drying while the HEMA concentration increases. Water has a much higher vapor pressure than HEMA. Eventually only HEMA should remain on the surface and in the subsurface region to the full depth of the demineralized dentin.[17,22] Little is known about the affinity of various adhesive monomers to collagen fibers in wet and dry states.

Because the density of tubules varies with dentinal depth, the water content of dentin is lowest in superficial dentin and greatest in deep dentin. In sensitive, vital dentin the outward flow of tubular fluid contributes to a continuous rewetting of the surface during clinical procedures.

Tissue Engineering the Collagen Fiber Network

Acid etching of dentin exposes the intertubular collagen fiber network. Several procedural errors can occur during such conditioning. With too little rinsing, residual acid may overetch the dentin or residual reaction products may block the narrow channels around the collagen fibers.

In superficial dentin, only 1% of the surface area is porous as a result of the dentinal tubules. After acid etching, 13.4% of the surface area consists of water-filled tubules that can serve as avenues for the infiltration of suitable monomers. The remaining 86.6% of the surface consists of demineralized intertubular dentin that has spaces around every collagen fiber. The fibers are separated by spaces 15 to 20 nm wide.[17]

More uniform monomer infiltration may occur in shallow demineralized layers than in deeper layers. It is better not to overetch dentin. If only the top half of etched demineralized dentin is infiltrated, a zone of unprotected demineralized matrix remains and will be vulnerable to hydrolysis over time.

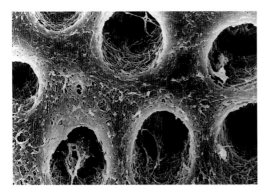

Fig 9-1 Dentin conditioned with phosphoric acid, exposing the intertubular collagen fiber network and partially dissolving the peritubular dentin cuff.[23] Note the intercollagen spaces of about 15 to 20 nm (original magnification × 18,300; Hexa-methyl-di-silazane [HMDS] processed).

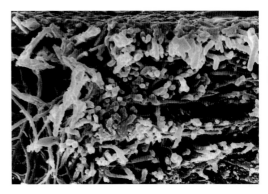

Fig 9-2 Intertubular and peritubular collagen meshwork after conditioning with phosphoric acid.[23] Note the transition between the collagen fiber arrangement and the underlying unaltered dentin at the demineralization front (original magnification × 36,600; HMDS processed).

The collagen fibers cannot be considered to consist of pure collagen because they are covered with proteoglycans and noncollagenous proteins. As these molecules are highly hydrated, the adhesive resins have to compete with water to make intimate contact with the collagen. The chemical reactivity of collagen is relatively low because it is a biologic polymer consisting of aggregates of collagen peptide chains. Most (70%) of the amino acids in collagen consist of glycine, proline, hydroxyproline, and alanine. As a consequence, chemical bonding with conventional dentinal adhesives is limited and makes only a minor contribution to resin-dentin bonds. Most of the retention is the result of the molecular entanglement of polymer chains with collagen fibers.[17]

Avoiding Collagen Collapse

Following acid etching, the inorganic mineral phase of the dentinal surface and some noncollagenous proteins are solubilized and some proteins are extracted, exposing the collagen fibers of the demineralized dentin matrix (Figs 9-1 and 9-2). The demineralized dentinal matrix becomes very soft and elastic, and can readily collapse if the organic matrix is denatured or destabilized during conditioning. As the water-supported collagen network is air dried, water is lost between the fibers and microfibrils, and surface tension forces operating at the air-collagen network interface may lead to collapse.[8] The collagen peptides may form intermolecular hydrogen bonds with the nearest neighboring collagen peptides, contributing to the further collapse of the network. This can cause a decrease in collagen interfiber spacing

Table 9-1 Theoretical composition of the limiting 2 to 3 μm of dentin (vol%) before and after bonding

	Mineralized dentin	Etched/rinsed dentin	Primed/infiltrated dentin	Self-etched/ unrinsed dentin
Mineral	45	0	0	10–20
Collagen	48	48	48	48
Water	7	52	0	0
Resin	0	0	52	32–42

Table 9-2 Physical properties of mineralized, demineralized, and resin-reinforced dentin

Property	Mineralized	Demineralized	Resin-infiltrated
Modulus of elasticity (MPa)	13,700	210	3,600
Toughness (MN/mm^{-3})	4.2	11.3	27.7
Percent elongation	2.3	22.3	6.8
Ultimate strength (MPa)	105.6	29.6	121.6

and a loss or reduction of permeability to resin monomers. It is a considerable challenge to maintain interfiber spacing and diffusion channels after the hydroxyapatite crystals have been removed. Overdrying of dentin can have undesirable effects because the collapsed collagen permits little diffusion of resin monomers around the collagen fibers, making it difficult to create uniformly hybridized dentin.[17] Pashley[17,19] calculated the theoretical composition of the limiting 2 to 3 μm of dentin (vol%) before and after bonding procedures, illustrating variability in the substrate (Table 9-1).

Pashley[17,19] also compiled data on the physical properties of mineralized, demineralized, and resin-reinforced dentin, revealing the changes that occur during bonding procedures (Table 9-2).

Along the collagen fibers, highly charged noncollagenous proteins, including dentinal sialoprotein and phosphoproteins may be found together with glycosaminoglycans. These create a hydrophilic gel-like polymer matrix network, draw water osmotically into the network, and bind large amounts of water. This hydrogel maintains the hydration of the wet substrate.[3,13]

The hydrophilic HEMA monomer and water are thought to break intermolecular hydrogen bonds, thereby softening the network and allowing it to expand.[15] Residual stresses created in the network when it shrinks may permit elastic recoil and active expansion. Using HEMA and water in the priming system can create a collagen-polyHEMA–hydrogel hybrid layer, which has weak mechanical properties and is hydrolitically unstable. It is unlikely that there is an intimate interface between collagen fibers and enveloping resin. It is more likely that there is an interface including hydrophilic resin glycosamino-glycans, collagen, and noncollagenous proteins.[13]

Also, acidic monomers such as 4-META and Phenyl-P diffuse into collapsed, de-mineralized dentin because their acidity can break the interpeptide hydrogen bonds of collagen fibers stuck together by solubilized noncollagenous proteins. This allows the collagen fibers to separate from each other, thereby restoring the spaces between adjacent fibers.[9]

Ten percent citric acid containing 3% ferric chloride is considered to be a good conditioning agent to remove the smear layer and demineralize the underlying intact dentin.[16] The ferric chloride serves as a polymerization promoter. It is also claimed that it prevents denaturing and collapse of the demineralized matrix. The ferric ions are adsorbed onto the demineralized dentin and cross-link peptides, thereby immobilizing them and preventing collapse when air dried. Depending on the acid concentration and the time of exposure, phosphoric acid denatures peptides exposed during the removal of the smear layer.[18]

A modern approach to the reduction in the number of bonding steps is the use of self-etching and self-priming systems (Clearfil Liner Bond 2, 2V, or Clearfil SE, Kuraray; FluoroBond, Shofu, Kyoto, Japan; the "all-in-one" Prompt L Pop, ESPE, Seefeld, Germany). These systems prevent collagen collapse and the loss of dentinal mass by leaving the smear layer in place and relying on acidic monomers to dissolve the smear layer and condition the underlying dentin. The liquid is applied, allowed to react for 30 seconds, and then air dried. There is no rinsing of the conditioned surface. Self-etching primers dissolve mineral crystals, but calcium phosphate may reprecipitate or become suspended in the resin. The hydroxy-apatite crystallites around the collagen fibers are sufficiently solubilized to permit infiltration of the adhesive monomers.[27] However, hybridized smear layers (dissolved smear layers reinforced by impregnated resin) may be intrinsically too weak to provide hydrolytic stability together with durable mechanical properties.[29] Slow hydrolysis of the organic portion of the dissolved and hybridized smear layer can occur. How well hybridized dentin bonds endure thermal cycling and masticatory stresses remains to be determined. If failure occurs, the hybrid layer would preferentially split at the junction of the hybridized layer with the resin-infiltrated dentin. Because this resin-infiltrated dentin is only 0.5 μm thick, there may be too little resin to form resin tags integrated with the surrounding hybrid layer, increasing the risk of the passage of microbial products to the pulp.[17]

"Condipriming" systems should be considered if conventional etching, rinsing, drying, and bonding steps could cause intensive hydrodynamic effects in hypersensitive dentin, including chemically eroded

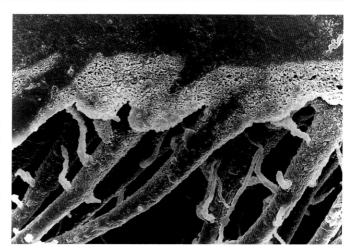

Fig 9-3 Intertubular and triangular peritubular hybridization in combination with resin tag formation and lateral branching obtained with Syntac Single-Component (Ivoclar, Schaan, Liechtenstein) (original magnification $\times$ 9,100; HCl-decalcified and NaOCl-deproteinized specimen).[23]

dentin in patients with bulimia. The ideal self-etching, self-priming bonding system should be able to diffuse by demineralization, penetrating a 2-μm thick smear layer and engaging the underlying intact dentin to a reasonable depth. The smear layer is a diffusion barrier for the acidic monomer mixture, with its effect depending on its thickness, density, and buffering capacity. The conditioning effect on enamel is still to be determined. Etching of enamel and the removal of the smear layer by a separate acid etching step before condipriming could produce more reliable and durable bonds to enamel and dentin.[27]

Optimizing the Hybrid Interdiffusion Zone

Hybrid layers are formed by resin-infiltration of enamel, dentin, and cementum. Hybridization can be considered a form of

"tissue engineering" because the mineral phase of a hard tissue is purposely dissolved and then infiltrated with resin monomer to intentionally change the physicochemical properties of the tooth surfaces and subsurfaces (Fig 9-3)

Dentinal primers have to maintain or recover the porosity induced by dentinal conditioning and demineralization. They also rewet the demineralized dentin and prevent collapse of the collagen fiber network. When primer monomers are dissolved in a water-miscible solvent and are placed on conditioned dentin, they diffuse into the demineralized dentin and act as precursors for bonding agents. Resin monomers are expected to infiltrate into the long, continuous, interconnected, and narrow channels or pores responsible for intertubular dentinal permeability.[28]

Hybridized dentin has a concentration gradient structure compromising a mixture of collagen and resin polymers formed by monomers that are diffused from the adhesive interface into the subsurface of the conditioned dentin and subsequently polymerized. The depth of penetration of the monomer into the delicate three-dimensional network of spaces between the collagen fibers should be equal to the depth of the demineralization. The physical and chemical properties of dentin are changed at the interface. It is to be expected that the physical properties of the hybrid layer are superior to those of demineralized dentin but inferior to those of mineralized dentin. Hybridized dentin is much less stiff but tougher than normal dentin. The hybrid layer is an artificial composite of resin and collagen fibers. Bonding to etched dentin should provide a shock-absorbing, stress-breaking inter-face that tends to resist the forces of poly-merization contraction and mastication. If the strength of the resin is increased, the resin-reinforced dentin will be stronger. It is also advisable to create a gradient in elastic modulus from the hybrid layer toward the composite.[21,28] When a thin (about 100-μm) layer of intermediate low viscosity composite with an intermediate modulus of elasticity is placed on top of a low-modulus adhesive layer, which over-lies a resin-infiltrated hybrid layer that has a low modulus of elasticity, it is very likely that there will be a very different stress concentration across the interphase than that which occurs when stiff resin composites are placed directly on a thin adhesive layer.

The substitution of resin for mineral in the subsurface of mineralized tissues is the essence of the creation of a hybrid layer. The exact interface between resin and dentin is obscure and should be regarded as a continuum. High-quality hybridized dentin resists both acid and proteolytic challenge and should resist the development of recurrent caries—a clinical goal of critical importance.

The clinical consequences of failure depend on where the failure occurs in the bonded interphase. If failure occurs between the composite resin and the adhesive layer, the clinical consequences will be limited because the dentinal seal remains intact. Similarly, if failure occurs between the top of the hybrid layer and the adhesive layer, the dentin will remain sealed. If the failure occurs within the hybrid layer, such as might occur between the hybridized smear layer and the under-lying resin-infiltrated dentin, the dentin should remain sealed and protected. Only if failure occurs between the bottom of the hybrid layer and the underlying dentin will the seal fail with the risk of demineraliza-tion, bacterial invasion, dentinal sensitivity, and pulpal irritation.[17]

Complete conversion of monomers to polymers is clinically impossible. At atmo-spheric pressure and normal body temper-ature, the curing of resin will be limited in the presence of the water and oxygen in dentinal fluids. Under such conditions, polymers and copolymers are probably far from achieving their optimal conversion, cross-linking, and theoretical physical properties. Given the importance of the conversion of monomers to polymers, clinicians and scientists should pay par-ticular attention to this aspect of bonding.[17]

The diffusion rate of monomers is proportional to the square root of their molecular weight. This means that if two comonomers such as HEMA and poly-alkenoic acid are combined as in Scotch-bond Multipurpose, the smaller molecules diffuse faster and deeper within the inter-fibrillar spaces (15 to 20 nm) than the larger ones. The monomer-solvent concentration, the viscosity and temperature of the solution, the intrinsic diffusivity and affinity of the solute (resin monomer) on the substrate, and diffusion time determine the uptake of the adhesive monomers.[17]

It is also important that impregnated monomers are well polymerized in order to complete the hybridization process before the composite resin is added and polymerized.

Taking Advantage of Resin Tags

Intratubular dentinal permeability is achieved if resin monomers penetrate into the dentinal tubules to form hybridized resin tags in the intratubular dentin. These tags form a small element of the resin-tooth interface in superficial dentin, but form an important element of the bond in deep dentin near the pulp.

Resin tags are not all hybridized peripherally over the full length of the tubule wall. Only in the top 2 to 5 μm, where the peritubular dentin is removed by conditioning, are the tags firmly attached by triangular hybridization (Fig 9-3). The exposed, circumferentially oriented collagen fibers in peritubular dentin increase the surface area of the tubule wall for radial resin infiltration. The integration of resin tags into the hybrid layer is essential in order to obtain a resin seal, to contribute to retention, and to prevent pulpal irritation. The contribution of these tags to bond strength is proportional to the cross-sectional area of the tags and the cohesive strength of the polymer. Therefore, it is essential to use high-strength, preferably particle-filled adhesives. Intertubular hybrid layer formation contributes to retention in proportion to the amount of intertubular dentin available for bonding. The overall bond strength varies with dentinal depth, given the variable contributions of the hybrid layer and resin tags to bonding. The varying wetness and the changing mechanical properties of dentin with depth complicate a theoretical calculation of bond strength.[17]

Classifying Dentinal Adhesive Systems

To make the correct choice of adhesive system, it is essential to base selection on a robust classification system as described by Van Meerbeek et al[28] (Table 9-3).

Table 9-3 Classification of modern adhesive systems according to their clinical application and the resultant mechanism of adhesion to dentin

Brand name	Manufacturer
One-step smear layer modifying adhesives	
Ariston Liner (Ariston)	Vivadent, Schaan, Liechtenstein
Compoglass SCA (Compoglass)	Vivadent
Everbond* (Hytac)	ESPE
Hytac OSB (Hytac)	ESPE
Prime&Bond 2.1 (Dyract)	DeTrey, Konstanz, Germany
Prime&Bond NT* (Dyract)	DeTrey
Solist (Luxat)	DMG, Hamburg, Germany
One-step smear layer dissolving adhesives/One-step self-etch adhesives	
Prompt L Pop	ESPE
Lp-2	ESPE
Syntac 3 (self-etch; exp)	Vivadent
Two-step glass-ionomer adhesives	
FujiBond LC*	GC, Tokyo, Japan
FujiBond LC Liq-Liq (exp)*	GC
Two-step smear layer modifying adhesive	
ProBOND	Caulk
Two-step smear layer dissolving adhesives/Two-step self-etch adhesives	
Clearfil Liner Bond 2*	Kuraray
Clearfil Liner Bond 2V*	Kuraray
Clearfil SE	Kuraray
Etch&Prime 3.0	Degussa, Hanau, Germany
Imperva FL-Bond* (Fluorobond)	Shofu
NRC & Prime&Bond NT*	Caulk
OptiBond (no-etch)*	Kerr, Glendora, CA
OptiBond FL (no-etch)*	Kerr
Sustel (F2000)	3M
Unifil BOND	GC
Coltène ART Bond[†]	Coltène, Altstätten, Switzerland
Denthesive II[†]	Hereaus-Kulzer, Wehrheim, Germany
Ecusit Primer-Mono[†]	DMG
Imperva Bond (no etch)[†]	Shofu
Scotchbond 2[†]	3M
Solid Bond[†]	Hereaus-Kulzer
Superlux Universalbond 2[†]	DMG
Syntac[†]	Vivadent
XR-Bond[†]	Kerr
Two-step smear layer removing adhesives/"One-bottle" total-etch adhesives	
Bond 1	Jeneric/Pentron, Wallingford, CT
EG Bond	Sun Medical, Kyoto, Japan
Everbond (exp)*	ESPE
Excite (exp)	Vivadent
Gluma 2000	Bayer, Leverkusen, Germany
Gluma One Bond	Heraeus-Kulzer
One Coat Bond*	Coltène

Table 9-3 (continued)

Brand name	Manufacturer
One-Step	Bisco, Itasca, IL
Optibond Solo*	Kerr
Optibond Solo Plus*	Kerr
Prime&Bond 2.1	DeTrey
Prime&Bond 2.1 Dual Cure	DeTrey
Prime&Bond NT*	DeTrey
Prime&Bond NT Dual Cure*	DeTrey
PQ1*	Ultradent, South Jordan, UT
Scotchbond 1 (Single Bond)	3M
Snapbond	Cooley & Cooley, Houston, TX
Solist	DMG
Solobond M	Voco, Cuxhaven, Germany
Stae	Southern Dental Industries, Victoria, Australia
Syntac Single-Component	Vivadent, Schaan, Liechtenstein
Syntac Sprint	Vivadent
Syntac 3 (total-etch; exp.)	Vivadent
Tenure Quik	Den-Mat, Santa Maria, CA
Tenure Quik with Fluoride	Den-Mat

Three-step smear layer removing adhesives/Three-step total-etch adhesives

ABC Enhanced	Chameleon, Kansas City, KS
Elitebond	Bisco
All-Bond 2	Bisco
Amalgambond Plus	Parkell, Farmingdale, NY
Clearfil Liner Bond*‡	Kuraray
Dentastic	Pulpdent, Watertown, MA
Denthesive	Hereaus-Kulzer
EBS	ESPE
EBS Multi	ESPE
Gluma Bonding System	Bayer
Gluma CPS	Bayer
Imperva Bond (total-etch)	Shofu
Mirage Bond	Chameleon
OptiBond (total-etch)*	Kerr
OptiBond FL (total-etch)*	Kerr
PAAMA2	Southern Dental Industries
Permagen	Ultradent
Permaquik*	Ultradent
Quadrant UniBond	Cavex Holland, Haarlem, Netherlands
Restobond 3	Lee Pharmaceuticals, South El Monte, CA
Scotchbond Multi-Purpose	3M
Scotchbond Multi-Purpose Plus	3M
Solid Bond	Heraeus-Kulzer
Super-Bond D Liner	Sun Medical, Kyoto, Japan
Tenure S	Den-Mat

*Adhesives providing filled adhesives.

†Early self-etch adhesives developed to be applied on dentin only, whereas enamel is etched separately with a phosphoric acid (> 30%) conditioner.

‡Because of the application of a silica-filled low-viscosity resin (Protect Liner) in addition to the application of the adhesive resin, Clearfil Liner Bond is applied in four steps.

147

Glass Ionomer–Based Adhesives for Mineralized Conditions

If glass ionomer–based adhesives are placed on enamel and dentin prior to their gelation, the chemical reactions are limited to the tooth surfaces. A binding reaction with the mineralized tissues is possible, however, by calcium chelation between the matrix of the glass ionomer and the mineralized tooth structure.[25] Local demineralization is not sufficient to dissolve all of the smear plugs, and the solubilized mineral is trapped between the glass ionomer and the subsurface. Glass-ionomer mixtures are adsorbed by bioaffinity to tooth structure and form intimate contact with the mineralized intertubular and peritubular dentin and the demineralized dentinal collagen matrix.

The measure of acid strength (pKa) of the polyacrylic acid conditioner, the degree of dissociation, the available concentration of acids, and the contact time all affect the conditioning effect on the substrate.[17,20] The pKa of phosphoric acid (2.12) is much lower than that of polyacrylic acid (4.25), hence the ability of phosphoric acid to demineralize dentin is potentially higher than that of polyacrylic acids. The local buffering capacity of the dentin and smear layer, given the presence of collagen and trivalent phosphate in hydroxyapatite, also plays a role.

When glass-ionomer adhesives are selected, one has to avoid removing most of the mineral phase during the conditioning process, otherwise the opportunity for ionic bonding to calcium and phosphate is lost. Using polyacrylic acid as a conditioner, plenty of minerals are exposed and are available for ion exchange at the collagen fiber periphery and at the interphase of demineralized and mineralized dentin.[30] The residual minerals may also prevent the collapse of the demineralized dentinal matrix following air drying, thereby bonding.

Clinical Consequences

Balancing the Configuration Factor and Shrinkage Stresses

During the polymerization of resin composites, shrinkage competes with dentin surface bonding. The configuration factor, or C-factor, describes the ratio of bonded to unbonded, or free, surface area.[4,5] Flat dentinal surfaces have a C-factor of 1, while occlusal Class I cavities have a C-factor lower than 5. The higher the C-factor, the higher the polymerization contraction forces operating on the cavity walls. The more the monomer is attached to peripheral surfaces, the more their flow is reduced during polymerization and the greater the stresses developed at the resin-tooth interfaces. During incremental insertion of a resin composite, the C-factor should be limited to 1. The real clinical relevance is still to be determined.

Performing Routine Hybridization of Dentin

Lundy and Stanley[14] suggested in 1969 that it is wise to hybridize all dentin exposed during restorative procedures to protect the pulp from restorative trauma. Resin tags and hybridized intertubular dentin should seal the dentin. Even if the resin composite is separated from the cavity wall by polymerization shrinkage, the hybridized dentin will keep the dentin sealed. Oral bacteria will populate marginal gaps but will not harm the pulp because the dentin remains sealed with a continuous layer of hybridized tags and dentin. Acids, bacteria, and bacterial products cannot penetrate this impermeable membrane. The sealing capacity of hybridized dentin is as important as the retention it affords composite resins.[2] Routine hybridization of dentin could greatly improve oral health-care outcomes.

Direct and Indirect Pulpal Capping with Dentin Bonding Systems

Indirect pulpal capping

Indirect pulpal capping of very deep dentin is a prudent measure to seal the tubules close to the pulp that are large, numerous, and close together. They may be considered to form a physiologic exposure given their high permeability. The pulp can be protected from bacterial microleakage through hybridization of deep dentin with adhesive resins.

Direct pulpal capping

Direct pulpal capping is indicated if there is a small pulpal exposure, identified by bleeding in a vital tooth. The healing potential and the degree of pulpal inflammation is often critical and misunderstood. Calcium hydroxide bases are well-known for their dentinogenesis, though the hard tissue barriers are often incomplete and show multiple tunnel defects. The key for success, however, is the prevention of

bacterial microleakage. Dentinogenesis will not take place in the presence of bacterial leakage or pulpal inflammation. Direct pulpal capping with adhesive bonding systems and their pulpal response has been studied. Katoh[12] reported good healing in humans when an adhesive resin was used for direct pulpal capping, although healing was slightly faster in calcium hydroxide controls. He advised the application of calcium hydroxide on the exposure, followed by coverage of the calcium hydroxide and the surrounding deep dentin with hybridized resin. A critical variable is the control of the bleeding. There are several treatment options. The pulpal exposure may be treated with 5% sodium hypochloride for 2 minutes to remove the clotted blood and clean the exposure site. One can also rinse with saline, 2% lidocaine containing epinephrine, or a calcium hydroxide solution until bleeding stops. The material placed over the exposed wound may not be as important as the peripheral seal and the control of hemorrhage from the exposure.[17] The practitioner still has to be aware of the toxicity of monomers in direct contact with pulpal cells and, because conversion will not be complete in such situations, residual monomers may be cytotoxic and allergenic.

Downsizing the Restoration

Recently, airborne particle abrasion techniques using aluminum oxide powder have been refined and shown to be of value in the cleaning of occlusal surfaces and, as minimally invasive techniques, in creating access to caries lesions. Such techniques facilitate the preservation of hard tooth tissue during cavity preparation.

Extreme care is necessary, however, to avoid extensive contamination of the dental practice with the ultrafine aluminium oxide particles (Figs 9-4 to 9-8).

The problems associated with rotary instrument preparation in the preparation of small approximal cavities are well-known and include both difficulties in preparing margins for enamel etching and iatrogenic damage to the adjacent tooth. Oscillating preparation instruments have been developed for a sonically driven handpiece (Sonicflex, KaVo). These instruments, available in a variety of forms, feature selective diamond coating on the working surfaces. The instrument surfaces contacting the adjacent tooth are smooth. The "microprep set" provides several instrument designs (lens and torpedo forms) that are especially useful for finishing margins in proximal cavities (Figs 9-9 to 9-17). The procedure is protective of the proximal surface of the adjacent tooth, which remains free of instrument damage. A large bevel with optimal enamel prism orientation for an adhesive restoration is obtained. This instrumentation may also be used in other types of preparations. These instruments permit what may be called "preventive restorative therapy." The ability to prepare margins in near contact with the adjacent tooth is only one feature. With these instruments, cavity preparations that correspond to irregular decalcification patterns, including small occlusal and lateral lesions can be created. In addition, the creation of fracture-free bevels improves bond strengths and enhances marginal adaptation and seal. This preparation technique is not limited to small direct restorations. Practically every form of proximal preparation, for both direct and indirect restorations, metal or metal-free, can be finished effectively with SonicSys instruments. Since ideal angles for proximal bevels vary with the restorative material and the cavity extension, a range of instruments is available for all situations, ranging from a tunnel to onlay and inlay preparations. Flowable, packable, moldable, and condensable composites offer new opportunities when used in conjunction with such preparation techniques.

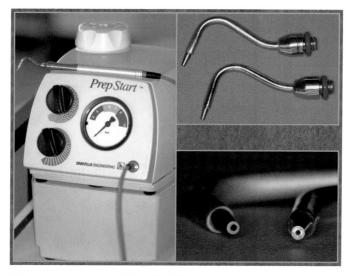

Fig 9-4 Air abrasion unit PrepStart (Danville Engineering, San Ramon, CA) with two different tip sizes using 27 μm aluminium oxide powder.

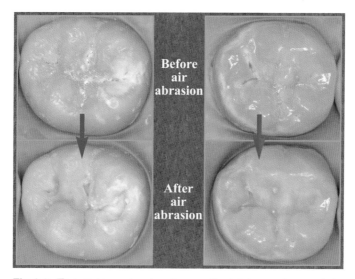

Fig 9-5 Two molar occlusal surfaces with staining and enamel demineralization before and following the use of air abrasion to minimize the removal of sound tooth tissue.

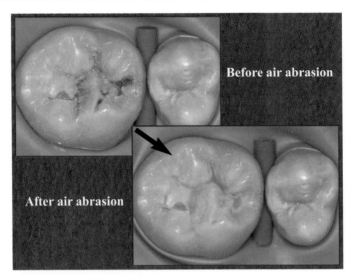

Fig 9-6 Molar and premolar occlusal surface before and after air abrasion. Note the minimally invasive preparation.

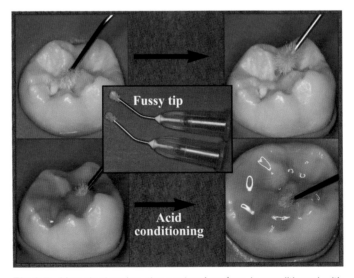

Fig 9-7 After air abrasion, the occlusal surface is conditioned with 35% phosphoric acid for at least 15 seconds.

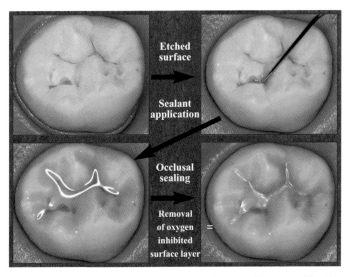

Fig 9-8 A sealant is applied to the etched occlusal surface. After light curing the oxygen-inhibited surface layer is removed.

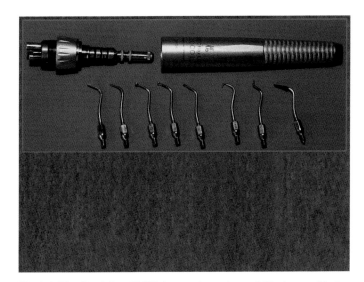

Fig 9-9 The SonicSys 2000L is an extremely useful instrument in the preparation and finishing of cavity margins in a very controlled and mineral-saving manner.

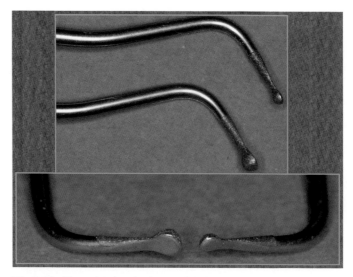

Fig 9-10 The microhemisphere exists in two sizes and in a mesial and distal design. They are coated with 45-μm diamond particles and polished at the inactive contralateral side.

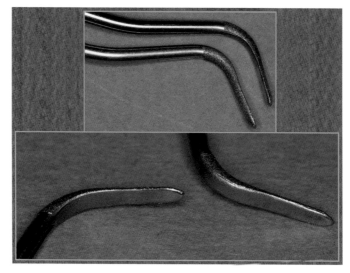

Fig 9-11 The torpedo tips exist in a mesial and distal design and also have an active and inactive side.

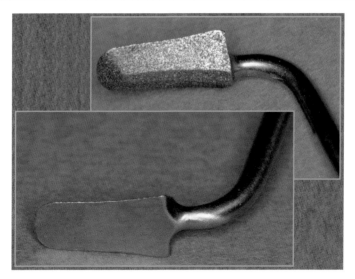

Fig 9-12 Specially designed space shuttle tip for proximal flattening and cervical uniform bevel finishing.

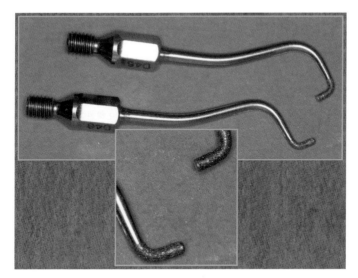

Fig 9-13 Specially designed hook and bajonet tip for tunnel preparations.

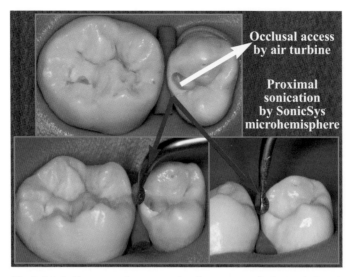

Fig 9-14 In the premolar, an occlusal access cavity is made by air turbine and the marginal ridge is futher eroded by sonication using the microhemisphere.

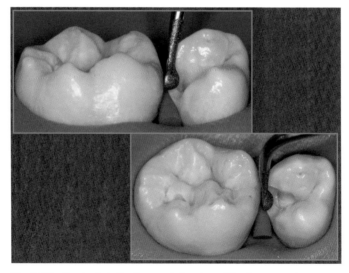

Fig 9-15 Gradual sonication and shaping of the box margins.

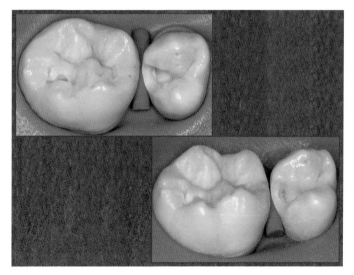

Fig 9-16 View of the finished peripheral bevel.

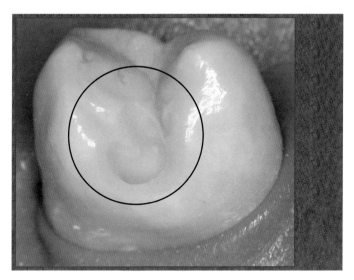

Fig 9-17 Direct view of the proximal finished bevel.

References

1. Barkmeier WW, Los SA, Triolo PT. Bond strengths and SEM evaluation of Clearfil Liner Bond 2. Am J Dent 1995;8:289–293.

2. Bertschlinger C, Paul SJ, Lüthy H, Schärer P. Dual applications of dentin bonding agents: Effect on bond strength. Am J Dent 1996;9: 115–119.

3. Cribb AM, Scott JE. Tendon response to tensile stress: An ultrastructural investigation of collagen: Proteoglycan interactions in stressed tendon. J Anat 1995;187:423–428.

4. Davidson CL, deGee AJ, Feilzer AJ. The competition between the composite-dentin bond strength and the polymerization contraction stress. J Dent Res 1984;63:1396–1399.

5. Feilzer AJ, deGee AJ, Davidson CL. Quantitative determination of stress reduction by flow in composite restorations. Dent Mater 1990; 6:167–171.

6. Gwinnett AJ. Bonded restorations; the critical link with the tissue. In: Global Restorative Symposium, Milford, DE: Dentsply/Caulk, 1996.

7. Gwinnett AJ, Tay FR, Wei SHY. Bridging the gap between overly dry and overwet bonding phenomenon optimization of dentin hybridization and tubular seal. In: Shimono M, Maeda T, Suda H, Takahashi K (eds.) Dentin/Pulp Complex. Tokyo: Quintessence, 1996:359–363.

8. Hulmes DJS, Wess TJ, Prockop DJ, Fratzl P. Radial packing, order, and disorder in collagen fibrils. Biophys J 1995;68:1661–1670.

9. Igarashi K, Toida T, Nakabayashi N. Effect of Phenyl-P/HEMA primer on bonding to demineralized dentin by phosphoric acid. J Jpn Dent Mater 1997;16:55–60.

10. Jacobson T, Söderholm KJ. Some effects of water on dentin bonding. Dent Mater 1995; 11:132–136.

11. Kanca J. Wet bonding: Effect of drying time and distance. Am J Dent 1996;9:273–276.

12. Katoh Y. Clinico-pathological study on pulpal irritation of adhesive resinous material. 1. Histopathological changes of the pulp tissue in direct capping. Adhes Dent 1993;11:199–211.

13. Lindén LA, Källskog O, Wolgast M. Human dentine as a hydrogel. Arch Oral Biol 1995;40: 991–1004.

14. Lundy T, Stanley HR. Correlation of pulpal histopathology and clinical symptoms in human teeth subjected to experimental irritation. Oral Surg Oral Med Oral Pathol 1969;27:187–201.

15. Maciel KT, Carvalho RM, Ringle RD, Preston CD, Russell CM, Pashley DH. The effects of acetone, ethanol, HEMA and air on the stiffness of human demineralized dentin. J Dent Res 1996; 75:1851–1858.

16. Nakabayashi N, Kojima K, Masuhara E. The promotion of adhesion by the infiltration of monomers into tooth substrates. J Biomed Mater Res 1982;16:265–273.

17. Nakabayashi N, Pashley D. Hybridization of dental hard tissues. Chicago: Quintessence, 1998:1–107.

18. Okamoto Y, Heeley JD, Dogon IL, Shintani H. Effects of phosphoric acid and tannic acid on dentine collagen. J Oral Rehabil 1991;18: 507–513.

19. Pashley DH. The clinical correlations of dentin structure and function. J Prosthet Dent 1991; 66:777–781.

20. Pashley DH. The effects of acid etching on the pulpodentin complex. Oper Dent 1992; 17:224–242.

21. Pashley EL, Talman R, Horner JA, Pashley DH. Permeabilitiy of normal versus carious dentin. Endod Dent Traumatol 1991;7:207–211.

22. Pashley EL, Zhang Y, Lockwood P, Rueggeberg F, Pashley DH. Effects of HEMA on water evaporation from HEMA-water mixtures [abstract 52]. J Dent Res 1997;76(special issue):20.

23. Perdigão J. An ultra-morphological study of human dentine exposed to adhesive systems [thesis]. Belgium: Catholic Univ of Leuven, 1995.

24. Perdigão J, Lopes L, Lambrechts P, Leitao J, Van Meerbeek B, Vanherle G. Effects of a self-etching primer on enamel shear bond strengths and SEM morphology. Am J Dent 1997;10:141–146.

25. Ruyter IE. The chemistry of adhesive agents. Oper Dent 1992;17(suppl 5):32S–43S.

26. Tay FR, Gwinnett, Pang KM, Wei SHY. Resin permeation into acid conditioned, moist and dry dentin: A paradigm using water-free adhesive primers. J Dent Res 1996;75:1034–1044.

27. Toida T, Watanabe A, Nakabayashi N. Effect of smear layer on bonding to dentin prepared with bur. J Jpn Dent Mater 1995;14:109–116.

28. Van Meerbeek B, Inoue S, Perdigão J, Lambrechts P, Vanherle G. Enamel and dentin adhesion. In: Summit JB, Robins JW, Schwartz RS, dos Santo J (eds). Fundamentals of Operative Dentistry. A Contemporary Approach. Chicago: Quintessence, 2001:178–235.

29. Watanabe I, Nakabayashi N. Bonding durability of photocured Phenyl-P in TEGDMA to smear layer-retained bovine dentin. Quintessence Int 1993; 24:335–342.

30. Yoshida Y, Van Meerbeek B, Nakayama Y, et al. Chemical bonding of polyalkenoate acids to hydroxyapatite [abstract 3397]. J Dent Res 1999;78:530.

Chapter 10

New Materials and Techniques

Carel L. Davidson

Introduction

During the last 40 years, the approach to restorative dentistry has dramatically changed from the excessive sacrifice of sound tooth structure to facilitate the placement of restorative materials, to minimal preparation and restoration. Changed thinking in the field of cariology aside, material science has contributed greatly to the new form of dentistry. Dental care, which consisted mainly of an extracting and cutting technology service, is now a bio-medically-based science that has preservation as a standard. The requirements for a satisfactory material are no longer high strength and low wear only, but a complex set of interrelated properties dominated by biocompatibility and esthetics. Appropriate mechanical characteristics are still required, but thanks to ingenious bonding mechanisms, new restorations are typically bonded to the remaining tooth structures. This contributes significantly to the longevity of the restored tooth unit. Average values for some mechanical properties of direct restorative materials are shown in Figs 10-1 and 10-2. Clearly the

introduction of bonding in restorative dentistry has realized the greatest achievements in the restoration of teeth in recent times. In addition to the benefits of adhesive techniques, the impact of esthetics has been considerable, with new materials able to mimic the optical characteristics of the tooth. The patient is increasingly aware of such possibilities and, as a consequence, is all the more demanding of esthetic restorations. Parallel with the introduction of new formulations for materials goes social awareness of the potential adverse effects on the environment and health. In this respect it is somewhat peculiar that the patient tends to have more distrust of a long established and relatively uncomplicated material such as silver amalgam, than the chemically complex resin-based composites. Notwithstanding a wealth of scientific literature that disproves any association between health problems and the mercury-containing filling materials, there is widespread acceptance of resin systems, some containing components that have been shown to cause dramatic biologic reactions.

Figs 10-1 and 10-2 A comparison of selected mechanical properties of different types of direct restorative materials (CGI, conventional glass ionomer; RMGI, resin-modified glass ionomer. Courtesy of Dr. A. J. de Gee).

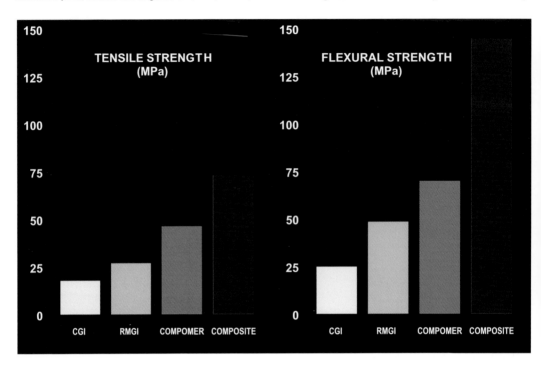

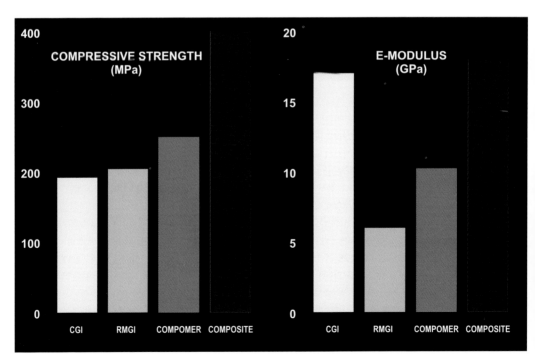

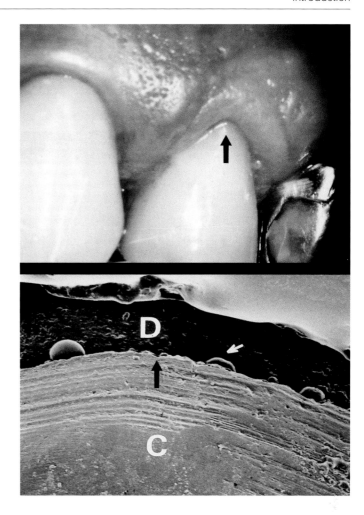

Fig 10-3 The acceptable clinical appearance of a Class V composite restoration is not necessarily an indication of the quality of the restoration. SEM reveals serious cervical marginal discrepancies. The arrow indicates the composite = dentin interface (C = composite, D = dentin).

A second contradiction pertaining to the move away from amalgam to resin-based composites relates to the clinician. Notwithstanding the ease of delivery of modern materials, typically the direct injection from a capsule of a single paste that only hardens after command-set light initiation, such procedures have proved to be so demanding that it requires a highly skilled dentist to place a satisfactory resin-based composite restoration. In contrast, a dentist needs to be lacking in skill and attention to place a poor quality restoration

of amalgam. A major problem with adhesive resin-based composite restorations is the generation of contractile forces during curing, causing separation at the margins as shown in Fig 10-3. In particular, light-cured, resin-based composites demand a profound understanding of the processes of adhesion, the creation of stresses on setting, and the nuances of the limits of light initiation.

After a period of quick succession introductions of new products with ever-higher quality claims, the developers of materials have come to realize that restorative dentistry based on sophisticated systems has become too complex for the clinician. This has led many dentists to become frustrated and lose interest in innovations instead of deriving satisfaction through the achievements of modern science.

To be more specific as to what is new and what is not, what has already been abandoned and what has been rediscovered among direct restorative materials and techniques, this chapter summarizes contemporary thinking.

Materials

Currently, new products are launched on the market more frequently than relevant research findings are published. Both scientists and practitioners are confused about new nomenclatures, compositions, properties, clinical performance, and biocompatibility. A series of essentially different materials are at our disposal for direct restorations. For convenience, they can be categorized into two groups, the metal-containing and the non–metal-containing materials. The first group is not tooth colored, the second one is.

Metal-Containing Direct Restorative Materials

Metal-containing direct restorative materials include:
- Direct-filling gold
- Amalgam
- Gallium alloys
- Metal-reinforced glass ionomers

With certain exceptions, cohesive gold restorations no longer have a place in everyday practice.

Silver amalgam has long been regarded as the ideal direct restorative material for the restoration of posterior teeth. The quality of dental amalgam has generally been judged on ease of handling and mechanical characteristics. Despite satisfying mechanical requirements, the application of amalgam has given rise to objections. There has been a continuous resistance to amalgam given its chemical properties, corrosion potential, and believed lack of biocompatibility. Corrosion suppression of mercury-based silver amalgam has been achieved through sophistication in the Ag_3Sn particle size and distribution, together with the substantial addition of copper into the alloy. Familiarity with the accomplishments of amalgam during placement and clinical performance ensures that this tried and tested material remains the No. 1 choice for many dentists. With modern dental technology, the sealing and durability of amalgam restorations can be improved, notably through the application of a resin-bonded layer between filling and preparation.

Although introduced to dentistry in the early 1990s, the gallium eutectic Ga-Sn-In-Ag that melts at 10°C was described for dental use in 1928[14] as mercury-free "amalgam." Such alloys, which are rather difficult to manipulate, yield to a compressive strength that is comparable to amalgam and share the sealing performance of amalgam when used as a retrograde filling material.[13] Gallium alloys may be an alternative for those who fear the presence of mercury in conventional amalgam; however, such alloys have been shown to cause cytotoxic reactions.[17]

Glass ionomers are the inorganic restorative materials that lie between the metal- and non–metal-containing restoratives. Their formulation comes the closest to that of tooth structure and they are unique in that they adhere directly to both enamel and dentin. Yet, like other restorative materials, glass ionomers are not ideal, and a series of changes in their formulation have been investigated to improve, in particular, their mechanical properties. Metal incorporation in glass-ionomer systems was an attempt to reinforce the structure in the early postplacement phase. Although the success of the so-called cermets placed in deciduous teeth was found to be slightly better than that of conventional glass ionomers,[12] the metal reinforcement of glass-ionomer systems failed to generate the widespread acceptance of glass ionomers as the material of choice for direct fillings in posterior teeth.

Non–Metal-Containing Direct Restorative Materials

Developments and interests in non-metallic, tooth-colored restorative materials have moved back and forth between resin-based composites and glass-ionomer cements. Resin-based composites are well-accepted stable materials but do not bond directly to tooth structure. In contrast, glass ionomers require extensive care during and directly after placement, but do bond directly to tooth structures and have a preventive potential through the release of fluorides. Complicated hybrid systems have been developed in the creation of hydrophobic resin composites able to bond to hydrophilic dentin, and glass ionomers have been modified by the addition of resins to improve handling and mechanical properties. Unfortunately, the latter more or less suppressed the potential for direct bonding and fluoride release.

Rubricating the non–metal-containing direct restorative materials is complicated by the overlap in formulation between the different types. In principle there exists a spectrum of tooth-colored materials ranging from the inorganic glass-ionomer cements to the mainly organic resin-based composites. Between these extremes lie hybrid mixtures, each incorporating some properties of both boundary materials. A complicating factor in combining the essentials of glass-ionomers cements and resin-based composites is that the former are hydrophillic and the latter hydrophobic. Consequently, a further way of differentiating the two groups from each other is that one is water containing and the other is not. The cements set by way of an acid-base reaction and the resins harden as a result of initiation of a polymerization process in a monomer system. The spectrum may be represented as follows:

Resin-based composite ↔ compomer ↔ resin-modified glass-ionomer ↔ glass-ionomer

In contrast to the overall characterization of amalgam, it is not possible to supply a general overview of the chemical properties of the various groups of materials within this spectrum of tooth-colored restoratives because they differ from brand to brand in formulation. Within this spectrum, however, the glass ionomer–based materials are the only ones that afford features lacking in amalgams and the resin-based composites. These features pertain to a sort of intelligence of the ionomers. Fluoride release, which provides opportunity for remineralization[2,16] at sites where demineralization may occur, is central to this quality. Moreover, glass ionomers are the only restorative materials that bond directly to enamel and dentin under humid conditions. Thanks to their low early strength, glass ionomers are not seriously affected by contractile setting shrinkage stresses, thus preserving the cavity seal. Because of their continuous chemical reaction, the glass ionomers have the potential for self-repair of acquired microcracks, while increasingly gaining strength and esthetics. It has been postulated that under certain conditions, glass ionomers may transform into a carbonized apatite.[15]

The limited requirements for cavity preparation for a glass-ionomer restoration underpin the concept of atraumatic restorative treatment (ART). This technique is indicated for dentistry in developing countries, where sophisticated equipment and optimal conditions do not exist and cavity preparation usually comprises only the excavation of caries with hand instruments.[9]

In contrast to the straightforward bonding of glass ionomers to tooth structure, the bonding of resin-based composites to tooth tissues is complex and technically demanding. Essentially the problem is related to the difference in nature of resin-based composites and tooth structure, composites being hydrophobic and the tooth structures hydrophillic, with the polymerization shrinkage of the resin-based composites being a confounding factor (Fig 10-4a).

Techniques

Bonding

The technique of successfully bonding to tooth structure is without doubt the No. 1 achievement in modern restorative dentistry. The differences in composition and chemistry of the various resin-bonding systems are enormous and beyond the scope of this chapter. In contrast, techniques for resin bonding share many similarities. Apart from a few products that are claimed to have retention that is chemical in nature, most resin-bonding systems interface with the tooth structures by way of infiltration of the (prepared) substrate, thus forming a micromechanical attachment. In this way the formation of a so-called hybrid layer is fundamental to most resin-bonding procedures. However, the quality of the bond relies not only on the successful hybridization of the substrate, but also on the resistance of the bond to stresses generated by the polymerization of the restoration.

Stress Control

If a restoration is adhesively attached to the cavity walls, it will be restrained in its response to contraction. Contractile forces set up by polymerization shrinkage generate stresses in the restored tooth (Fig 10-4a). If the stresses exceed the adhesive or cohesive strength of the materials involved, fracture and separation will occur (see Fig 10-3). With a flexible adhesive lining, the restoration is able to withstand the shrinkage stresses without losing its bond to the tooth structure. To bridge the gap between the restoration and the walls of the cavity, the lining material should be

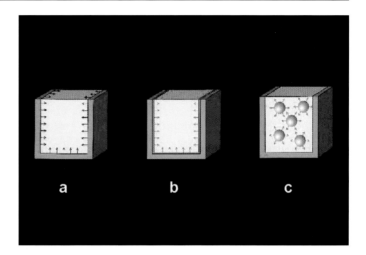

Fig 10-4 As a consequence of curing shrinkage, the adhesive restoration is subject to considerable contractile stresses (a). An elastic interfacial lining acts as a stress reliever (b). Porosity adds to the free surface required for stress relief by flow (c).

present in a substantial thickness to act as a stress absorber (Fig 10-4b). The bonding material should have an intrinsic thickness dictated by its composition and structure. The larger the molecules of the monomer system and the higher the filler-loading, the more viscous the material will be and the thicker the layer will appear when applied on the cavity. Because high viscosity can negatively affect the potential of a fluid to infiltrate the micropores of a substrate, some bonding systems are delivered in the form of two separate materials, a bonding agent and a liner, so that both requirements can be satisfied. Different bonding agents do not always form a continuous layer on conditioned dentin at the first application. Low-viscosity bonding agents may effectively infiltrate dentinal tubules, but may not form a continuous lining of sufficient thickness on the substrate. It has been shown[4] that for those bonding agents that do not form a continuous layer of appropriate thickness, a second application is recommended. Garberoglio[10] demonstrated that the successful application of un-

filled resin layers and linings of resin-modified glass ionomers reduces stresses in the restoration. Today, lightly filled dentin bonding agents are available that ensure both excellent hybridization of the dentinal substrate and the formation of a continuous layer across the cavity surface. Moreover, the filler particles render the lining opaque. Assuming that all materials at the interface between the restoration and the cavity walls are coherently attached to each other, the interfacial layer will be able to function effectively as a stress absorber.

Volume change brings about additional problems. Materials can reshape, but are unlikely to change in volume. Because of their loosely bound molecules, gasses can contract or expand, but the structure of liquids and solids does not permit isothermal volume changes. When gas is entrapped in the solid or liquid material, however, the volume can alter. Some materials are intrinsically porous, which enables them to take up diverse volumes; foam and sponge are good examples. Thus, if a dental lining or filling material contains pores or internal cracks, the substance is able to expand and occupy an enlarged space, as in the case of a sponge (Fig 10-4c). In this context, it is noteworthy that the mixing of two pastes will invariably introduce air bubbles into the material, such that the requirement for porosity in an autocuring material is automatically solved. This mechanism might very well be the explanation of the observation that the placement of an initial increment of self-curing composite between adhesive and light-curing composite leads to improved marginal adaptation.[10]

It could also be demonstrated that there is a substantial reduction in polymerization contraction stresses in self-curing resins when compared with light-curing resins.[1] If the shrinking restoration consists of a totally dense material, forced stretching will cause cracks or complete fracture of the interfacial bond. At a certain density of cracks, the internal free surface may be sufficiently large to allow stress relief, but the coherence of the material, and thus its strength, will be negatively affected. After some time, when resins absorb water from the environment and swell, the internal spaces might again allow volume compensation. This may restore the original volume, but it will not restore the lost coherence.

In the case of glass-ionomer cements, a different behavior has been observed. Glass ionomers also shrink during setting and thus face the same problems with contraction stress as resin-based composites. On the other hand, traditional glass ionomers initially exhibit a lower cohesive strength than their bond strength to tooth structure. For this reason, they are liable to fracture cohesively when forced to compensate for lost volume. It has been shown that, under restrained conditions, a setting glass ionomer develops internal microcracks.[3] When sufficient water is available, however, the glass ionomer will rapidly swell, thus closing the cracks. Because of the relatively long-lasting setting reaction of glass ionomers, some of the cracks are repaired through further chemical reaction, which restores some of the lost cohesive strength. In this way, glass-ionomer cements are the most functional materials in respect of stress reduction and volume adaptation. It is uncertain as to whether the mechanisms described are also effective in resin-modified glass ionomers.

For all direct restorative materials, setting of the viscous mass is based on chemical reactions, which, for materials other than photo-initiated materials, usually commences following the mixing of two components. Appropriate mixing is not easy. One cannot avoid the incorporation of air bubbles, and on mixing the chemical reaction commences, transforming the visco-elastic material into a solid mass. A direct consequence of the slow reaction of glass ionomers is the initial low strength of the material. Enormous effort has gone into techniques that quicken the setting reaction without negatively affecting the working time and handling properties of ionomers. One of the most promising solutions to these inconveniences was the introduction of new mechanisms for initiation of the setting reaction.

Setting Control

An important development in direct restorative techniques was the ability to control the setting of the filling material. A first step was control of the chemical reaction in two-component systems with accelerators and retarders. The really important break-through, however, came with the intro-duction of photocuring. The key was the use of light initiators incorporated in the resin system that were activated when irradiated with light of a certain wave-length. Subsequent to the initial euphoria surrounding the simplicity of use and ease of handling of single-paste, light-cured fill-ing materials, concerns grew regarding the quality of the conversion of these resins after irradiation.

To work effectively with resin-based composites and resin-modified glass ion-omers requires a profound understanding of the setting of these materials and the factors that influence this process. Besides the initiation of the polymerization reac-tion, the setting depends on characteris-tics such as composition (type of resin), construction (microfill, hybrid, or small particle), and the condition of the material (age and temperature). When initiation is achieved through the mixing of two com-ponents, one containing the initiator and the other the activator, one can be certain that the level of conversion is high and homogeneously distributed throughout the material. In contrast, when initiation is based on the activation of the initiator by adding energy to the system in the form of visible light, serious problems may arise.

Light Initiation

For the purpose of light initiation, the dentist has to select a light source from a variety of instruments; each based on a different concept. The choice is between halogen, plasma-arc, laser, or LED lamps with energy levels that range from 150 mW/cm^2 to well above 1,000 mW/cm^2. A

problem with the high intensity lamps, de-signed for irradiation times as short as 3 seconds, is that energy reduction factors become more critical than when the prac-titioner has time to control the position of the tip. Clinical requirements for curing are short irradiation times in combination with high and uniform conversion throughout the whole restoration and low shrinkage stress. Unfortunately, conversion of resin-based composites is usually proportion-ally associated with both shrinkage and stiffening. This gives substance to the paradox that improvements to the degree of conversion negatively affect the preser-vation of marginal continuity.[5]

Light Sources

Traditionally, the blue light of wavelength 470 nm necessary to photo-initiate resins is generated with halogen lamps mounted in various instruments. The emission spec-trum of a halogen lamp is much wider than the narrow 470-nm band necessary for camphorquinone. The light activation units are equipped with a filter, which ab-sorbs most of the superfluous wave-lengths. According to the ISO specification for polymerization light sources, the ener-gy output has to be measured over the spectral band of 470 to 500 nm. It has to be emphasized that camphorquinone is not the initiator for all resin-based com-posite products. This means that a wide spectrum of wavelengths might be a safe approach if many different product brands are used.

One of the main differences between the various types of light source is the energy level. This can be as low as 150 to 200 mW/cm^2 or as high as 650 to 800

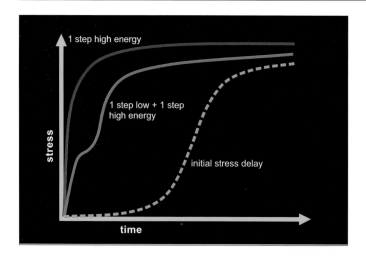

Fig 10-5 The stiffening of a resin-based composite with time using three different curing modes: one-step high energy irradiation, two-step irradiation (initial low energy followed by high energy), and slow start with continuously increasing energy.

mW/cm². To counter the advantages of command set, a recognized disadvantage of light curing is the sudden stiffening of the material together with the unavoidable curing contraction of the restorative material.[6] It is now generally accepted that the combination of stiffening and shrinkage will stress the restored tooth, possibly causing damage. One way to control sudden stress build-up is reduction in the initial degree of curing by commencing with low energy irradiation (Fig 10-5). The advantage of slowing down the (initial) conversion has been demonstrated experimentally.[7] The risk of incomplete conversion and, as a consequence, reduced longevity of the restoration, is tackled by additional prolonged irradiation at a higher energy level. To facilitate this so-called ramped curing, manufacturers have recently developed two step light sources. It has been shown experimentally that, although the stress ultimately reaches the same level, two-step curing leads to superior marginal integrity of the restoration.[8,11]

To use such instruments to best effect, the practitioner needs to know the precise curing requirements of the resin-based composite being used and to adjust the technique according to the particular situation. This makes the technique most procedure sensitive. To tackle this drawback of modern restorative dentistry, high-energy plasma-arc and LED light sources have been marketed. These devices offer various settings, such as 1s, 2s, 3s, full energy, or step-cure, which is initial half energy with subsequent full energy.

High-energy plasma-arc light sources provide a short burst of continuous light in a narrow wavelength band of 470 nm at an energy level > 1,000 mW/cm². Such a narrow band might miss the absorption of certain initiator agents other than camphorquinone. To avoid expensive, sophisticated energy sources, as required for plasma-arc lamps, the latest development is the use of LED technology. The advantages are numerous, including favorable energy supply associated with cordless hand pieces, negligible heat generation, programmable light spectrum and intensity and low costs for the renewal of lamps. The life expectancy of halogen lamps is approximately 50 hours. Plasma arc lamps may work for 500 to 5,000 hours and LED sources have an almost indefinite lifetime.

As previously noted, each material and shade of materials as well as different clinical situations require specific irradiation according to spectral distribution and light intensity. A programmable light source, which may eventually be programmed with the aid of bar coding of the syringe, might provide a solution to ease the practitioner's dilemma.

Conclusions

Although the dental profession is continuously flooded with newly formulated products, often before they have been properly assessed, the range of truly different materials remains limited. Given environmental and cosmetic considerations, the trends for direct restorative materials is away from amalgam toward tooth-colored alternatives. Of the tooth-colored restoratives, the resin-based composites are most widely used, notwithstanding their demanding technique. Aids to the use of resin-based composites, including bonding and command set, require further consideration because practitioners presently require a profound understanding of the processes involved to achieve optimum results. Bonding only offers retention and sealing if applied strictly according to stringent rules, while light curing often means working in the dark. On the other hand, glass-ionomer cements deserve more widespread acceptance given that the quality of restorations of these materials is less dependent on the skill and understanding of the dentist than is the case with resin-based composites. The formulation of glass-ionomers provides a series of properties that collectively designate such materials as intelligent. Glass-ionomers therefore hold most promise for the future.

References

1. Alster D, Feilzer AJ, De Gee AJ, Mol A, Davidson CL. The dependence of shrinkage stress reduction on porosity concentration in thin resin layers. J Dent Res 1992;71:1619–1622.

2. Arends J, Christoffersen J, Ruben J, Jongebloed WL. Remineralization of bovine dentin in vitro. The influence of F content in solution on mineral distribution. Caries Res 1989;23:309–314.

3. Davidson CL. Glass-ionomer bases under posterior composites. J Esthet Dent 1994;6:223–226.

4. Davidson CL. Lining and elasticity. In: Dondi dall'Orologio G, Prati C (eds). Factors influencing the quality of composite restorations. Carimate, Italy: Ariesdue Srl, 1997:87–93.

5. Davidson CL. Resisting the curing contraction with adhesive composites. J Prosthet Dent 1986;55:446–447.

6. Davidson CL, De Gee AJ, Feilzer AJ. The competition between the composite-dentin bond strength and the polymerization contraction stress. J Dent Res 1984;63:1396–1399.

7. Davidson-Kaban SS, Davidson CL, Feilzer AJ, de Gee AJ, Erdilek N. The effect of curing light variations on bulk curing and wall-to-wall quality of two types and various shades of resin composites. Dent Mater 1997;13:344–352.

8. Feilzer AJ, Dooren LH, de Gee AJ, Davidson CL. Influence of light intensity on polymerization shrinkage and integrity of restoration-cavity interface. Eur J Oral Sci 1995;103:322–326.

9. Frencken JE, Songpaisan Y, Phantumvanit P. An atraumatic restorative (ART) treatment technique evaluation after one year. Int Dent J 1994;44:460–464.

10. Garberoglio R, Coli P, Brännström M. Contraction gaps in Class II restorations with self-cured and light-cured resin composites. Am J Dent 1995;8:303–307.

11. Goracci G, Mori G, Casa de'Martinis L. Curing-light intensity and marginal leakage of resin composite restorations. Quintessence Int 1996; 27:355–362.

12. Hickel R, Manhart J. Glass-ionomers and compomers in pediatric dentistry. In: Davidson CL, Mjor IA (eds). Glass-ionomer cements. Berlin: Quintessence, 1999:201–226.

13. Hosoya N, Lautenschlager EP, Greener EH. A study of the apical microleakage of a gallium alloy as a retrograde filling material J Endod 1995;21:456–458.

14. Puttkamer A. Quecksilberloses Amalgam. Zahnarztl Rundsch 1928;35:1450.

15. Shimokobe H. Properties as a pit and fissure sealant. In: Katsuyama S, Ishikawa T, Fuji B (eds). Glass-Ionomer Dental Cement: The Materials and their Clinical Use. St. Louis: Ishiyaku EuroAmerica, 1993.

16. Ten Cate JM, Van Duinen RNB. Hyper mineralization of dentinal lesions adjacent to glass-ionomer cement restorations. J Dent Res 1995; 74:1266–1271.

17. Wataha JC, Nakajima H, Hanks CT, Okabe T. Correlation of cytotoxicity with element release from mercury- and gallium-based dental alloys in vitro. Dent Mater 1994;10:298–303.

Chapter 11

Efficiency of New Enamel-Dentin Bonding Systems: Assessment by General Practitioners

Michel Degrange, Laïla Hitmi, Denis Bouter,
Samuel Gonthier, Fanny Basset, and Julien Bijaoui

Introduction

Sustained progress in the field of adhesive technology has provided clinicians with products and systems that allow increasingly conservative approaches to the esthetic restoration of teeth. The enamel-dentin bonding systems (DBSs) developed during the last decade are all based on the total-etch concept. They are capable of creating strong, impervious bonds to remaining tooth tissues. Conditions for optimal bonding to enamel are now standard practice; however, bonding to dentin remains dependent on an understanding of the variations of the complex structure and properties of the substrate. The present concept of dentinal adhesion is based on the removal of the smear layer and dissolution of the mineral phase from the superficial dentin. This exposes and opens the dentinal tubules and creates intertubular microporosities sufficient to allow monomer infiltration into the exposed collagen network and patent tubules.[8,12,17] This is achieved by acid-conditioning of the dentin, priming of the etched surface with hydrophilic monomers and solvents, and infiltration of the primed dentin with resin monomers which copolymerise with the composite matrix. This process can be performed clinically in various ways according to the presentation of the adhesive system. The so-called fourth generation adhesive systems, developed in the early 1990s, are applied using a multistep procedure. Recently two further types of adhesive systems have been developed to simplify and reduce the stages of application. One-bottle systems, which include the primer and the adhesive resin in one liquid can be applied in two steps. Self-etching systems can be applied in either one or two steps.

To compare the effectiveness of different adhesive systems, many laboratories use dentin shear or tensile bond tests as an initial screening evaluation. Currently, reports of dentin bond strengths as high as 25 MPa are not uncommon. Such high

173

bond strength values are often exploited for commercial gain, with claims that the adhesive is as effective on dentin as on enamel. Generally, bond strength testing is undertaken by well-trained experts working under standardized conditions. However, results obtained with the same adhesives in different laboratories may differ widely. Previous studies have identified some of the most important experimental variables influencing bond strength data.[2,9,13] Nonuniform stress distribution within the bonded specimens may also help to explain some of the observed variations.[10,18,19]

The assessment of new adhesive systems and techniques is complicated by the frenetic pace of introduction of new materials in the dental market. Moreover, adhesive systems are technique-sensitive, with the most recent one- or two-step adhesives being paradoxically no more reliable than the multistep alternatives.[3] When using a one-bottle system, the extent of moisture on the dentinal surface is a critical factor in allowing good infiltration of monomers into the etched dentinal surface.[4-6] A dentinal surface that is either too wet or too dry can have undesirable effects on dentinal hybridization.[7,14-16] Operator familiarization and variability is therefore an important issue in investigations on dentin bonding.[1,11] Practical training is essential to optimize the handling of the adhesive system. This approach was adopted by Prof Holz some 5 years ago in the Department of Restorative Dentistry at the University of Geneva. Over a period of 3 days, more than 2,500 shear bond strength tests were carried out by 92 Swiss dentists using bovine dentin.[1] Nine different adhesive systems were evaluated. The differential between the most and the least

effective adhesives was around 60%; the discrepancy between dentists was found to be 28%. This experiment confirmed that the experience, skill, and care taken by the operator are more important to the outcome of shear bond testing than the nature of the adhesive. Moreover, mean bond strength values, irrespective of the adhesive system, was around 12 MPa. Such values are considerably lower than the values obtained in laboratory investigations.

This chapter describes an experience, similar to that described above, based on recent investigations in different regions of France. The approach was to develop a new type of multi-operator test with the following aims:

- To control how the adhesive technique is employed in general practice
- To evaluate the effect of directions for use and principles of application provided to the practitioners during training
- To rank the performance of the adhesive systems investigated under the test conditions and to assess the technique sensitivity of each of the adhesives
- To measure the discrepancy among the bond strength values according to operator variability

Materials and Methods

The author's department of biomaterials undertook to organize a series of practical training sessions on dentin bonding. The selected test was a simple shear test to give an immediate assessment of the quality of bonding and direct feedback to the participants.

The testing was undertaken in either the Paris V Dental School or in provincial meeting rooms specially equipped for the purpose. The preparation of the bonded specimens required only water and compressed air in three-in-one syringes, light-curing units, and a grinding/polishing machine. The Paris-based testing was undertaken using the department's tensile testing machine (JJ Lloyd T30K, Lloyd Instruments, Fareham, UK). For the provincial testing, a smaller portable machine (JJ Lloyd RSX) was used.

Sufficient dentinal substrate specimens were prepared in advance of each series of tests. Permanent molar teeth, stored immediately after extraction in 1% chloramine solution for a maximum of 3 months, were used throughout. The teeth were cleaned of soft tissue debris and then embedded in acrylic resin (Plexil, ESCIL, France). Flat dentinal surfaces were produced by wet grinding on SiC paper #800. Each sample was identified by a number carved in the embedding material.

Each operator was asked to bring the adhesive system in use in their practice. Using at least two prepared tooth specimens, the task set was to produce a series of dentin-bonded composites appropriate for mechanical testing. First the participants were informed about the scope of the trial and provided with the instructions necessary to carry out the required procedures. They were instructed to use a Teflon split mold (Figs 11-1a to 11-1c) with a central hole (3 mm in diameter and 5 mm deep). Following application of the adhesive, the participants were asked to fix the mold to the dentinal substrate specimen by means of a double aluminium ring and then fill it with two increments of composite, each light cured for 20 seconds. To minimize the experimental variables, only one composite material was used (Z100,

3M, St. Paul, MN). The output of the light curing units was required to be > 600 mW/cm^2. No instruction was given at this stage regarding the handling of the dentin bonding system. Following the bonding of an initial specimen (sample 1) using their own adhesive system, the participants, who were supervised but allowed to work without comment, stored sample 1 in water for approximately 10 minutes. They then measured the shear bond strength using a guillotine-type device on the tensile testing machine operating at a crosshead speed of 5 mm/minute until fracture occurred.

The participants then received brief oral instruction regarding the principles of the different classes of available dentin bonding systems, including details of the respective modes of application. Each participant then proceeded to test different adhesive systems used according to the relevant directions for use, with direct supervision and correction of any deviations in the appropriate operative technique. At the end of the program, each participant was invited to retest their own dentin bonding system on the original tooth specimen, taking account of observations made during the course.

The shear bond strength values were recorded in a spreadsheet as the tests were conducted. The spreadsheet included the operator's name, trial number, sample reference, and brand of dentin bonding system.

The following analysis includes results from the first five programs, which were organized in Aix-les-Bains, Paris (1), Marseille, Paris (2), and Lille. Five hundred fifty tests were completed by 121 dentists using 22 dentin bonding systems, only 10 of which were used by a sufficient num-

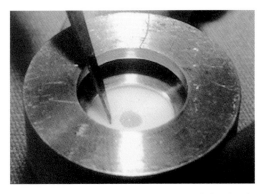

Fig 11-1a Once the specimen is formed, the ring is removed.

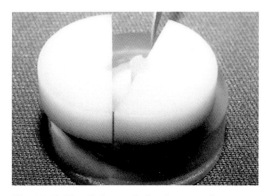

Fig 11-1b The Teflon split ring is opened.

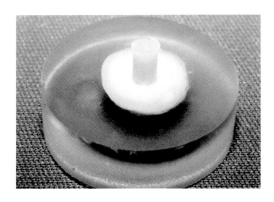

Fig 11-1c The sample is ready for testing.

ber of participants for the purposes of data analysis. The distribution of the materials tested according to the trial center is detailed in Table 11-1. Shear bond data were analysed using a one-way analysis of variance (ANOVA). Comparison between pairs were made using the Student-Newman-Keuls test at a level of significance of $P < .05$. The difference between the first and the last test completed using the participants' own dentin bonding system was analyzed using the paired t test.

Results

The mean shear bond strength values for the 10 selected dentin bonding systems are summarized in Table 11-2 and Fig 11-2. The outcome of the statistical analysis is set out in Table 11-3. The interval between the lowest (6.2 MPa) and the highest (13.5 MPa) mean shear bond strength is 118%.

The mean shear bond strength for Optibond Solo Plus (Kerr, Romulus, MI), an ethanol-based one-bottle system, was the highest value obtained, although not statistically greater than the values obtained for Clearfil SE Bond (Kuraray,

Table 11-1 Distribution of the materials tested according to trial center

Product	Manufacturer	Class	Code	Trial				Total
				Aix-les-Bains	Lille	Marseille	Paris (1+2)	
Excite	Vivadent	Ethanol-based one-bottle	Excite	20	17	19	9	59
One Coat	Coltène Whaledent	Water-based one-bottle	One Coat	0	11	10	6	27
One Step	Bisco	Acetone-based one-bottle	One Step	7	13	22	0	42
Optibond Solo Plus	Kerr	Ethanol-based one-bottle	Opt Solo+	10	19	13	13	55
Permaquick 1	Ultradent	Ethanol-based one-bottle	PQ1	11	2	8	5	26
Prim & Bond NT	Dentsply	Acetone-based one-bottle	P&BNT	2	11	5	9	27
Prompt L Pop	Espe	One-step self-etching	PLPop	5	0	18	8	31
Scotchbond Bond One	3M	Ethanol-based one-bottle	SB1	10	34	32	15	91
Scotchbond Multipurpose	3M	Mutistep	SBMP	8	5	7	17	31
Clearfil SE Bond	Kuraray	Two-step self-etching	SE Bond	17	20	27	1	65
Total				90	132	155	77	454

Table 11-2 Summary of the mean shear bond strength (SBS) for the 10 selected dentin bonding systems

Adhesives	Mean SBS (MPa)	SD (MPa)
Excite	9.5	4.6
One Coat	12.3	3.6
One Step	9.8	4.3
Optibond Solo Plus	13.5	3.4
Permaquick 1	11.0	3.5
Prim & Bond NT	10.3	3.6
Prompt L Pop	6.2	6.0
Scotchbond Bond One	11.2	3.8
Scotchbond Multipurpose	10.8	3.6
Clearfil SE Bond	12.5	4.1

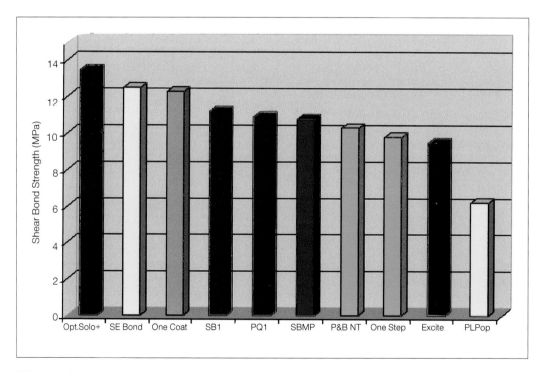

Fig 11- 2 Mean shear bond strength mean values for the 10 selected adhesive systems.

Table 11-3 Statistical comparison between pairs according to the Student-Newman-Keuls test*

	Excite	One Coat	One Step	Optibond Solo Plus	Perma-quick 1	Prim & Bond NT	Prompt L Pop	Scotchbond Bond One	Scotchbond Multipurpose	Clearfit SE Bond
Excite	–	S	NS	S	NS	NS	S	NS	NS	S
One Coat	S	–	NS	NS	NS	NS	S	NS	NS	NS
One Step	NS	NS	–	S	NS	NS	S	NS	NS	NS
Optibond Solo Plus	S	NS	S	–	S	S	S	NS	S	NS
Permaquick 1	NS	NS	NS	S	–	NS	S	NS	NS	NS
Prim & Bond NT	NS	NS	NS	S	NS	–	S	NS	NS	NS
Prompt L Pop	S	S	S	S	S	S	–	S	S	S
Scotchbond Bond One	NS	NS	NS	NS	NS	NS	S	–	NS	S
Scotchbond Multipurpose	NS	NS	NS	S	NS	NS	S	NS	–	NS
Clearfil SE Bond	S	NS	NS	NS	NS	NS	S	S	NS	–

*S, significant (P < .05); NS, not significant (P > .05)

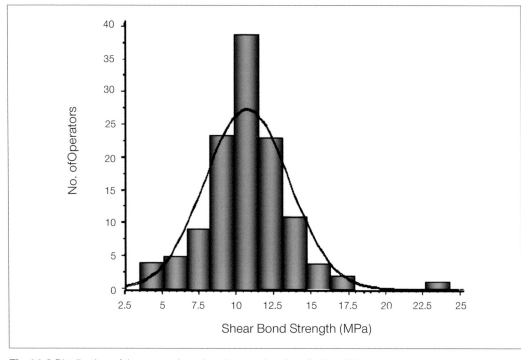

Fig 11-3 Distribution of the mean shear bond strength values for the 121 operators.

Osaka, Japan), One Coat (Coltène Whaledent), and Scotchbond One/Single Bond (3M). A further group of systems that were found to be statistically similar were then identified. This group included Permaquick 1 (Ultradent, South Jordan, UT) to Excite (Vivadent, Schaan, Liechtenstein) in Fig 11-2. The one-step, self-etching adhesive Prompt L Pop (ESPE, Seefeld, Germany) was found to have a significantly lower mean shear bond strength with a wide standard deviation. Variation in the standard deviation was found to be a feature of differences in the dentin bonding system.

Variation in the mean values for shear bond strength obtained by each operator is illustrated in Fig 11-3. The mean, median, mode, and standard deviation according to operator are set out in Table 11-4. The variation among the 121 operators was found to be around 350% with a random distribution. Consequently, the mean, median, and mode are equivalent with a value close to 10.7 MPa. This is less than half the value obtained with the same dentin bonding systems under laboratory conditions. As a consequence, operator variability was considered to be an important factor in the effectiveness of dentin bonding.

In addition to the above, this study highlighted the importance of instruction in the use of dentin bonding systems. A significant improvement ($P < .001$) was found between the mean values for initial (9.2 MPa) and final (11.7 MPa) specimen shear bond strengths.

Table 11-4 Features of the mean values obtained by each operator

Mean	10.7
SD	2.8
Minimum	3.5
Maximum	24.3
Variance	7.9
Median	10.8
Mode	10.8

Discussion

It was the purpose of the present study to demonstrate that adhesive bonding is technique sensitive and strongly operator related. This multicenter approach was adapted from the Swiss "Battle of the Bond."[1] Cuicchi et al reported a variation of 60% among the values obtained for the dentin bonding systems tested, with an operator variability of 280%. The present results are similar, albeit that operator variability has a more dramatic effect (118% vs 350%). In laboratory studies, operator variability is generally controlled and then masked because only one person, often an expert technician, makes the bonded samples. Nevertheless, the importance of operator variability must be taken into account in future studies to give users of dentin bonding systems more reliable information regarding shear bond strengths that may be obtained in clinical use. In clinical use, shear bond strengths may be found to be closer to 10 MPa than 20 MPa. The quality of enamel bonding will, however, remain the standard with the likelihood of a strong (> 20 MPa) impermeable bond.

The shear bond strength values obtained in the present study correspond to values obtained in early laboratory investigations 24 hours after bonding and usually following thermocycling. The clinical relevance of this type of aging remains to be established. However, a strong initial bond is required to resist polymerization stresses.

Other studies have demonstrated variability between practitioners but not variability according to the type of adhesive as found in the present investigation. Of the one-bottle systems tested, those containing ethanol as a solvent gave higher bond strengths than the acetone-based systems. Previous studies have reported the acetone-based products to be more sensitive to variations in the wetness of the dentinal substrate. Similarly, it has been suggested that self-etching materials are less sensitive to variations in the wetness of dentin. This helps to explain the findings regarding Clearfil SE Bond in the present study. Further studies are required to investigate other variables that may significantly influence shear bond strength values.

Conclusion

The present study confirms that operator variability is more important than the nature of the dentin bonding system in the development of shear bond strength. Lack of knowledge and understanding of dentin bonding systems among practitioners was observed. As a consequence, it is suggested that practitioners must have opportunity to learn more and acquire practical experience of the effective application of dentin bonding systems. A good starting point is reference to manufacturers' directions for the use for such systems.

The method of the present study was found to be capable of discriminating between the sensitivities and performance of different dentin bonding systems. Further studies of this type are indicated.

References

1. Ciucchi B, Bouillaguet S, Holz J. The battle of the bonds 1995. Schweiz Monatsschr Zahnmed 1997;107:33–36.

2. Finger WJ. Dentin bonding agents. Relevance of in vitro investigations. Am J Dent 1988;1: 184–188.

3. Finger W, Balkenhol M. Practitioner variability effects on dentin bonding with an acetone-based one-bottle adhesive. J Adhes Dent 1999; 1:311–314.

4. Gwinnett AJ. Dentine bond strength after air drying and rewetting. Am J Dent 1994;7: 144–148.

5. Gwinnett AJ. Moist versus dry dentin: Its effect on shear bond strength. Am J Dent 1992;5: 127–129.

6. Kanca J. Effect of resin primer solvents and surface wetness on resin composite bond strength to dentin. Am J Dent 1992;5:213–215.

7. Kanca J. Wet bonding: Effect of drying time and distance. Am J Dent 1996;9:237–276.

8. Pashley DH, Ciucchi B, Sano H, Horner JA. Permeability of dentin to adhesive resins. Quintessence Int 1993;24:618–631.

9. Rueggeberg FA. Substrate for adhesion testing to tooth structure—Review of the literature. Dent Mater 1991;7:2–10.

10. Samsri S, Van Noort R. Do dentin bond tests serve a useful purpose? J Adhes Dent 1999; 1:57–67.

11. Sano H, Kanemura N, Burrow MF, Inai N, Yamada T, Tagami J. Effect of operator variability on dentin adhesion: Students vs dentists. Dent Mater J 1998;17:51–58.

12. Sano H, Shono T, Takatsu T, Hosoda H. Microporous dentin zone beneath resin-impregnated layer. Oper Dent 1994;19:59–64.

13. Söderholm KJM. Correlation of in vivo and in vitro performance of adhesive restorative materials. A report of the ASC MDI156 Task Group on test methods for the adhesion of restorative materials. Dent Mater 1991;8:10–15.

14. Tay F, Gwinnett JA, Pang KM, Wei SHY. Resin permeation into acid-conditioned, moist and dry dentin: A paradigm using water-free adhesive primers. J Dent Res 1996;75:1034–1044.

15. Tay F, Gwinnett JA, Wei SHY. Micromorphological spectrum overdrying to overwetting acid-conditioned dentin in water-free, acetone-based, single-bond primer/adhesives. Dent Mater 1996;12:236–244.

16. Tay F, Gwinnett AJ, Wei SHY. The overwet phenomenon: A transmission electron microscopic study of surface moisture in the acid-conditioned, resin-dentin interface. Am J Dent 1996; 9:161–166.

17. Van Meerbeck B, Inokoshi, S, Braem M, Lambrechts P, Vanherle G. Morphological aspects of the resin-dentin interdiffusion zone with different adhesive systems. J Dent Res 1992; 71:1530–1540.

18. Van Noort R, Noroozi S, Howard IC, Cardew G. A critique of bond strength measurments. J Dent 1989;17:61–67.

19. Versluis A, Tantbirojn D, Douglas WH. Why do shear bond tests pull out dentin? J Dent Res 1997;76:1298–1307.

Chapter 12

Improving Outcome: Anterior Restorations

Bernd Klaiber, Burkhard Hugo, and Norbert Hofmann

Introduction

Resin-based composites have been used for 30 years to replace missing enamel and dentin in anterior teeth. These restorations enjoy high rates of clinical success, provided the requirements of the adhesive restorative technique have been met, a good shade match has been achieved, and the tooth has been restored to its original shape. Moreover, resin-based composites can be used to change the appearance, size, color, spacing, and positioning of the teeth. Bonding to teeth, possibly together with selective grinding of other teeth, allows esthetic corrections that formerly required full-crown restorations or orthodontic treatment (Table 12-1). For example, direct esthetic restorations can be used to correct inherited and acquired developmental defects (Fig 12-1), rotated teeth (Fig 12-2), and exposed root surfaces and black triangles (Fig 12-3).

Fundamentals of Dental Esthetics

Any changes to the shape of a tooth, eg, widening, lengthening, rotation, or correction of misalignment, will only have an esthetically pleasing result when certain fundamental principles are obeyed. The rules of dental esthetics have been reported in the literature.[1-3,5,6] In particular, Rufenacht[5] has illustrated the importance of cohesive and segregative forces, symmetry, proportion, dominance, and negative spaces for a successful dental composition.

Changing the shape of teeth requires careful planning. Often this can be accomplished chairside by adding resin-based composite to a tooth and shaping it. This procedure, the mock-up, helps to outline the goal and gives the patient and the dentist an appreciation of the anticipated result.

Table 12-1 Indications for direct esthetic restorations in anterior teeth

Maintaining and restoring the original shape of the tooth
– Restoration of enamel and dentin lost because of caries, trauma, erosion, attrition, and abrasion (eg, Fig 12-8)
– Placement of direct resin veneers to restore labial surfaces that have become unsightly because of multiple fillings, especially when margins are defective and color match is poor (Fig 12-5)
– Restoration of stained, hypocalcified, and fluorotic teeth

Changing the original shape of the tooth
– Treatment of inherited and acquired developmental defects (Fig 12-1)
– Closure of diastemas as an adjunct to or a substitute for orthodontic treatment (Fig 12-7)
– Closure of a diastema created by a single missing lower incisor
– Widening of teeth prior to full-crown restoration of adjacent teeth
– Transformation of canines into lateral incisors to compensate for missing laterals
– Changing the appearance of inclined teeth
– Changing the appearance of rotated teeth (Fig 12-2)
– Creation of a more juvenile smile (Fig 12-3) by:
    a) Covering exposed root surfaces to mimic a new cementoenamel junction located more apically
    b) Reduction of black triangles resulting from interproximal gingival recession

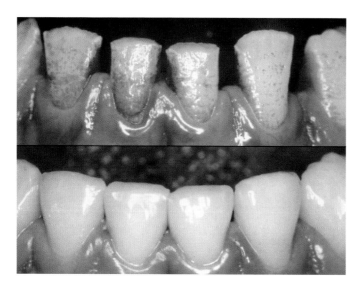

Fig 12-1 Mandibular anteriors affected by enamel hypoplasia prior to (top) and after (bottom) direct esthetic restoration.

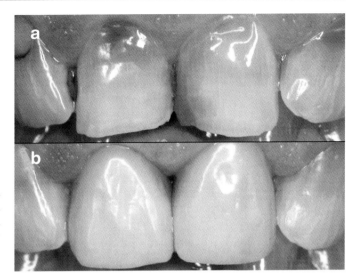

Fig 12-2 Direct esthetic restorations for the correction of two rotated and axially malpositioned central incisors. Note the alignment of the marginal ridges (a, baseline; b, final result).

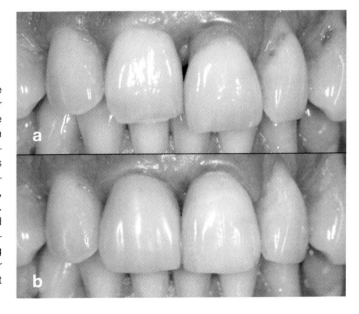

Fig 12-3 The exposed root surface of the left maxillary central incisor and the black triangle convey the impression of an "aged" dentition (a). To create a more youthful appearance, the exposed root was covered, creating a new cementoenamel junction apically located, and the black triangle was reduced. In addition, the left maxillary central incisor was reduced along the incisial edge. The palatal positioning of the right maxillary central incisor was disguised by placing a direct composite resin veneer (b).

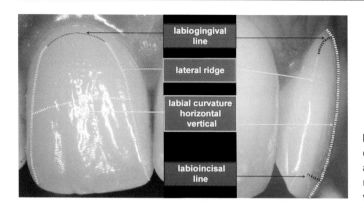

labiogingival
line

lateral ridge

labial curvature
horizontal
vertical

labioincisal
line

Fig 12-4 The shape of a tooth is determined by the labiogingival and labioincisal line angles, the marginal ridges, and horizontal and vertical curvature.

Creating Optical Illusion

The beauty of a single tooth emanates from the natural appearance of its outline form, proportion, and shade. The contour of a tooth is largely defined by its lateral ridges (Fig 12-4). Their shape needs to be clearly discernible. When the shape of a tooth is changed, the ridges must be reestablished in the new position. They need to be clearly accentuated and their course must not be twisted or angulated in an unnatural fashion. The labial surface between the lateral ridges and the labiogingival and labioincisal line angles are more or less curved in both the horizontal and vertical planes. Irrespective of length and width, the appearance of a tooth depends to a large extent on the position of the labiogingival and labioincisal line angles and on the labiofacial curvature. Another aspect influencing the perceived width of a tooth is the position of the proximal contacts. Labially located contacts make the tooth look wider, whereas lingually located contacts create the impression of a narrower tooth.

Gingivoincisal developmental grooves and perikymata on the labial surface further modify the appearance of a tooth. Dominance of the horizontal structures makes the tooth look wider and shorter, whereas emphasis on vertical structures creates a narrower and longer appearance.

Shade selection for the interproximal and cervical areas creates further opportunity to create an optical illusion. Selection of a darker shade for the interproximal or cervical area makes the tooth appear narrower or shorter, respectively. In contrast, a lighter shade in the respective areas will create the impression of a wider or longer tooth (Figs 12-5 and 12-6).

One of the most important parameters controlling the perceived width of a tooth is the size of the interincisal triangles. Large interincisal triangles make teeth appear narrow. Small triangles make teeth look wide.

In Tables 12-2 and 12-3 the different ways of creating an optical illusion are listed. These possibilities should be deliberately applied, for example, in cases where the width of a tooth must be increased to close a diastema, while at the same time avoiding the impression of a disproportionately wide tooth.

Fig 12-5 Central incisors prior to *(a)* and after *(b)* placement of direct esthetic restorations. Selection of a darker shade for the cervical and a lighter shade for the interproximal areas make the teeth appear wider and shorter. The distance between the thin blue lines on both images is identical, demonstrating that the length of the teeth has not been changed.

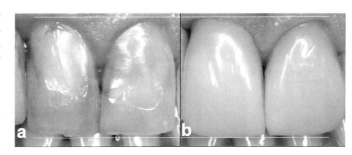

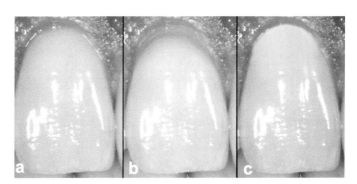

Fig 12-6 Computer-based image processing showing the baseline situation *(a)*, a darker shade in the cervical area making the tooth look shorter and wider *(b)*, and a lighter shade giving the impression of a longer, narrower tooth *(c)*.

Table 12-2 Creating optical illusions of width

Feature	Widening	Narrowing
Labial curvature in horizontal (mesiodistal) plane	Decrease	Increase
Lateral ridge	Move in lateral direction	Move in medial direction
Interproximal contact	More labial	More lingual
Shade selection for the interproximal area	Select a lighter shade	Select a darker shade
Incisocervical developmental grooves and perikymata	Emphasize perikymata	Emphasize incisocervical developmental grooves
Size of interincisal triangles	Reduce	Increase

Table 12-3 Creating optical illusions of length

Feature	Shortening	Lengthening
Labial curvature in vertical (incisocervical) plane	Increase	Decrease
Cervicolabial line angle	Move in incisal direction	Move in apical direction
Shade selection for the cervical area	Select a darker shade	Select a lighter shade
Incisocervical developmental grooves and perikymata	Emphasize perikymata	Emphasize incisocervical developmental grooves

Matrix Technique for Creating Individual Interproximal Molds

Routine clinical procedures for restoring Class III and Class IV cavities include the interproximal placement of a straight length of transparent matrix strip. In such situations, the proximal shape of the tooth will not be changed, therefore the matrix strip can be adapted to the tooth and held in place by inserting interproximal wedges. The wedges separate the adjacent teeth and facilitate the creation of a tight interproximal contact. The same procedure is used when a direct veneer that leaves the proximal shape of the tooth unchanged is to be placed.

In contrast, the complete or partial closure of diastemas is a more complicated situation with various conflicting demands. On the one hand, the matrix should be tightly adapted to the cervical area of the tooth to avoid the formation of interproximal overhangs. On the other hand, it must allow the buildup of a new proximal contour to close, or at least reduce, the interproximal space, with or

without a tight interproximal contact as appropriate. In many cases, attempts to adapt the matrix to the tooth by the placement of a wedge will prevent sufficient material being added to the cervical area to create a well-proportioned, harmonious lateral contour. After removal of the wedge, large black triangles are left. To make things more complicated, the creation of tight interproximal contacts is often difficult using this technique.

To overcome these difficulties, the creation of individual interproximal molds is suggested (Figs 12-7a to 12-7f). First, a matrix strip is inserted interproximally extending into the gingival sulcus. A light-curing composite for provisional purposes (eg, Fermit N, Vivadent, Schaan, Liechtenstein or Clip, Voco, Cuxhaven, Germany) is placed between the back of the matrix and the adjacent tooth. Prior to light curing, these low-viscosity materials stick to the matrix, the adjacent tooth, and gingivae, provided saliva has been blown away using compressed air prior to application. Starting from the incisal edge, the matrix is pushed toward the adjacent

190

Figs 12-7a to 12-7f Creation of an individual interproximal mold using the matrix technique.

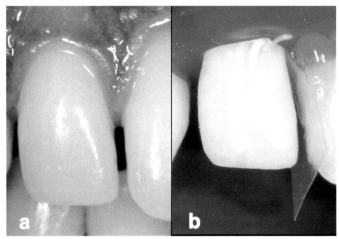

Fig 12-7a Maxillary lateral incisor with diastemas mesially and distally.

Fig 12-7b Contouring of the mesial matrix strip according to the desired proximal contour. The strip is attached to the adjacent tooth using a provisional material (Fermit N).

Fig 12-7c A thin layer of flowable composite has been injected between the matrix and the cervicopalatal area of the tooth. Subsequently, this layer is extended toward the incisal edge. The teeth are separated by placing and twisting a plastic instrument between them. The instrument acts as a lever and separates the teeth, creating opportunity to form tight interproximal contacts.

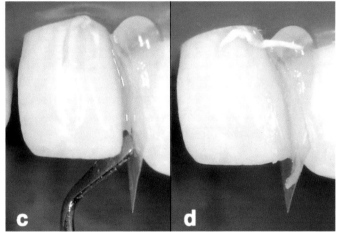

Fig 12-7d The interproximal buildup is completed using high viscosity dentin and enamel shades.

Fig 12-7e Restoration of the distal aspect of the tooth according to the same principles.

Fig 12-7f At the recall visit, the restoration displays harmonious contours, good color match, tight interproximal contacts, and a favorable tissue reaction.

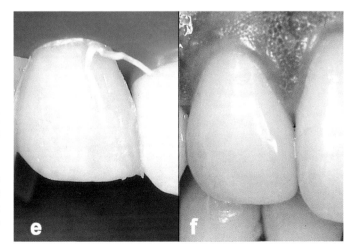

tooth using a thin plastic instrument. Proceeding in a cervical direction, the required proximal contour is created by working provisional material out of the interproximal space. Because of the stickiness of the provisional material, the matrix is held in the desired form and position. The resulting proximal mold is "frozen" by light curing the provisional material for 30 seconds from either side.

After appropriate conditioning and bonding, a flowable composite is injected into the cervical angle between the tooth and the matrix. For this purpose, it may be found preferable to use a thin metal cannula. The bulk of the restoration is placed in several layers using dentinal shades of a high-viscosity composite.

At this point, a tight interproximal contact may be created in one of two ways. Either a wedge is inserted interproximally to separate the teeth or a plastic instrument is pushed between the dentinal core and the matrix and twisted to act as a lever to separate the teeth. In the latter case, a translucent, flowable composite is injected between the core and the matrix and light cured while the teeth are kept separated by the plastic instrument.

The restoration is completed using the enamel shades of the composite. Once the lateral shape of the tooth has been created by the proximal mold, only the labial and lingual surfaces remain to be contoured.

The technique described facilitates the management of difficult clinical situations and provides predictable results.

Layering Technique Following the Anatomic Contouring of the Tooth

The color of a natural tooth results from reflection and diffraction of light within its different components—enamel, dentin, and the pulp. These tissues vary considerably in color and translucency. Conventional brands of composites come in a range of shades, but generally fail to provide different translucencies. In the case of small restorations, for example, Class III or Class V fillings, limitations in translucency are not very important. The color of direct restorations results from the combined effect of the underlying hard tissue and the shade of the overlying composite. Often restorations have feather-edged margins that will not be apparent even in highly visible areas.

Large esthetic anterior restorations will not, however, emulate the natural tooth when only one shade of restorative material has been used. In contrast, it seems logical to use different shades of composite that match as closely as possible the tissue that has to be restored. Dentinal shades should provide very intense colors (high chroma according to Munsell[4]) and a relatively low translucency. The core of the restoration, built up using dentinal shades, plays a prominent role in the final result. Enamel shades should, in contrast, provide enhanced translucency together with relatively low intensity of color. Only a few brands of composites satisfy these requirements (eg, Herculite XRV, Kerr, Orange, CA and Enamel plus HFO, Micerium srl, Avegno, Italy).

For a successful anterior restoration, it is necessary to analyze the chromatic composition of the tooth. This permits, during placement of the restoration, imita-

Figs 12-8a to 12-8l Case presentation demonstrating the anatomic layering techniques.

Fig 12-8a Discoloration of an old composite restoration in the right maxillary central incisor. The chromatic composition of the contralateral incisor serves as a model for the new restoration. Size and shape of the incisal mamelons and the translucent effects of the incisal edge should be analyzed and documented at this point.

Fig 12-8b Placement of rubber dam conceals any information on the chromatic composition of the contralateral incisor.

Fig 12-8c After removal of the old restoration, a chamfer was prepared along the labial enamel margins.

Fig 12-8d The lingual aspect shows the extent of the defect.

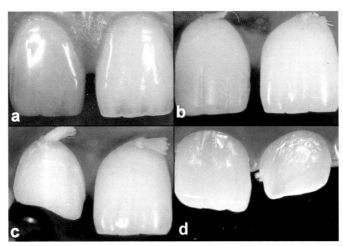

tion of the different tissues and their optical properties by placing the appropriate types and shades of composite while mimicking the anatomic composition of the tooth—the anatomic layering technique.[7] The case presented in Figs 12-8a to 12-8l and the schematic drawing Fig 12-9 illustrate this technique.

The concept of an anatomic layering technique may also be applied to direct resin veneers if the chromatic composition of the tooth is to be maintained. For example, enamel and dentin lost through erosion can be restored by application of composite featuring the appropriate translucency.

Changing the chromatic composition of a tooth requires modifications to the anatomic layering technique. Staining or discoloration of the underlying dentin may be masked using opaque shades or compensated for by the application of lighter dentinal shades of the composite. Such dentinal layers are relatively thick and are at the expense of the overlying enamel layer. Polychromatic layers of 0.5- to 1-mm thickness may be required, consisting of thin overlapping layers of different dentinal shades (from dark to light) covered by a thin enamel layer. Even if labial space is limited, incisal mamelons and other characteristics of the incisal edge can be imitated.

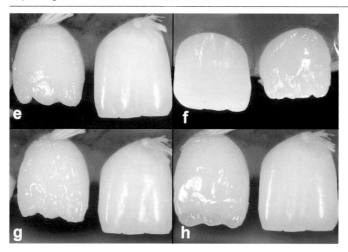

Fig 12-8e Following conditioning of the surface, the dentinal core was placed using a dark (A3) dentinal shade.

Fig 12-8f Lingual aspect.

Fig 12-8g The dentinal core was extended toward the incisal edge using a lighter (A2) dentinal shade to create the required length and shape.

Fig 12-8h Reconstruction of the enamel core using a translucent (clear) enamel shade.

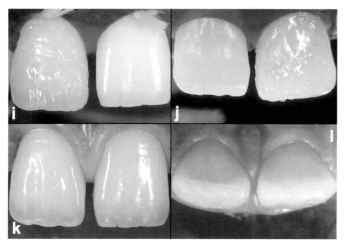

Fig 12-8i Restoration of the labial surface and the incisal edge to include the desired features using a generic enamel shade ("White I").

Fig 12-8j Lingual aspect.

Fig 12-8k Direct esthetic restoration at a recall visit. The chromatic composition and translucent effects of the incisal edge correspond to the contralateral tooth.

Fig 12-8l Lingual aspect.

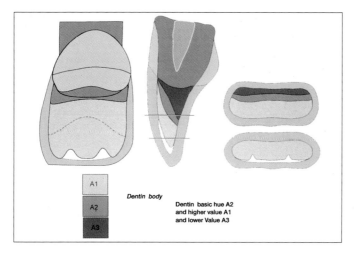

A1

Dentin body

A2

Dentin basic hue A2
and higher value A1
and lower Value A3

A3

Fig 12-9 Schematic presentation of the anatomic layering technique used in the case presented in Figs 12-8a to 12-8l.

Materials and Instruments

The materials and instruments used for esthetic corrections include:

- Fine hybrid composites of different shades and translucencies
- Flowable fine hybrid composites
- Bonding agents
- Resin tints and opaques (for occasional use)
- No. 12 scalpel blade for interproximal separation prior to light curing, trimming overhangs, and performing minor shape corrections after light curing
- Transparent matrix strips and light-curing provisional material for creating proximal molds
- Small double-ended flat-plastic instrument for the application and contouring of composite, for separating teeth to create tight proximal contacts, and to gain access to the interproximal surfaces for contouring and finishing
- Flame-shaped fine-particle diamond-coated finishing burs, reciprocating files for contouring after light-curing, and finishing disks and strips
- Medium and fine particle abrasive rubber points for polishing, together with silicon-carbide–containing brushes for final polishing
- Airborne particle abrasion unit for creating a retentive surface for composite repair

Conclusions

Composites and adhesive techniques have improved tremendously over the years. As a consequence, it is possible to perform esthetic corrections by placing direct restorations that previously would have required indirect restorations. The advantages and disadvantages of direct esthetic restorations are listed in Table 12-4. Formerly, esthetic corrections typically required the provision of full-crown or veneer restorations on otherwise healthy teeth. In many cases, esthetic corrections were not carried out because the risk of the possible adverse effects of full-crown preparations was regarded as too high and they often were not a financially viable option. Opportunities to improve the appearance of teeth by placing direct restorations will have an increasing impact on many aspects of dentistry and provide an alternative to traditional, more invasive procedures. Minimally invasive techniques offer the chance to perform esthetic treatments with an acceptable risk-benefit ratio.

Table 12-4 Advantages and disadvantages of esthetic corrections using direct restorations

Advantages:
- Minimal loss of dental hard tissue, no trauma from preparation
- Final result mostly achieved in one visit
- Subsequent corrections and repair are possible at any time
- Largely reversible procedure
- May serve as a compromise treatment for questionable teeth
- Independence from the dental laboratory
- Less expensive for the patient
- Exploits the dentist's sense of esthetics

Disadvantages:
- Very demanding for the dentist
- More plaque accumulation compared with that associated with dental porcelain
- Relatively rapid degradation of the surface of resin-based composites
- Less than ideal outcome given, for example, occasional inclusion of air bubbles in resin-based composites

References

1. Chiche G, Pinault A. Esthetics of Anterior Fixed Prostodontics. Chicago: Quintessence, 1994.

2. Dong JK, Jin TH, Cho HW, Oh SC. The esthetics of the smile: A review of some recent studies. Int J Prosthodont 1999;12:9–19.

3. Lombardi RE. The principles of visual perception and their clinical application to denture esthetics. J Prosthet Dent 1973;29:358–382.

4. Munsell AH. A Color Notation, ed 11. Baltimore: Munsell Color, 1961.

5. Rufenacht CR. Fundamentals in Esthetics. Chicago: Quintessence, 1990.

6. Schärer P, Rinn LA, Kropp FR. Ästhetische Richtlinien für die rekonstruktive Zahnheilkunde. Berlin: Quintessenz, 1985.

7. Vanini L. Light and color in anterior composite restorations. Pract Periodontics Aesthet Dent 1996;7:673–682.

Chapter 13

Conservative Treatments in the Esthetic Zone

Didier Dietschi and Ivo Krejci

Introduction

There are different standards or levels of quality in dental care. Standard 1 includes the arrest of any pathologic process and provides for the protection of the remaining tissues. Standard 2 additionally addresses the shape and function of the dentition. Esthetics is of concern only in Standard 3, which prevails in western countries[18] and has become the main priority for many patients. As prevention of caries and periodontal diseases becomes an essential part of the everyday approach to effective care, fewer extractions will be necessary and restorations will require maintenance over extended periods in clinical service.

Facing this new reality will have a tremendous impact on the vision of and approach to restorative treatments in the esthetic area. In contrast to now outdated ways of practicing dentistry, relatively non-invasive treatment options must be considered. Conceptually, this should guarantee the most favorable long-term biomechanical behavior of restored teeth and at the same time keep overall fee levels relatively low. Although these considerations appear obvious, they are unfortunately far from being widely recognized,

largely through ignorance of the indications and potential of minimally invasive procedures.

The purpose of this chapter is to present modern concepts for treating esthetic, restorative, and functional deficiencies in the anterior segments, with emphasis on the most conservative techniques, including chemical treatments of dental discolorations and direct freehand bonding.

Treatment Concepts

The so-called "progressive treatment concept" involves a comprehensive biologic, functional, and esthetic diagnosis of conditions and presenting problems and the application of all known forms of appropriate treatment and specialist dental care in a sequential order[7]:

- Orthodontics
- Periodontics
- Chemical and chemomechanical treatments of discolorations
- Enamel recontouring
- Freehand composite restorations
- Veneers
- Adhesive bridges
- Implants

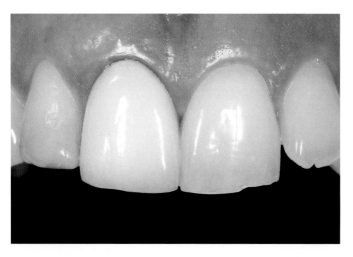

Figs 13-1a to 13-1c Esthetic failure and retreatment of an anterior metal ceramic crown.

Fig 13-1a The failed metal ceramic crown (on the right maxillary central incisor). Some of the most common esthetic problems are apparent, including lack of translucency, visible margin, and gingival darkening.

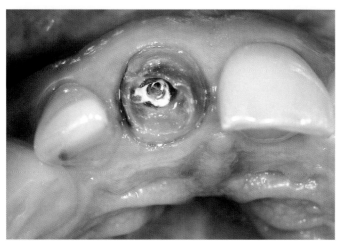

Fig 13-1b In addition to the esthetic deficiencies, the lack of remaining coronal tissue compromises the long-term biomechanical prognosis of the tooth.

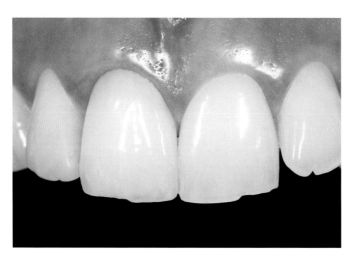

Fig 13-1c Only a new crown could address the esthetic failure (prosthetics courtesy of Michel Magne, CDT).

- Fixed prosthodontics
- Removable prosthodontics

The short- and long-term incidence of pulpal complications, gingival recession, periodontal lesions, recurrent caries, and mechanical failures suggest caution in providing crowns in young patients (Figs 13-1a to 13-1c). Such patients should be considered as very special and most deserving of particular efforts when planning and realizing any form of treatment.[26]

Chemical and Chemomechanical Treatment of Dental Discolorations

The most common types of dental discoloration that may be conservatively treated are listed in Table 13-1. It is important to identify the cause of the discoloration because this helps determine its location, the treatment to be applied, and the possible outcome.[8]

Techniques, including the bleaching of vital and nonvital teeth and microabrasion, may result in a dramatic and possibly stable esthetic improvement in the appearance of discolored teeth.[14,25] It is therefore possible to preclude the need to prepare affected teeth for restorations such as veneers and crowns.

Microabrasion

This is the least conservative of the chemical treatments for discolored teeth. Microabrasion is intended to eliminate hypoplastic areas of light to mild fluorosis and some superficial white spots.[3,4] The discolored tissue will be selectively removed by the active application of a slurry of hydrochloric acid and pumice. The slurry can be prepared chairside or is available as a "ready to use" product (eg, Opalustre, Ultradent, Salt Lake City, UT). With each 15- to 20-second application, 20 to 30 μm of enamel tends to be removed. As a consequence, the technique should be applied with caution and only in the management of superficial discolorations (Figs 13-2a and 13-2b).

Vital Bleaching

This is the most commonly applied chemical treatment for dental discolorations. It has been used for several decades and is presently available in various forms (Figs 13-3a to 13-3c). These different forms of vital bleaching have specific indications and the efficacy of the different systems remains to be determined.[12] Vital bleaching is indicated in the treatment of various forms of hypoplastic lesions, teeth darkened as a result of aging, unsightly tooth shades, and discolorations caused by systemic illness. "Home bleaching" is the most widely applied treatment for dental discoloration because it is the most powerful and least expensive approach.[15] The active agent is carbamide peroxide, which eliminates discoloration by oxidation of organic pigments. All other chairside or so-called "in-office" bleaching methods are based on the same principle but make use of stronger bleaching agents with rapid release of oxidizing ions. However, reduced application times probably reduce effectiveness in deep layers of the tooth.

Table 13-1 Dental discolorations and related treatments

Condition	Tissue concerned	Treatment
Generalized discoloration		
Fluorosis (I–III)*	Enamel (mainly surface)	Microabrasion
Tetracycline discoloration (I–III or I–IV)**	Dentin	Vital bleaching (I–II) or veneers (II–IV)
Generalized enamel dysplasia	Enamel	Microabrasion or veneers
Severe systemic disorders	Enamel/dentin	Microabrasion, vital bleaching, or veneers
Localized discoloration		
Infection/trauma of primary teeth (Turner's teeth)	Enamel/dentin	Vital bleaching, composites, or veneers
Systemic disorders	Enamel/dentin	
Acquired discoloration of vital teeth		
Tissue aging/maturation	Enamel/dentin	Vital bleaching
Pulpal calcification/obliteration	Dentin	Vital bleaching
Organic pigment deposition:		
– In fissures	Enamel/dentin	Vital bleaching
– Dentinal exposure	Dentin	
Inorganic pigment deposition:		
– Metal corrosion	Enamel/dentin	Restoration
Acquired discoloration of nonvital teeth		
Pulpal hemorrhage	Dentin	Internal bleaching
Pulpal necrosis	Dentin	Internal bleaching
Endodontic treatment	Dentin	Internal bleaching
Organic pigmentation:		
– Fissures	Enamel/dentin	External bleaching
– Dentinal exposure		

*Severity degree according to Black and McKay, 1916; McKay, 1936; and Fejerskov et al, 1977.[1,13,22]
**Severity degree according to Boksman and Jordan, 1983 and Feinman et al, 1987.[2,12]

Figs 13-2a and 13-2b Treatment of fluorosis.

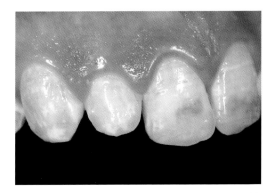

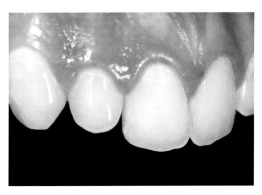

Fig 13-2a The dentition of a young patient with mild to severe fluorosis. The discoloration significantly compromises the appearance of the teeth.

Fig 13-2b The problem was addressed by conservative procedures, including microabrasion and vital (home) bleaching.

Figs 13-3a to 13-3c Vital bleaching.

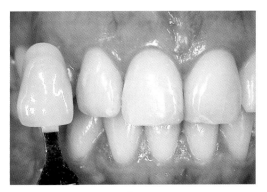

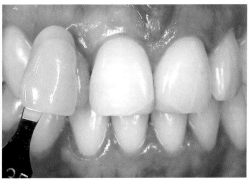

Fig 13-3a This young woman was dissatisfied with the color of her teeth. Some minor irregularities are present.

Fig 13-3b Home bleaching resulted in a significant improvement in the color of the teeth, without any loss of hard tissue.

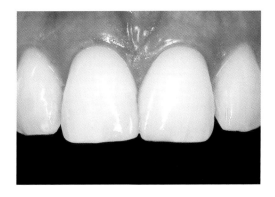

Fig 13-3c The small Class IV restorations in the central incisors were replaced 8 weeks after completion of the bleaching. The translucency of the teeth was restored.

Nonvital Bleaching

This technique has established effectiveness and safety, based on several decades of clinical use.[12,14] The traditional technique for the bleaching of a nonvital tooth (the so-called "walking bleach technique") consists of placing a mixture of 30% hydrogen peroxide solution and sodium perborate in a clean pulp chamber. Bleaching occurs through the slow release of perhydroxyl and oxygen free radicals. The bleaching agents are retained under a provisional restoration for 7 to 14 days and are replaced repeatedly, possibly up to six times, until a satisfactory shade is achieved (Figs 13-4a to 13-4d).

The intracoronal use of carbamide peroxide as part of patient-applied bleaching, employing a soft plastic guard, has recently been proposed as an alternative technique.[19] The potential of this method remains to be established in terms of limiting root resorption and bacterial contamination within the root canal.

Freehand Composite Restorations

Direct composites are indicated for any type of Class III, IV, and V restoration and for esthetic corrections of tooth form, size, and color.[5] The "cosmetic" use of composites is growing rapidly with improvements in the physical and optical properties of resin-based materials. Although ceramics still have distinct advantages, their use relative to modern composite materials continues to diminish (Figs 13-5a to 13-5c).[6]

The popular use of composites involves the so-called "natural" (anatomic) layering concept,[9] in which dentin and enamel are replaced using different materials. Such techniques require comprehensive knowledge and understanding of the spatial arrangement and optical properties of the natural tissues to be replaced using a two- or three-layer technique. The simplest and most effective approach is to apply different materials to mimic dentin and enamel. Although some manufacturers lend some support to this concept, very few composite systems to date provide suitable enamel shades. The surface materials often have inadequate translucency, opalescence, and range of shades. The composite systems based on a "single shade/single material" concept may only provide acceptable results in small Class III and Class V restorations.

The sophistication of the "multishading" method depends on the cavity configuration. The simplest configuration occurs in Class V situations and the most challenging in Class IV restorations. In Class IV restorations a full range of dentin and enamel-incisal shades is required. In addition, some opaque and intensive hue tints may be useful in replicating anatomic peculiarities, such as dysplastic discolorations, cracks, and microfractures.

Surface qualities play a significant role in the long-term behavior of restorations. Esthetic appearance is directly influenced by the composition of the composite.[27] To maintain an acceptable surface smoothness clinically, the mean filler particle size should not exceed 1 µm, with the maximum particle size being limited to 5 µm. Other important filler characteristics include composition and hardness, which influences surface qualities and wear resistance. Microfilled composites still surpass most fine-particle hybrid composites in

Figs 13-4a to 13-4d Nonvital bleaching.

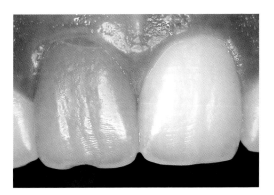

Fig 13-4a Preoperative view of the discoloration of a right maxillary central incisor devitalized by trauma. Such discoloration is the most frequent indication for internal bleaching.

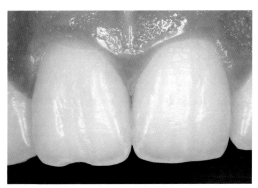

Fig 13-4b Appearance of the tooth following completion of nonvital bleaching.

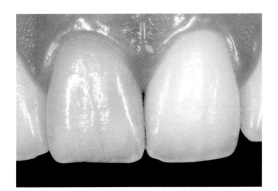

Fig 13-4c The discoloration recurred after 4 years. Such recurrence is common with nonvital bleaching, but varies greatly between patients.

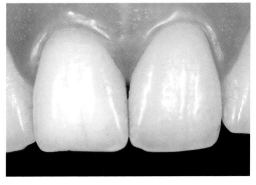

Fig 13-4d The tooth following repeat (two-visit) bleaching.

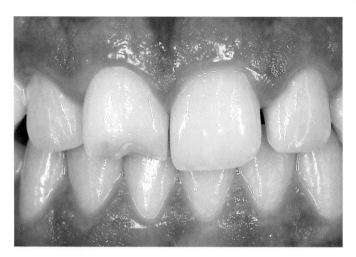

Figs 13-5a to 13-5c Freehand anterior composite restoration.

Fig 13-5a The right maxillary central incisor was fractured but had remained vital.

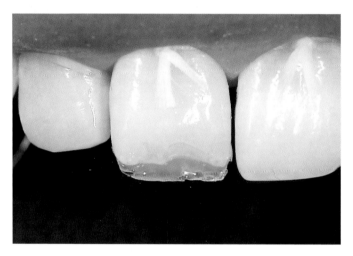

Fig 13-5b Given the young age of the patient, the tooth was restored using a direct composite technique.

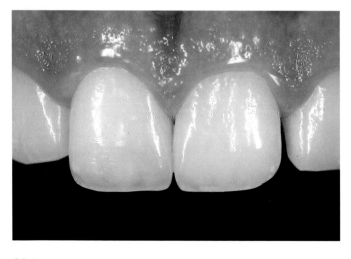

Fig 13-5c View of the completed esthetically pleasing restoration placed using an anatomic composite buildup technique.

terms of surface qualities, but at the expense of wear resistance. Microfilled composites are also relatively brittle and frequently suffer chipping or fractures in areas of functional loading. The present trend remains toward reduced particle size in fine particle hybrids to match the surface qualities of microfilled composites, but without loss of physical properties.

Combined Use of Chemical Treatments and Composite Restorations

Distressing sequelae of dental trauma are often encountered in young patients, notably the discoloration of nonvital fractured incisors. This problem should no longer be managed using traditional techniques. In contrast, conservative management consisting of bleaching and the replacement of missing tissues using a layered composite technique should be favored (Figs 13-6a to 13-6c).[9] The critical advantage of this approach is opportunity for the completion of tooth development and eruption with minimal, if any, biologic disturbance and no esthetic complications.

Advanced Adhesive Restorations

Ceramic veneers and bonded fixed partial dentures are available for the management of unsightly teeth and partial edentulism (Figs 13-7a to 13-7c and 13-8a to 13-8c).[8,20,21] Such restorations are conservative options to full crowns and traditional fixed partial dentures, involving extensive tooth preparation. Notwithstanding implant therapy, which offers advantages over conventional techniques for the replacement of missing teeth, modern adhesive techniques undoubtedly solve many problems.[23,24,28] Promising results may be obtained with metal-free ceramic and new fiber-reinforced composite materials.[10,11,16,17]

Conclusion

There is a learning curve with every new product and material. Composites and ceramics are superior to traditional restorative materials but are less user friendly. In the new millennium, biologic and adhesion-driven treatments have replaced mechanistic dentistry. It is hoped that preservative treatment modalities will be increasingly used by general practitioners for the benefit of, in particular, younger patients.

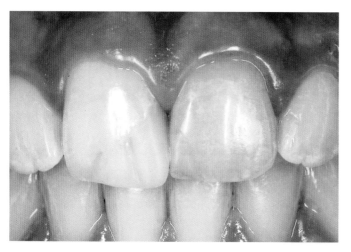

Figs 13-6a to 13-6c Combined treatment using bleaching and the placement of a composite restoration.

Fig 13-6a Clinical situation following trauma that resulted in the fracture of both central incisors. The right tooth is nonvital; the left tooth has darkened as a result of dentinal deposition. The teeth are to be treated for esthetic reasons.

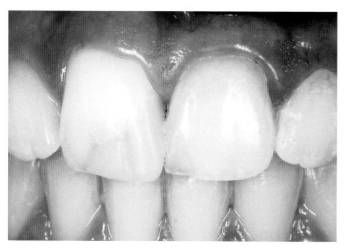

Fig 13-6b Both teeth were first bleached (right internally, left externally) using modified home bleaching.

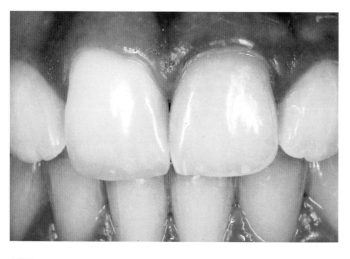

Fig 13-6c The teeth were restored with direct composite restorations placed using a multilayer technique to optimize form and esthetics.

Figs 13-7a to 13-7c
Ceramic veneers.

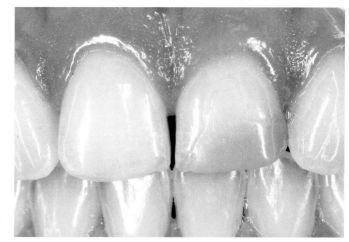

Fig 13-7a The wear of the right maxillary central incisor and the discoloration and fractured incisal angle of the adjacent central incisor were unacceptable to the patient.

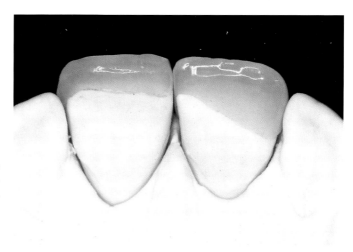

Fig 13-7b In adult patients requesting long-term restorations, ceramic veneers provide a very esthetic but still conservative option, even when major changes are to be made to tooth form (palatal view.

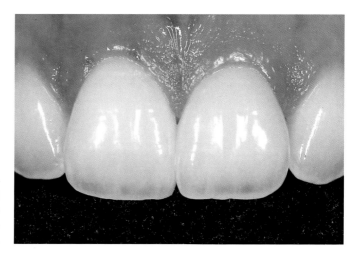

Fig 13-7c Postoperative view illustrating the successful management of the central incisors by the provision of ceramic veneers (prosthetics courtesy of Michel Magne, CDT).

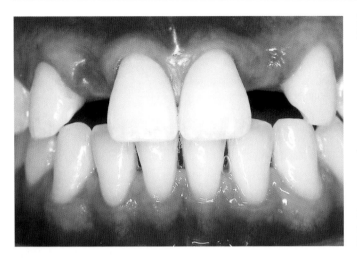

Figs 13-8a to 13-8c Adhesive fixed partial denture.

Fig 13-8a Young adult with bilateral absence of the maxillary lateral incisors.

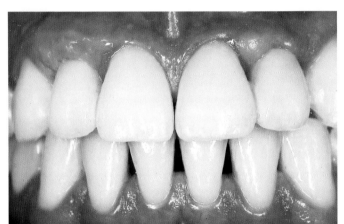

Fig 13-8b The missing teeth were replaced with bonded fixed partial dentures subsequent to connective tissue grafts to prepare the pontic sites (prosthetics courtesy of Michel Magne, CDT).

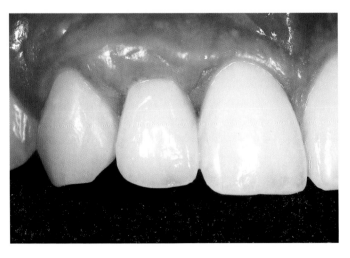

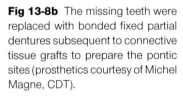

Fig 13-8c Lateral view. Such restorations do not interfere with the normal maturation of abutment teeth and, as a consequence, are a valuable alternative to conventional fixed partial dentures and implants (prosthetics courtesy of Michel Magne, CDT).

References

1. Black GV, McKay FS. Mottled enamel: An endemic developmental imperfection of the enamal of the teeth heretofore unknown in the literature of dentistry. Dent Cosmos 1916;58: 129–156.

2. Boksman L, Jordan RE. Conservative treatment of the stained dentition: Vital bleaching. Aust Dent J 1983;28:67–72.

3. Croll TP. Enamel Microabrasion. Chicago: Quintessence, 1991.

4. Croll TP, Cavanaugh RR. Enamel color modification by controlled hydrochloric acid-pumice abrasion: (I) Technique and examples. Quintessence Int 1986;17:81–87.

5. Dietschi D. Free-hand bonding in the esthetic treatment of anterior teeth: Creating the illusion. J Esthet Dent 1997;9:156–164.

6. Dietschi D. Free-hand composite resin restorations: A key to anterior esthetics. Pract Periodontics Aesthet Dent 1995;7:15–25.

7. Dietschi D, Dietschi JM. Current Developments in composite materials and techniques. Pract Periodontics Aesthet Dent 1996;8:603–613.

8. Dietschi D, Krejci I. Traitements chimiques des dyschromies dentaires. Real Clin 1999;10:7–24.

9. Dietschi D, Schatz JP. Current restorative modalities for young patients with missing anterior teeth. Quintessence Int 1997;28: 231–240.

10. Edelhoff D, Spiekermann H, Rübben A, Yildirim M. Kronen-und Brückengerüste aus hochfester Presskeramik. Quintessenz 1999;50:177–189.

11. Feinman RA. The aesthetic composite bridge. Pract Periodontics Aesthet Dent 1997;9:85–89.

12. Feinman RA, Goldstein RE, Garber DA. Bleaching Teeth. Chicago: Quintessence, 1987: 9–32.

13. Fejerskov O, Thylstrup A, Larsen M. Clinical and structural features and possible pathogenic mechanisms of dental fluorosis. Scand J Dent Res 1977;85: 510–537.

14. Goldtsein RE, Garber DA. Complete Dental Bleaching. Chicago: Quintessence, 1995.

15. Haywood VB, Heymann HO. Night guard vital bleaching. Quintessence Int 1989;20:173–176.

16. Kern M, Strub JR. Klinische Anwendung und Bewährung von Adhäsivbrücken aus der Aluminiumoxidkeramik In-Ceram. Dtsch Zahnärtzl Z 1992;47:532–539.

17. Krejci I, Boretti R, Giezendanner P, Lutz F. Adhesive crowns and fixed partial dentures fabricated of ceromer-FRC: Clinical and laboratory procedures. Pract Periodontics Aesthet Dent 1998;10:487–498.

18. Krejci I, Lutz F. Zahnfarbene Adhäsive Restaurationen in Seitenzahnbereich. Zürich: Verlag PPK, 1998:1–10.

19. Liebenberg WH. Intracoronal lightening of discolored pulpless teeth: A modified walking bleach technique. Quintessence Int 1997;28: 771–777.

20. Magne P, Magne M, Belser U. Natural and restorative oral esthetics. Part III: Fixed partial dentures. J Esthet Dent 1994;6:15–22.

21. Magne P, Magne M. Facettes en céramique à l'aube de l'an 2'000: Une fenêtre ouverte sur la bio-mimétique. Real Clin1998;9:329–343.

22. McKay FS. Mottled enamel. In: Black GV (ed). Pathology of the Hard Tissues of the Teeth—Oral Diagnosis (revision by AD Black). Chicago: Medico-Dental, 1936:255.

23. Samama Y. Fixed bonded prosthodontics: A 10-year follow-up report. Part II: Clinical assessments. Int J Periodontics Restorative Dent 1996;16:53–59.

24. Thompson VP, Wood M, De Rijk WG. Longevity of resin-bonded fixed partial dentures. In: Degrange M, Roulet JF (eds). Minimally Invasive Restorations with Bonding. Chicago: Quintessence, 1995:185–199.

25. Touati B, Miara P, Nathanson D. Esthetic dentistry and ceramic restorations. London: Dunitz, 1999:81–100.

26. Valderhaug J. A 15 years clinical evaluation of fixed prosthodontics. Acta Odontol Scand 1991;49:35–40.

27. van Noort R, Davis LG. The surface finish of composite resin restorative materials. Br Dent J 1984;157:360–364.

28. Zitzman N, Marinello C. Anterior single-tooth replacement: Clinical examination and treatment planning. Pract Periodontics Aesthet Dent 1999;11:847–858.

Chapter 14

Improving Outcome: Posterior Restorations

Javier García Barbero

Introduction

Improvements in the performance of posterior restorations, notably esthetic restorations, have occurred very rapidly in recent times. Problems, including effective bonding to enamel and the wear resistance of composite restoratives, essentially have been solved. Nevertheless, there are many aspects of esthetic posterior restorations that remain less than ideal. Some of these limiting features, such as polymerization shrinkage, have to be addressed by the manufacturers of materials. Other problems, although related to inherent limitations of materials, can be compensated for by good clinical technique, for example, the formation of proximal contact points. Certain problems related to material properties may be overcome by indirect techniques, but given the high cost and clinical complications of indirect restorations, direct restorations are most commonly used.

This chapter outlines aspects of the use of composite resins for posterior restorations that may be improved, given existing knowledge and understanding. An attempt has been made to differentiate the challenges that face manufacturers from those to be addressed by clinicians.

Adhesion

The adhesion of materials to dentin is irregular, very technique sensitive, and, in certain respects, unreliable. Frequently, within one restoration there may be areas where effective adhesion has been achieved with the formation of a reliable hybrid layer, and adjacent areas where the adhesive procedure has failed and a gap has formed (Fig 14-1). Limitations in adhesive techniques and variations in substrates probably account for most failures, with minor defects leading to clinically significant effects.

Remedies

Manufacturers should be encouraged to develop filled adhesives with a degree of elasticity, increasing adhesion capability and limiting technique sensitivity. The elasticity of adhesives is an important property in cushioning volume changes in filling materials. Filler in an adhesive acts as a thickening agent, resulting in thicker layers of adhesives between tooth and restoration.[1] Some studies show that thicker layers of adhesive are associated with lower

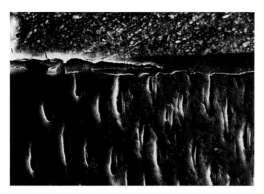

Fig 14-1 SEM image showing an area where adhesion has failed (middle left), beside another area where the adhesion is correct (middle right). In the area where the adhesion has failed, there are no resin tags in the dentinal tubules.

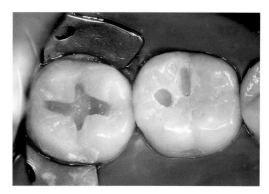

Fig 14-2 At present, leaving dentin slightly moist is considered important. It is difficult clinically to control surface moisture on prepared dentin. The surface should be glistening but not awash with fluid.

interfacial stresses.[17] The effect of filler loading on the rigidity of adhesives is not yet known nor is the capacity of filled adhesives to behave as elastic buffers.[28]

A strategy to reduce technique sensitivity is to minimize the number of clinical steps, and thereby limit the possibility of errors. Therefore the use of self-etching adhesives that do not involve the use of orthophosphoric acid to etch dentin is gaining favor. Research indicates that such adhesives behave in a similar manner to conventional adhesives, have similar bond strengths, and suffer limited technique sensitivity. However, self-etching adhesives do not remove the smear layer and as a consequence tend to leave the prepared surfaces of the preparation contaminated with bacteria.

A major turning point will be the availability of adhesives capable of forming bonds able to withstand the stresses generated by the polymerization shrink-

age of composites. In the meantime, the practitioner must use adhesives carefully while controlling the moisture content of the limiting surface of the dentinal substrate (Fig 14-2). Excess moisture prevents effective adhesion and excessive drying of dentin results in the collapse of the collagen network, precluding the formation of a properly formed hybrid layer. In addition, solvents must be removed with the utmost care (Fig 14-3).

A common mistake is not to allow sufficient time for evaporation of solvents. If all the solvent has not been evaporated prior to bonding, it is highly likely that the adhesive interface will fail. In addition, if there is excessive use of compressed air, the adhesive may be blown into excessively thick layers, mainly in cavity angles, with other parts of the cavity being left devoid of adhesive. The best approach to achieve solvent removal is to gently blow the adhesive film on a preparation from a dis-

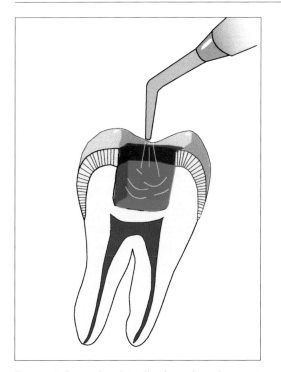

Fig 14-3 Removing the adhesive solvent is essential for adhesion. A soft but continuous blow with the air syringe is the best way to evaporate solvents.

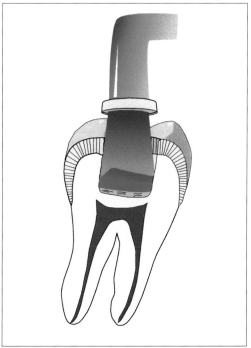

Fig 14-4 Polymerization shrinkage can be compensated for by the softening effect of a flowable composite resin layer placed on the cavity floor.

tance of several centimeters over a period of 10 to 15 seconds. Whatever the technique employed, adhesion and marginal seal will be greatly enhanced if all the margins of the preparation are in enamel.

An initial layer of flowable composite can be placed as a base to diminish the effects of polymerization shrinkage. The elastic modulus of flowable composites is such that a thin layer of material will provide a cushion for polymerization stresses. However, the polymerization shrinkage of flowable composites is higher than that of hybrids. It could therefore be deduced that the interfacial stress would be high. However, this would not appear to be the case, albeit that the stress-limiting effect remains unpredictable (Fig 14-4).[18]

Incremental placement and polymerization lessens the effects of the shrinkage of composites. Indirect composite restorations and ceramic inlays should be used as necessary in larger cavities.

Figs 14-5a and 14-5b The use of metallic precontoured matrices helps to create contact points. However, such matrices can be difficult to place.

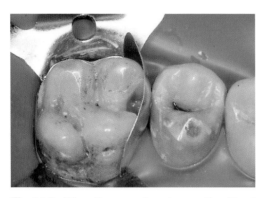

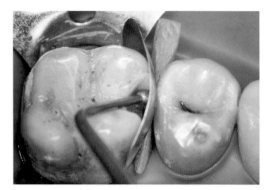

Fig 14-5a When they are placed correctly without having been distorted, the anatomic form will be restored.

Fig 14-5b After placing the matrix, a round-ended instrument is used to refine the contour of the matrix.

Contact Points

The challenge of achieving appropriate contact points—still one of the greatest difficulties in the handling of composite resins belongs mainly to the practitioner. Unlike many defects in restorations in posterior teeth, an open contact gives patients cause to complain, compounded by symptoms associated with food packing.

Remedy

Although some schools of thought believe that manufacturers should strive to produce truly condensable composite resins, the practitioner can minimize contact point problems by using contoured matrices (Figs 14-5a and 14-5b).

Conventional matrix systems (Tofflemire, Automatrix, etc) tend to leave restorations with flat approximal surfaces and coronally located contact areas that suffer certain limitations. Precontoured matrices (Palodent, 3M, St. Paul, MN) allow good approximal anatomy and the correct positioning of the contact point. However, a significant problem with precontoured matrices is the difficulty in placing them correctly without causing distortions in their form. Once placed, a precontoured matrix must be carefully assessed as to the adequacy of the contour that the restoration will assume.

A condensable composite and a range of procedures, such as force forming the contact with a suitably shaped light-guide tip pressed against the matrix, can be used to help form contacts (Fig 14-6). Alternatively, a small porcelain insert may be used as illustrated in Fig 14-7. Difficult cases may be best managed with indirect restorations in which the contact point is formed in the laboratory, precluding the need to form the restoration against a matrix.

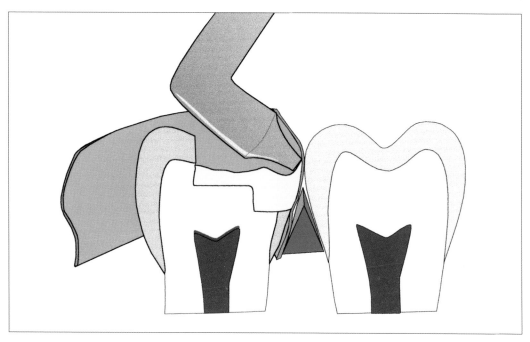

Fig 14-6 During polymerization, the matrix can be pushed against the adjacent tooth using a specially shaped curing light tip, thus ensuring a good contact.

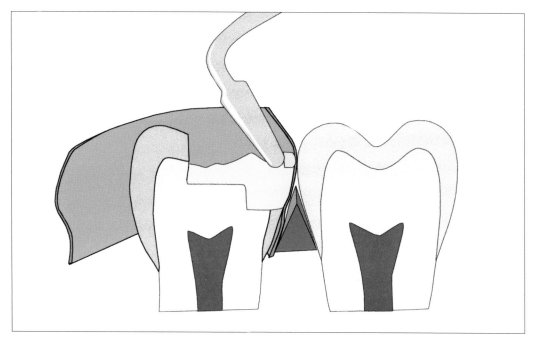

Fig 14-7 A small porcelain insert can be used to force the matrix against the adjacent tooth. If the porcelain is etched with hydrofluoric acid, it will bond to the composite resin.

215

Polymerization Shrinkage

The unsolved problem of polymerization shrinkage has led to uncertainties as to the most favorable method of light curing and continues to place certain limitations on the use of composites in restoring posterior teeth.[7] When composite resins are polymerized clinically, the degree of conversion of monomers to polymers may be a fraction of that which may be achieved under pressure and at elevated temperatures in vitro.

Remedy

Further improvements in the reliability and efficiency of light-activating units, as well as changes to the composition and construction of composite resins to enhance conversion on polymerization, would be invaluable. At present there are developments on two fronts in relation to curing units. One approach is the use of argon-xenon plasma lamps with the capacity to cure an increment of material in 2 seconds. While speed of cure is an advantage, high-speed curing can result in limited conversion rates and high residual stresses. The other principal development relates to lamps of variable intensity. Such lamps initiate polymerization with low-intensity light that increases gradually with the curing time. Although the use of variable intensity units is slower than plasma units, they result in more favorable polymerization. Slow rates of polymerization have been shown to generate relatively little stress and acceptable interfacial integrity.[8] Further research is necessary to determine the most beneficial form of light curing capable of achieving high rates of conversion yet minimal residual stress.[9]

In the meantime, the practitioner must:

1. Not exceed recommended layer thicknesses for different materials and shades (Fig 14-8). Exceeding recommended thicknesses for curing results in the deepest layers of restorations being incompletely polymerized as a consequence of reduced intensity with light scattering. Unfortunately, incomplete polymerization tends to pass unnoticed beneath the hard polymerized surface of a restoration.[22] Correct polymerization of deep layers is a must, not only to ensure the optimun properties of the composite,[2] but also to avoid adverse pulpal effects.[6] Some studies indicate that increments should not be thicker than 2 mm to ensure appropriate uniform polymerization,[30] even if the manufacturer's directions for use specify 4 to 5 mm (bulk placement composites). Furthermore, thick layers of composite result in high internal stresses and poor marginal integrity, given that the greater the volume of the composite to be polymerized, the greater the polymerization shrinkage.[25]

2. Ensure that the distal end of the tip of the light-activating unit is placed as close as possible to the composite (Figs 14-9 and 14-10), avoiding shadowing (Fig 14-11). The distance between the distal end of the light guide and the composite surface is an important factor.[3,26] Because light travels in straight lines, it is very easy for a matrix or undercut sections of the preparation to cause shadowing. Material in shadow will, at best, be poorly polymerized by reflected light. The conversion rate in these areas will be low and will be undetected clinically. Good practice includes supplemental

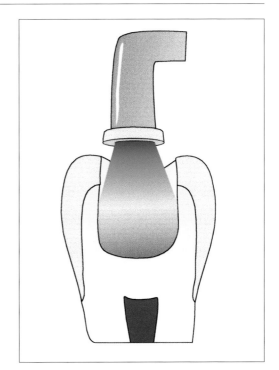

Fig 14-8 If a thick layer (> 2 mm) of composite is placed, light will not pass through and the deepest part of the restoration will remain unpolymerized. This gives rise to the so-called "soggy bottom," which may be a reason for early failure of the restoration.

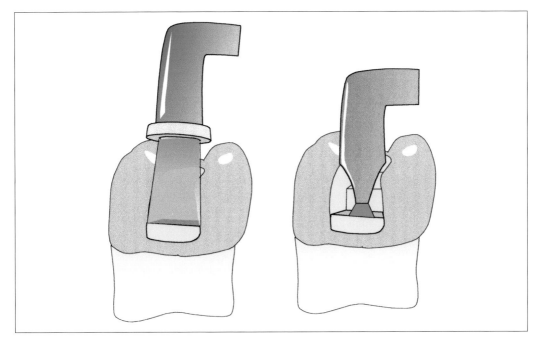

Fig 14-9 The distance between lamp and composite is an important factor. If the distance increases, the degree of conversion is reduced. It is advisable to use light guides with narrow tips that may be positioned close to the deepest layer of composite in a preparation.

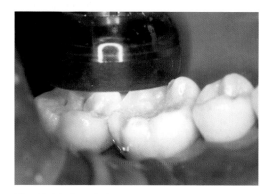

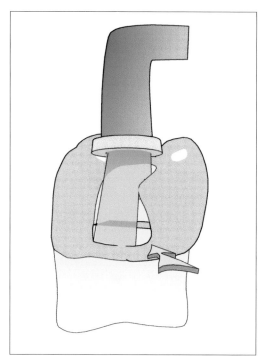

Fig 14-10 Certain items such as clamps for rubber dam, matrix retainers, and light-guide protectors may prevent placing the light close to the restoration. This illustration gives an indication of the separation between tooth and light caused by a light-guide protector.

Fig 14-11 It is not uncommon for part of the remaining tooth to cause shadowing on the composite during curing, limiting polymerization. To cure the section of composite indicated by the arrow in the illustration, it would be necessary to repeat the curing from a different angle.

Figs 14-12a and 14-12b If the tip of the light guide touches uncured composite in a cavity, some composite will stick to the light-emitting surface. This adherent material will subsequently limit the passage of light and thereby reduce the efficiency of the lamp. Composite debris on the tip of a light guide must be removed with acetone without scratching the surface, which, if damaged, will become increasingly difficult to clean.

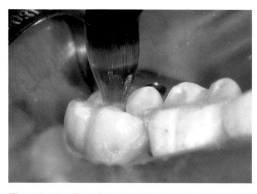

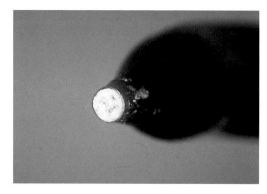

Fig 14-12a Tip of light guide touching uncured composite in a cavity.

Fig 14-12b Uncured composite has adhered to the surface of the light guide.

light curing from both buccal and lingual directions following the removal of the wedge and matrix.

3. Resist the temptation to scan the composite with the curing light during polymerization.

4. Ensure that the distal end of light guides is kept free of adhesive and composite debris. Light activating units with small-diameter tipped light guides afford the clinician the opportunity to minimize the distance between the light and the surface of the composite resin. However, if the light guide touches uncured composite, the tip becomes at least partially covered with material, which hinders full-light exposure (Fig 14-12).

Antibacterial Properties

The elimination of microorganisms in the tooth-restoration interface is of great importance. Bacteria and their toxins present in the tooth-restoration interface are responsible for the pulpal irritation and death frequently associated with composite resins. Knowledge of such effects stems from the work of Qvist, Brännström, and others.[5,24] Bacteria are commonly found beneath composite restorations[4,16] and to date there are no restorative materials with potent antibacterial properties. Attempts to develop such properties by including fluoride or chlorhexidine in a composite have been reported.[15,31] However, fluoride release from composites is limited and chlorhexidine is not well tolerated by the pulp. It has been demonstrated that some primers and bonding agents have certain antibacterial properties[21,23] and the etching of dentin to remove the smear layer also eliminates bacterial contamination.[27]

With modern self-etching adhesives, the cavity is not rinsed with water and, as a consequence, the smear layer remains and sustains live bacteria. However, some self-etching adhesives have certain antibacterial properties.[19,20] Also, some trials of adding bactericidal monomers to resins such as MDBP (methacryloyloxydodecyl-pyridinium bromide) are taking place.[12,14] An experimental primer with MDBP has been shown to be active against oral bacteria without a reduction in bond strength.[11] Studies on the cytotoxicity of such a new monomer as a component of self-etching adhesives have been encouraging.[13] In the meantime, it must be assumed that the antibacterial properties of existing adhesive systems are limited.

Remedy

Manufacturers should further explore possible means to add antibacterial substances to adhesives to be applied to dentin. The practitioner can, however, accomplish good bacterial control of dentin prior to placing a restoration. Bacterial control may be achieved with cavity cleansers containing chlorhexidine or sodium hypochlorite. However, the application of such cleansers after the etching of dentin significantly reduces bond strengths.[10,29]

An interesting option is to treat cavity preparations with caries solvents with a base of sodium hypochlorite. Such solvents are able to selectively remove carious dentin without harming intact healthy dentin and, if applied following the completion of cavity preparation, ensure the removal of bacteria from the walls of the cavity (Fig 14-13). Because such solvents

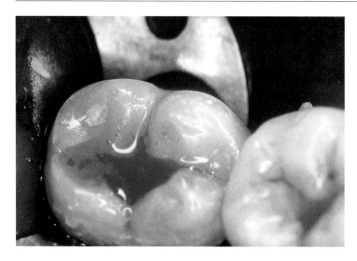

Fig 14-13 Caries may be elimiated by filling the cavity with an appropriate caries-dissolving gel and gently rubbing the carious surfaces with specially designed instruments. Besides removing denatured dentin, hypochlorite in the gel may have an antibacterial effect.

are relatively now, the evidence supporting their use is limited. Notwithstanding difficulties in using such solvents in the management of large lesions, they may be found to have advantages in certain situations, notably given that they contain hypochlorite and do not appear to cause pulpal damage.

Defects in Restorations

Defects are frequently formed in restorations placed clinically and may go unnoticed by the clinician (Fig 14-14). Such defects are generally related to difficulties encountered during restoration placement. Voids are formed in a restoration when there is air entrapment between increments. This happens when using composites that adhere to instruments and are difficult to place in small preparations. If air is trapped between two layers of composite, the effect may be limited to weakening of the restoration. In contrast, if air is trapped between composite and dentin, there is a strong possibility of bacterial growth and subsequent pulpal damage.

Remedy

Manufacturers should be encouraged to produce composite resins of appropriate viscosity that do not adhere to instruments. Even with such materials, the practitioner must ensure that air is not trapped between and within increments of material when placing restorations (Fig 14-15). If a plastic instrument is used to insert the material, care is required to ensure appropriate adaptation along one wall or surface at a time. If a syringe is used, the tip should be positioned close to the floor of the preparation and withdrawn slowly as material is injected and adapted.

Irregularities in floors of cavity preparations may be managed by placing an initial layer of a flowable composite, which minimizes the risk of air entrapment below the restoration (Fig 14-16).

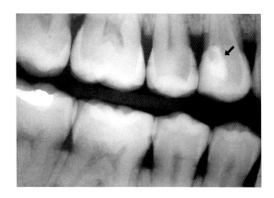

Fig 14-14 Important defects in restorations can go unnoticed. In this radiograph the arrow points to a large, previously unnoticed defect in a composite restoration.

Figs 14-15a and 14-15b Air may be readily trapped when placing composite in a cavity.

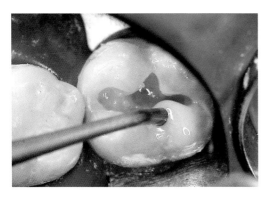

Fig 14-15a Photograph of a cavity illustrating how air may be trapped by composite sticking to the margins of the preparation.

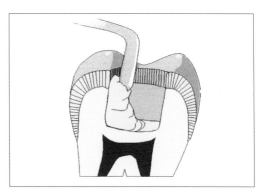

Fig 14-15b Illustration showing how composite should be built up along one wall at a time to avoid the trapping of air.

Figs 14-16a and 14-16b If a thin layer of a flowable composite is placed to eliminate irregularities in the floor of the cavity, the risk of trapping air in the subsequent placement of the restoration is greatly reduced.

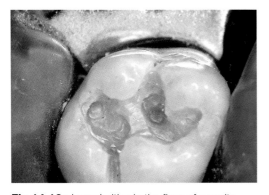

Fig 14-16a Irregularities in the floor of a cavity.

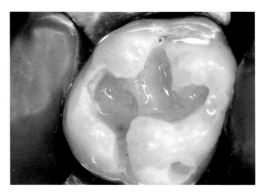

Fig 14-16b After placement of a restoration.

Conclusion

Despite many recent developments in materials and techniques for the use of composites in the restoration of posterior teeth, there remain many aspects of this important and growing part of present-day operative dentistry that require further investigation and refinement.

References

1. Alster D, Feilzer AJ, de Gee AJ, Davidson CL. Polymerization contraction stress in thin resin-composite layers as a function of layer thickness. Dent Mater 1998;13:146–150.

2. Asmussen E. Restorative resins: Hardness and strength vs quantity of remaining double bonds. Scand J Dent Res 1982;90:484–489.

3. Bayne SC, Heyman, Swift EJ. Update on dental composite restorations. J Am Dent Assoc 1994;125:687–701.

4. Bergenholz G, Cox CF, Loesche WJ, Syed SA. Bacterial leakage around dental restorations: Its effect on the dental pulp. J Oral Pathol 1982; 11:439–450.

5. Brännstrom M, Nordenval KJ. Bacterial penetration, pulpal reaction and the inner surface of Concise enamel bond. Composite fillings in etched and unetched cavities. J Dent Res 1978;57:3–10.

6. Caughman WF, Caughman GB, Shiflett Ra, Rueggeberg F, Schuster GS. Correlation of cytotoxicity, filler loading and curing time of dental composites. Biomaterials 1991;12:737–740.

7. Dietschi D, Dietschi JM. Current development in composite materials and techniques. Pract Periodontics Aesthet Dent 1996;8:603–613.

8. Feilzer AJ, De Gee AJ, Davidson CL. Quantitative determination of stress reduction by flow in composite restorations. Dent Mater 1990;6:167–171.

9. Feilzer AJ, De Gee AJ, Davidson CL. Setting stresses in composites for two different curing modes. Dent Mater 1993;9:2–5.

10. Frankenberger R, Krämer N, Oberschachtsiek H, Petschelt A. Dentin bond strength and marginal adaptation after NaOCl pretreatment. Oper Dent 2000;25:40–45.

11. Imazato S, Ehara A, Torii M. Antibacterial activity of dentin primer containing MDBP after curing. J Dent1998;26:267–271.

12. Imazato S, Russel RRB, McCabe JF. Antibacterial activity of MDPB polymer incorporated in dental resin. J Dent 1995;23:177–181.

13. Imazato S, Tarumi H, Ebi N, Ebisu S. Cytotoxic effects of composite restoratios emplying self-etching primers or experimental antibacterial primers. J Dent 2000;28:61–67.

14. Imazato S,Torii M,Tsuchltani Y, McCabe JF, Russel RRB. Incorporation of bacterial inhibitor into resin composite. J Dent Res 1994;73: 1437–1443.

15. Jedrichowski JR, Caputo AA, Kerper S. Antibacterial and mechanical properties of restorative materials combined with clorhexidines. J Oral Rehabil 1983;10:373–381.

16. Kaketa A. Anaerobic bacteria isolated under composite resin fillings. Jpn J Conservative Dent 1984;27:534–548.

17. Kemp-Scholte CM, Davidson CL. Complete marginal seal of Class V resin composite restoration effected by increased flexibility. J Dent Res 1990; 69:1240–1243.

18. Labella R, Lambrechts P, Van Meerbeck B, Vanherle G. Polymerization shrinkage and elasticity of flowable composites and filled adhesives. Dent Mater 1999;15:128–137.

19. Ohmori K, Maeda N, Kohono A. Evaluation of antibacterial activity of three dentin primers using an in vitro tooth model. Oper Dent 1999; 24:279–285.

20. Onoe N, Nakajima M, Fujitani M, Kaketa A, Inoue M, Hosoda H. Antibacterial activity of newly designed adhesive primers containing salicylic acid derivative. Jpn J Conservative Dent 1993;36:13–24.

21. Palenik CJ, Setcos JC. Antimicrobial abilities of various dentine bonding agents and restorative materials. J Dent 1996;24:289–295.

22. Pilo R, Cardash HS. Post-irradiation polymerization of different anterior and posterior visible light-activated resin composites. Dent Mater 1992;8:299–304.

23. Prati C, Fava F, Gioia D, Selighini M, Pashley D H. Antibacterial effectiveness of dentin bonding systems. Dent Mater 1993;9:338–343.

24. Qvist V, Qvist J. Marginal leakage along concise in relation to filling procedure. Scand J Dent Res 1977;85:305–312.

25. Roulet JF. Benefits and disadvantages of tooth-colored alternatives to amalgam. J Dent 1997; 25:459–473.

26. Rueggeberg FA, Jordan DM. Effect of light-tip distance on polymerization of resin composite. Int J Prosthodont 1993;6:364–370.

27. Settembrini L, Boylan R, Strassler H, Scherer W. A comparison of antimicrobial activity of etchants used for a total etch technique. Oper Dent 1997;22:84–88.

28. Van Meerbeek B, Willems G, Celis JP, et al. Assessment by nano-indentation of the hardness and elasticity of the resin dentin bonding area. J Dent Res 1993;72:1434–1442.

29. Vichi A, Ferrari M, Davidson CL. In vivo leakage of an adhesive system with and without NaOCl as pretreatment [abstract 3077]. J Dent Res 1997;76(special issue):398.

30. Yap AUJ. Effectiveness of polimerization in composite restoratives claming bulk placement: Impact of cavity depth and exposure time. Oper Dent 2000;25:113–120.

31. Yap AUJ, Khor E, Foo SH. Fluoride release and antibacterial properties of new-generation tooth-colored restoratives. Oper Dent 1999; 24:297–305.

223

Chapter 15

Posterior Esthetics with Composite Resins

Roberto Spreafico and Jean-François Roulet

Introduction

The philosophy of restorative dentistry has been transformed over the last two decades. Two principal factors may be considered to account for the change:

1. The dramatic decline in caries observed in industrialized countries[24]
2. The availability of reliable dental adhesives[3,27]

As a consequence of the decline in caries, clinicians are usually confronted with relatively small lesions. Furthermore, guidelines for cavity preparation are no longer dictated by the properties of the restorative material but, in contrast, by the extent of the lesion. Employing the minimally invasive approach, thereby conserving as much sound tooth substance as possible, is the key to success. Where operative intervention is indicated, the removal of sound tooth substance is limited to gaining access to the lesion to allow inspection and management of the caries.[29]

The reinforcing effects of adhesive technology enable the dentist to restore the tooth to its original strength.[11,36] For the patient, esthetics are the most obvious advantage of minimally invasive adhesive dentistry, with high levels of satisfaction being reported with tooth-colored restorations.[17,31,32] In the restoration of posterior teeth, good esthetics can be readily achieved with composite resins; there are, however, certain requirements and limitations to be respected. In this chapter, consideration is given to the keys to success with direct posterior composite restorations.

Keys to Success

Use the Most Conservative Approach

Nothing is better than natural tissue. It is, therefore, very important to conserve as much sound tooth tissue as possible. With advances in adhesive technology, it is no

---

longer necessary to configure the cavity, with the exception of the margins, according to the properties of the restorative material. Therefore, as little as possible sound enamel and dentin should be sacrificed to allow the inspection of the lesion and the removal of caries. This is the major advantage of the direct approach. Because there are no paths of insertion to be prepared, as is necessary in the provision of indirect restorations, the form of the preparation can be limited to the shape of the caries lesion. As a consequence, there is opportunity to adopt a highly conservative approach.

Routinely Employ Adhesive Procedures

Modern dental adhesives may be found to be reliable.[3] However, it is of paramount importance to precisely follow the manufacturers' directions for use. Errors during application will significantly reduce the quality of the bond.[28] To obtain an effective bond, especially to dentin, it is essential to avoid desiccation of the tooth prior to the application of the bonding system, and to completely cure the adhesive prior to the application of the composite.[18,33,35] Poorly bonded restorations not only have inferior margin quality, and are therefore prone to recurrent caries,[25] but may be highly susceptible to postoperative sensitivity. Even the most esthetically pleasing restorations are disliked by the patient if function and temperature changes elicit pain. Restoration of a tooth to its original strength requires a high-quality bond, both in the marginal area and throughout the internal interfaces.[10] This underlines the importance of meticulous adhesive techniques together with the incremental application

of the composite material as discussed below.

Bevel the Enamel Margins

Placing bevels in enamel serves two purposes. First, beveling leaves enamel prisms cut more or less perpendicularly,[4] enhancing the quality and effectiveness of the integration of the composite with the enamel, thereby improving margin quality. Second, esthetics are improved by a gradual shift from the color of the tooth to the color of the composite. Because composite materials are translucent, this effect is most pronounced with lighter shades of material. When there is little to no enamel along the cervical margin, the dentist is faced with a problem. It is known that margin quality is relatively poor cervically.[21,23] As a consequence, there is a choice of two options clinically: Option one is to select an indirect approach, which is known to give good margin quality along a cervical margin in dentin.[30] With this approach, however, more sound tooth tissue must be sacrificed to create a path of insertion for the restoration. The second option is to line the cervical step of the preparation with a resin-modified glass-ionomer cement[7,9,22,23] or with a flowable composite,[20,26,34] which may be found to provide an acceptable margin quality. To date, there is no clinical evidence based on long-term controlled studies that distinguishes the most reliable way to manage this problem.

Use a Layering Technique

Composites shrink during polymerization. Irrespective of using a minimally invasive approach, the volume of composite required to restore a posterior tooth is invariably greater than that used in the restoration of an anterior tooth. If the material is effectively bonded to all the cavity walls, its shrinkage will be restricted, thus generating stress at the interface.[6] The amount of stress generated depends on several factors: the mass of the polymerised composite, the speed of polymerisation, as determined by the output of the lamp and the time of polymerisation, the e-modulus of the composite material, and the cavity configuration.[5,12–16] To minimize the effects of polymerization contraction, it is essential to place the material incrementally using horizontal or oblique layering techniques. With the oblique (diagonal) layering technique, it is possible to produce gap-free occlusal restorations, even if the cavity is large.[1] Managing a proximal restoration is more complex. The objective of any approach should be to convert a complex Class II configuration into a simple Class I configuration.[15] This may be readily achieved.

Following cavity preparation, a sectional matrix band is inserted and a wooden wedge is placed to adapt the matrix to the cervical margin. Careful adaptation of the matrix to the cervical margin avoids overhangs and facilitates proximal finishing and polishing. A metallic matrix retainer is then placed and the teeth separated. It is important to check the adequacy of the contact between the matrix and the adjacent tooth.

The adhesive procedures are then completed and the restoration placed using a centripetal technique.[2,19] The first step in this technique is to build up the box wall, transforming the Class II configuration into a Class I configuration. A single increment of an "enamel" composite is applied against the matrix and across the cervical step. Particular care should be taken to prevent air inclusions and voids along the cervical cavosurface margin. The thickness of this shell-like wall should not exceed 0.5 mm. The "C factor" of this layer is very advantageous; in effect, there are two surfaces (one facing onto the matrix and the other onto the cervical step) free to deform and distribute the contraction stresses. Furthermore, the thin proximal wall is probably not able to deform the cusps of the tooth during setting.

Following removal of the retainer, matrix, and wooden wedge, the restoration is completed with a number of increments of dentinal and enamel composite, applied in an oblique fashion.

Obtain a Tight Proximal Contact

For a posterior restoration to function correctly, a tight contact point and harmonious proximal morphology is essential. Restorations with inadequate proximal contacts tend to suffer food impaction with associated lesions of the gingival papillae. This is both inconvenient and uncomfortable for the patient and destructive to the periodontium. For small- and moderate-sized cavities, sectional matrix bands and metallic retainers (Palodent and Compositight, 3M, St. Paul, MN) have been shown to give the best results. A tight contact point is obtained because of good separation of the teeth during placement of the composite, followed by the return of the tooth to its original position subsequent to removal of the matrix. Furthermore, as a result of their convex shape, sectional matrices facilitate the creation of correct proximal anatomy, with a rounded marginal ridge.

Restore Functional Occlusal and Proximal Anatomy

In general, function follows the form of the occlusal anatomy. Therefore, to avoid excessive occlusal corrections after the placement of a restoration, it is important to restore the occlusal anatomy as close as possible to its original form during the placement of the restoration. This is best achieved using a layering technique, with reference to the remaining cusp inclines as a guide. The best esthetic results are obtained if missing dentin is replaced with a relatively opaque ("dentin") composite and missing enamel is replaced with a more translucent ("enamel") composite. The larger the defect, the less anatomic information is present and the greater the difficulty in restoring the tooth using a direct technique. Therefore, for large restorations, or when cuspal coverage is indicated, a more favorable outcome may be achieved by providing indirect, luted restorations. In such situations one can expect to achieve good margin quality, especially in the cervical area as discussed above.

Achieve Good Internal Adaptation

For posterior composite restorations, questions remain as to whether pulp protection is necessary, including the use of glass-ionomer base to achieve selective bonding. For the protection of the pulp from invading microorganisms, reliable sealing of the dentinal tubules is best. This can be accomplished with dentin bonding agents; a cement base is no longer necessary. Furthermore, placing a cement base does not improve the margin quality.[8,9] Whether the total bonding technique is able to provide good internal adaptation to help reinforce the tooth and simultaneously provide good margin quality remains debatable.[8,34] However, it is the opinion of the authors that total bonding is reliable.

Create a Good Integration with Periodontal Tissues

Besides the occlusal surface, which is subjected to functional stresses and wear, the weak link of posterior composite restorations is the cervical area. For many reasons, including anatomy, cavity configuration, and difficulty of access, it is a challenge to obtain good marginal quality in the cervical area. To minimize plaque accumulation, it is important to obtain the best possible cervical marginal quality. Therefore, everything possible must be done to improve cervical marginal quality. To this end and, in turn, to improve the longevity of a restoration, it is important to have good access to the cervical area during restoration placement. This facilitates optimal finishing and polishing using oscillating instruments followed by finishing/polishing strips. In addition, a well-finished cervical margin provides the patient with the opportunity to practice effective self-care of the restoration. To achieve such an outcome, it is, on occasion, necessary to undertake a papillectomy or even surgical crown lengthening prior to the insertion of a composite restoration, notably when the cervical margin is located subgingivally.

Two cases demonstrating the application of the above principles are illustrated in Figs 15-1a to 15-1q and 15-2a to 15-2h.

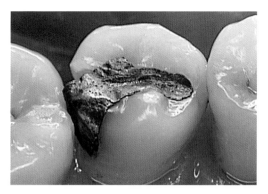

Fig 15-1a Preoperative view of a failed amalgam.

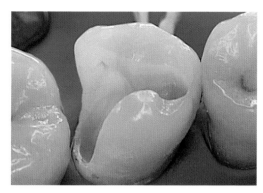

Fig 15-1b The cavity is prepared.

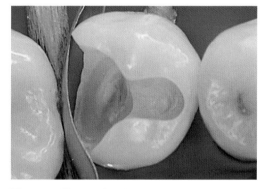

Fig 15-1c The sectional matrix and wooden wedge are applied.

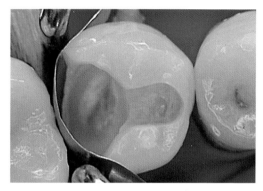

Fig 15-1d The metallic retainer facilitates both good proximal contact and harmonious anatomic form.

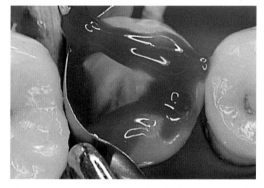

Fig 15-1e The enamel is selectively etched for 20 seconds.

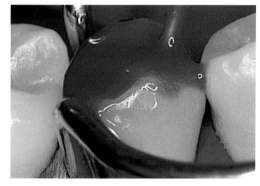

Fig 15-1f The dentin is etched for no more than 15 seconds using the same etchant.

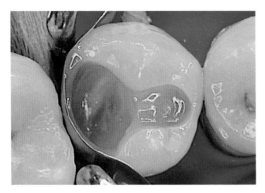

Fig 15-1g At the end of the adhesive procedures, the box wall is built up with a single, thin increment of composite.

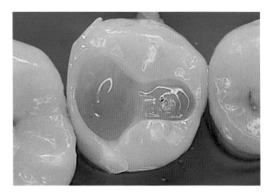

Fig 15-1h The Class II cavity is, in effect, converted into a Class I cavity. The cavity floor is lined with a small amount of flowable composite.

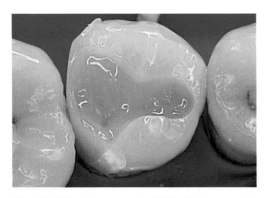

Fig 15-1i Two increments of "dentin" composite are layered obliquely.

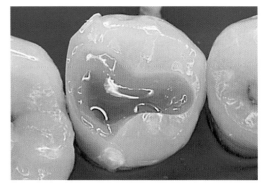

Fig 15-1j Some brown colorant is applied to the dentinal layer.

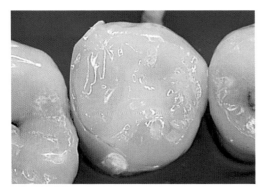

Fig 15-1k The remaining portion of the cavity is then filled with a small amount of enamel composite.

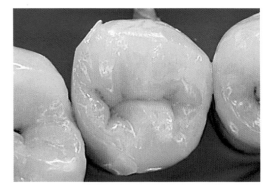

Fig 15-1l The occlusal anatomy is created prior to polymerization.

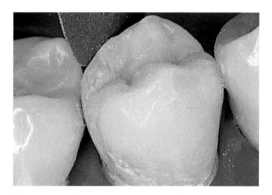

Fig 15-1m The buccal and lingual margins are refined with abrasive disks.

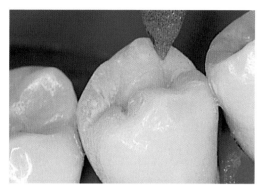

Fig 15-1n The occlusal margin is refined using a rubber point with abundant water irrigation.

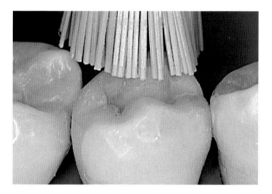

Fig 15-1o The final luster finish is obtained with a finishing brush.

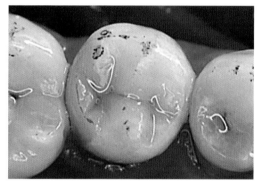

Fig 15-1p The completed restoration after rubber dam has been removed. If particular care is taken in creating natural occlusal anatomy, the need for occlusal adjustments is limited.

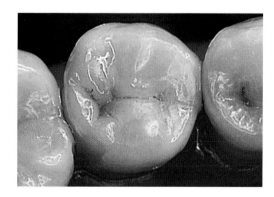

Fig 15-1q The same tooth 2 weeks later.

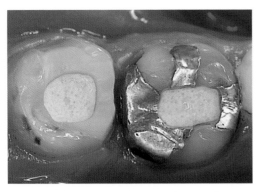

Fig 15-2a The two mandibular molars require core buildups and full crown restorations.

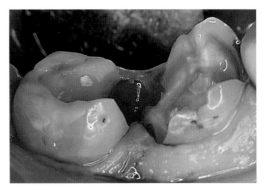

Fig 15-2b The cervical margins are subgingival, necessitating crown lengthening.

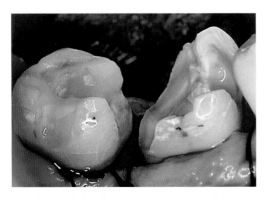

Fig 15-2c Following osseous surgery, the periodontal tissues are apically repositioned and sutured.

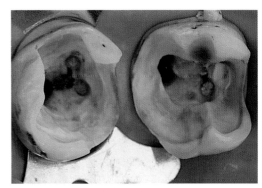

Fig 15-2d Two weeks later the teeth are prepared for the composite buildups.

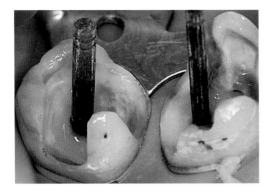

Fig 15-2e Two carbon posts are adhesively cemented.

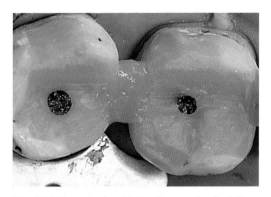

Fig 15-2f In order to stabilize the proximal relationship, two small amounts of composite are bonded to the buildups.

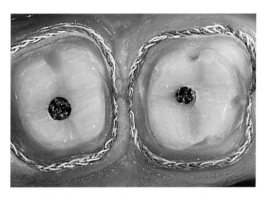

Fig 15-2g Tissue healing after 9 months, immediately prior to recording the final impression.

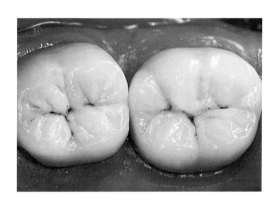

Fig 15-2h The porcelain-fused-to-metal restorations a few weeks after placement.

Conclusions

Based on data from laboratory investigations, it may be concluded that high quality posterior restorations can be placed using composite resins. However, the clinician must be precise in the use of operative techniques, meticulous in following the manufacturers' directions for use for the bonding system, and thorough in the application of the selected technique for insertion of the composite resin. Furthermore, to be successful it is essential to have an effective method of moisture control. Clinical experience supports the view that well-placed posterior composites may be found to fulfil patients' needs for esthetics and durable restorations. Long-term clinical studies have revealed excellent in-service behavior among composite restorations. With an annual failure rate of only 0.5% to 5.0%, posterior composites may be found to perform as well as alternative forms of direct restoration (see chapter 16).

References

1. Bergmann P, Noack M, Roulet J-F. Marginal adaptation with glass ceramic inlays adhesively luted with glycerine gel. Quintessence Int 1991;22:739–744.

2. Bichacho N. The centripetal build-up for composite resin posterior restorations. Pract Periodontics Aesthet Dent 1994;6:17–23.

3. Blunck U, Haller B. Klassifikation von Bondingsystemen. Quintessenz 1999;50:1021–1033.

4. Carvalho RM, Santiago SL, Fernandes CAD, Suh BI, Pashley OH. Effects of prism orientation on tensile strength on enamel. J Adhes Dent 2000;2:251–257.

5. Davidson CL, de Gee AJ. Light-curing units, polymerization, and clinical implications. J Adhes Dent 2000;2:167–173.

6. Davidson CL, de Gee AJ, Feilzer AJ. The competition between the composite-dentin bond strength and the polymerisation contraction stress. J Dent Res 1984;63:1396–1399.

7. Dietrich T, Lösche AC, Lösche GM, Roulet J-F. Marginal adaptation of Class II sandwich restorations using different light cured GICs and compomers [abstract 47]. J Dent Res 1997;76(special issue):19.

8. Dietrich T, Lösche AC, Lösche GM, Roulet J-F. Marginal adaptation of direct composite and sandwich restorations in Class II cavities with cervical margins in dentine. J Dent 1999;27:119–128.

9. Dietrich T, Lösche AC, Lösche GM, Roulet J-F. Microleakage of based, bonded and sandwich Class II restorations [abstract 2074]. J Dent Res 1998;77:891.

10. Dietschi D, Moor L. Evaluation of the marginal and internal adaptation of different ceramic and composite inlay systems after an in vitro fatigue test. J Adhes Dent 1999;1:41–56.

11. Douglas WH. Methods to improve fracture resistance of teeth. In: Vanherle G, Smith DC (eds). Posterior Composite Resin Dental Restorative Materials. St. Paul: Minnesota Mining and Mfg, 1985:433–441.

12. Feilzer AJ, de Gee AJ, Davidson CL. Increased wall-to-wall curing contraction in thin bonded resin layers. J Dent Res 1989;68:48–50.

13. Feilzer AJ, de Gee AJ, Davidson CL. Quantitative determination of stress reduction by flow in composite restorations. Dent Mater 1990;6:167–171.

14. Feilzer AJ, de Gee AJ, Davidson CL. Relaxation of polymerisation contraction shear stress by hydroscopic expansion. J Dent Res 1990;69:36–39.

15. Feilzer AJ, de Gee AJ, Davidson CL. Setting stress in composite resin in relation to configuration of the restoration. J Dent Res 1987;66:1636–1639.

16. Feilzer AJ, de Gee AJ, Davidson CL. Setting stress in composites for two different curing modes. Dent Mater 1993;9:2–5.

17. Goldstein RE. Change Your Smile. Chicago: Quintessence, 1984.

18. Hansen SE, Swift EJ. Microleakage with Gluma: Effects of unfilled resin polymerization and storage time. Am J Dent 1989;2:266–268.

19. Hassan K, Mante F, List G, Dhuru V. A modified incremental filling technique tor Class II composite restorations. J Prosthet Dent 1987;58:153–156.

20. Labella R, Lambrechts P, Van Meerbeek B, Vanherle G. Polymerization shrinkage and elasticity of flowable composites and filled adhesives. Dent Mater 1999;15:128–137.

21. Lösche GM, Hilbig WH, Roulet J-F. The margin quality of direct posterior composite restorations close to the CEJ [abstract 1889]. J Dent Res 1992;71:752.

22. Lösche GM, Lösche AC, Roulet J-F. In vitro marginal analysis in Class II (MOD) cavities. Industrial Report for the 3M Company. Berlin: Department of Operative and Preventive Dentisty and Endodontics, 1995.

23. Lösche AC, Lösche GM, Roulet J-F. The effect of prolonged water storage on marginal adaptation of Class II fillings [abstract 3013]. J Dent Res 1996;75:394.

24. Marthaler TM. The prevalence of dental caries in Europe 1990-1995. Caries Res 1996;30: 237–255.

25. Mjör IA. Amalgam and composite resin restorations: Longevity and reasons for replacement. In: Anusavice KJ. Quality evaluations of dental restorations: Criteria for placement and replacement. Chicago: Quintessence, 1989:61–72.

26. Payne JH. The marginal seal of Class II restorations: Flowable composite resin compared to injectable glass ionomer. J Clin Pediatr Dent 1999;23:123–130.

27. Perdigao J, Lopes M. Dentin bonding—Questions for the new millennium. J Adhes Dent 1999;1:191-209.

28. Peschke A, Blunck U, Roulet J-F. Influence of incorrect application of a water-based adhesive system on the marginal adaptation of Class V restorations. Am J Dent 2000;13:249–256.

29. Roulet J-F. Buonocore memorial lecture—Adhesive dentistry in the 21st century. Oper Dent 2000;25:355–366.

30. Roulet J-F, Lösche GM. Long term performance of aesthetic posterior restorations. In: Hunt FR (ed). Glass Ionomers: The Next Generation [Proceedings of the 2nd International Symposium on Glass Ionomers, 16–19 June 1994, Philadelphia]. Gulph Mills, PA: British Technology Group USA, 1994:181–192.

31. Roulet J-F, Mettler P, Friedrich U. Die Abrasion von Amalgam und Komposits im Seitenzahnbereich. Dtsch Zahnarztl Z 1978;33:206–209.

32. Roulet J-F, Mettler P, Friedrich U. Studie über die Abrasion von Komposits im Seitenzahnbereich—Resultate nach 3 Jahren. Dtsch Zahnarztl Z 1980;35: 493–497.

33. Tay FR, Gwinnett AJ, Pang KM, Wei SHY. Variability in microleakage observed in a total-etch wet-bonding technique under different handling conditions. J Dent Res 1995;74: 1168–1178.

34. Unterbrink GL, Liebenberg WH. Flowable resin composites as "filled adhesives": Literature review and clinical recommendations. Quintessence Int 1999;30:249–257.

35. Van Meerbeek B, Peuman M, Verschueren M, et al. Clinical status of ten dentin adhesive systems. J Dent Res 1994;73: 1690–1702.

36. Weiß E. Der Einfluß adhäsiv befestigter mod-Inlays auf das Bruchverhalten menschlicher Zahne [thesis]. Berlin: Freie Universität, 1993.

235

Chapter 16

Longevity of Restorations

Juergen Manhart and Reinhard Hickel

Introduction

Effective preventive programs, enhanced dental care, and growing interest in caries-free teeth have changed the prevalence and pattern of caries. Patients are living longer and retaining more of their natural teeth.[115] Changes in dental restorative treatment patterns, combined with the introduction of new and improved restorative materials and techniques, has greatly influenced the longevity of dental restorations.[180] Marked changes in the use of restorative materials have occurred during the past 10 to 20 years[82,83,156,181] and esthetic considerations are growing in importance for the restoration of posterior teeth.[23,228] Alleged adverse health effects and environmental concerns associated with the release of mercury gave rise to controversial discussions about the use of amalgam as a contemporary restorative material.[83,84,140,142,150,200,224,226,229] Moreover, there is a growing concern about the use of metallic alloys in general.[227] Besides cast gold inlays, esthetic alternatives to amalgam restorations include glass ionomers, resin-modified glass ionomers, compomers, direct composite restorations, composite inlays, and ceramic inlays.[228] Tooth-colored adhesive inlays can be made by a dental technician in the laboratory or chairside as a direct composite inlay or CAD/CAM ceramic restoration (eg, Cerec, Sirona, Bensheim, Germany).[81,151,185,186,232]

Cross-sectional clinical studies differ in many aspects from controlled prospective longitudinal clinical trials on the performance of dental restorations.[171,180] In the design of a controlled longitudinal study, a very limited number of excellent dentists, specially trained and standardized for the specific procedure, place the restorations under almost ideal conditions. The patient population is often selected from reliable, easily accessible individuals, such as dental students and dental school staff and faculty, with good compliance and highly motivated in relation to oral health and hygiene.[224] The lesions treated are usually carefully selected and limited to the indications of the materials investigated. The recall criteria are defined and, ideally, the calibrated recall assessments are performed by dentists different from those inserting the restorations.[180] Replicas and color photographs may be recorded on a regular basis to assist in the evaluation of the restorations over time.[227]

Cross-sectional clinical investigations of dental restorations are less strictly defined than longitudinal studies. Important factors such as the restorative materials used can usually only be differentiated as types of materials, while the technical procedure employed, details of the cavity preparation, and the use of a base material are unknown factors.[180] In most cases it is difficult if not impossible to determine the exact age of the restorations.[226] Cross-sectional clinical studies offer some major advantages. For example, a large number of restorations can be assessed in a relatively short time and the type of dental care the patients receive is typical rather than ideal as it is in longitudinal studies.

Failure of dental restorations is a major problem in dental practice, especially in the treatment of adults. Placement and replacement of restorations still constitutes the major workload in general dental practice, although preventive programs and an increased awareness of oral health have had positive effects on the DMFT index in many countries.[118,171,226] About 60% of all operative work done is attributed to the replacement of restorations.[170] The clinical assessment of restoration failure differs according to the diagnostic criteria applied and will reflect the interpretative variability of different operators. The examination of patients for treatment needs frequently reveals restorations that do not meet precise criteria for success but are capable of further clinical service and do not necessarily require replacement. In view of the high costs of delivering restorative dentistry to the community, it is of particular interest to know how long dental restorations may be expected to survive.[31,197]

The aim of this chapter is to analyze the literature, predominantly of the last decade, regarding the longevity of dental restorations in permanent teeth, and to identify factors contributing to the survival of these restorations.

Longevity of Direct Posterior Restorations (Class I and II)

Amalgam Restorations

Amalgam was the material of choice for the restoration of Class I and II cavities for more than 100 years.[224] Many clinical studies report the long-term clinical performance of amalgam restorations. The results of selected clinical studies are summarized in Table 16-1. Annual failure rates range between 0% to 7% for non–gamma-2– and gamma-2–containing alloys with observation periods of up to 20 years.[4,5, 29,31,100,102,118,124,132,133,144,178,194,197,203,204, 219,224,225,236–239,242,263,273]

Several authors have reported a longer survival time and a lower annual failure rate for Class I compared to Class II amalgam restorations.[4,31,104] Robinson[219] found a 10-year median survival time for amalgam restorations in a 20-year survey. Interestingly, he reported a relatively high percentage of mesio-occlusal and disto-occlusal restorations surviving the 20-year period, while a high percentage of occlusal restorations did not. This seemed to be a result of the development of new approximal caries during the lifetime of occlusal restorations.

Dahl and Eriksen indicated that the causes of replacement of 200 amalgam restorations were recurrent caries (53%), fractures (33%), and restoration overhangs

(10%).[34] Lavelle[124] described recurrent caries (> 50%), fractures (> 26%), and dimensional defects (> 20%) as being the main problems, resulting from a large cross-sectional survey of 6,000 amalgam restorations. Pulpal irritations accounted for only 1% of the restoration failures. In a second part of the same study, reporting the data of a further longitudinal survey, Lavelle reports a mean annual replacement or loss of 7% for amalgam restorations.

The findings of a retrospective study of 2,344 Class I and II amalgam restorations in a NHS (National Health Service) practice in northeast England demonstrated no statistically significant difference between the median survival time of Class I (8 years) and Class II (7 years) restorations.[197]

The survival prediction analysis published by Smales et al in 1991 showed an annual failure rate of 6.3% for Shofu Spherical alloy (Shofu, Kyoto, Japan) while the three competitive amalgam products failed with an annual rate of between 1% and 1.7%.[238]

Osborne et al[194] compared the clinical performance of five gamma-2 alloys with seven non–gamma-2 alloys after 14 years of clinical service and found a loss rate of 16% for the gamma-2–containing group compared with 8.4% for the non–gamma-2 alloys. Furthermore, his findings demonstrated a significantly greater rate of marginal failure for traditional low-copper alloys.

As a result of a cross-sectional survey, Mjör[180] reported in 1997 a median longevity of 9 years for 282 amalgam restorations placed by general practitioners in Sweden. The clinical diagnoses, secondary caries (50%) and bulk fracture of the restoration (29%), were the main reasons for replacement. The median survival

time of 10 years for small and 8 years for large restorations showed that cavity size influenced the longevity of amalgam restorations.[172]

Qvist et al[208] reported an 8-year median survival rate for all amalgam restorations with the rate being slightly lower for Class II and slightly higher for single-surface restorations. Klausner and Charbeneau[109] showed that 51% of replaced restorations surveyed were more than 10 years old. Other studies indicated an average lifetime for large amalgam restorations of about 6 years compared with 11 years for small restorations.[161] The 50% survival time of amalgam restorations in Denmark was reported to be approximately 7 years.[209]

In controlled clinical trials, Doglia et al[38] found a 5-year survival rate of 83% to 100% for restorations of four different amalgam alloys and Osborne et al[193] reported an 8-year survival rate of 49% to 84% for three different alloys. The selection of the alloy significantly influenced the clinical outcome in both studies.

Moffa[182] demonstrated a survival rate of 90% for Class I and 75% for Class II amalgam restorations after 5 years. In another patient population, a survival rate of 65.5% after 12 years of clinical service was reported, with fracture (31.5%), recurrent caries (29%), and defective margins (25.7%) being the main reasons for failure. Jokstad et al[102] found a median age of 14 years for Class I amalgam restorations, while the results for Class II restorations ranged between 7 and 11 years. Two-surface restorations exhibited a greater longevity than three- or four-surface Class II amalgam restorations.

In a recent publication, Burke et al[24] reported a mean age of 7.4 years for Class I and 6.6 years for Class II restorations of

Table 16-1 Longevity of amalgam restorations in posterior teeth

Year of publication	First author	Observation period (y)	Black class	Restorative materials	Restorations (n)	Patients (n)
1969	Allan[4]	10	I II	Amalgam (alloys not specified, gamma-2 alloys)	78 92	
1971	Robinson[219]	20	I and II	Amalgam (alloys not specified, gamma-2 alloys)	145	
1976	Lavelle[124]	20	I and II	Amalgam (alloys not specified, gamma-2 alloys)	6,000	
1976	Lavelle[124]	20	I and II	Amalgam (alloys not specified, gamma-2 alloys)	400	
1977	Allan[5]	20	I and II	Amalgam (alloys not specified, gamma-2 alloys)	148	
1981	Crabb[31]	10	I II	Amalgam (alloys not specified, gamma-2 alloys)	269 530	
1984	Paterson[197]	15	I II	Solila	854 1,490	
1989	Letzel[132]	5–7	I and II	Conventional and high-copper alloys	2,341	
1989	Moffa[182]	5	I II	Amalgam (alloys not specified)	314	
1990	Qvist[210]		I II	Amalgam (alloys not specified)		
1990	Smales[236]	3	I	Dispersalloy	13	
1990	Welbury[263]	5	I	Amalcap	150	103
1991	Jokstad[100]	7–10	II	4 non–gamma-2 alloys 1 conventional alloy	256	141

Method	Study design	Survival rate (%)	Annual failure rate (%)	Median survival time (y)	Remarks
Defined criteria for clinical failure	Cross-sectional	54 39	4.6 6.1		Slightly better performance in Class I cavities
Defined criteria for clinical failure	Cross-sectional	22.8	3.9	10	75% of the amalgam restorations lasted > 5 years
Defined criteria for clinical failure	Cross-sectional		4.8		Main reasons for replacement: secondary caries, fracture, dimensional defects
Defined criteria for clinical failure	Longitudinal		7	> 10	
Defined criteria for clinical failure	Cross-sectional	14	4.3	8	
Defined criteria for clinical failure	Cross-sectional	59.5 37.2	4.1 6.3	> 10 8	Slightly better performance in Class I cavities
Defined criteria for clinical failure	Cross-sectional			8 7	No statistical difference between Class I and II amalgams
Defined criteria for clinical failure	Longitudinal	88–91			
Modified USPHS criteria		90 75	2 5		
Defined criteria for clinical failure	Cross-sectional			9.5 8	
Defined criteria for clinical failure	Longitudinal	100	0		Small restorations
Modified USPHS criteria	Longitudinal	92.7	1.5		All amalgams failed because of recurrent caries
USPHS criteria		73.5	2.7–3.8		Main reasons for replacement: secondary caries and bulk fracture; no significant difference between gamma-2 and non–gamma-2 alloys

Table 16-1 (continued)

Year of publication	First author	Observation period (y)	Black class	Restorative materials	Restorations (n)	Patients (n)
1991	Osborne[194]	14	I and II	5 gamma-2 alloys and 7 non–gamma-2 alloys	367	40
1991	Pieper[203]	9–11	I II	Amalgam (alloys not specified)	129 413	
1991	Smales[238]	11–18	I and II	New True Dentalloy, Dispersalloy, Indiloy, Shofu Spherical	1,680	
1991	Smales[237]	18	I and II	New True Dentalloy, Shofu Spherical, Dispersalloy, Tytin, Indiloy	1,801	
1991	Smales[239]	15	II		768	
1992	Mjör[173]			Amalgam (alloys not specified)	360	
1993	Mjör[178]	5	II	Dispersalloy	88	
1994	Jokstad[102]	> 10	I II	Amalgam (alloys not specified)	803 > 3,000	
1994	Mahmood[143]	> 14	I and II	Amalgam (alloys not specified)	245 (P) 455 (A)	
1996	Smales[241]	15	II	Amalgam (alloys not specified)	160	
1996	Wilson[273]	5	I and II	High-copper amalgams (Sybralloy, Dispersalloy, Tytin)	172	
1997	Hawthorne[72]		I and II	Amalgam (alloys not specified)	1,371	

Method	Study design	Survival rate (%)	Annual failure rate (%)	Median survival time (y)	Remarks
Defined criteria for clinical failure and photographs	Longitudinal	87.2	0.9		Gamma-2 amalgams had 84% success rate, non–gamma-2 alloys had 91.6% success rate
Modified USPHS criteria	Cross-sectional	85.3	1.3–1.6		
	Cross-sectional		1.0–1.7 and 6.3		Shofu Spherical had an annual failure rate of 6.3%; the other alloys had an annual failure rate of 1.0%–1.7%
Defined criteria for clinical failure	Cross-sectional	70	1.7		
		72	1.9		No difference in survival time between cuspal-coverage Class II amalgam restorations and restorations without cuspal coverage
Defined criteria for clinical failure	Cross-sectional			4.7	
Modified USPHS criteria	Longitudinal	95	1		Estimated survival function; small Class II cavities
	Cross-sectional			14 7.1	Increased number of surfaces in Class II restorations resulted in a lower median longevity
Defined criteria for clinical failure	Cross-sectional			7.9 9	Study conducted in Pakistan (P) and Australia (A)
	Cross-sectional	47.8	3.5		Cuspal-coverage amalgam restorations
Defined criteria for clinical failure	Longitudinal	94.8	1		Deterioration was greatest in molars and large-sized restorations
Defined criteria for clinical failure	Cross-sectional			22.5	Life-table method

Table 16-1 (continued)

Year of publication	First author	Observation period (y)	Black class	Restorative materials	Restorations (n)	Patients (n)
1997	Letzel[133]	13	I and II	Conventional zinc-free Conventional zinc-cont High-copper zinc-free High-copper zinc-cont (alloys)	3,119	
1997	Mjör[180]	> 25	I and II	Amalgam (alloys not specified)	282	
1997	Roulet[225]	6	I and II	5 high-copper amalgams (Amalcap plus, Contour, Permite C, Dispersalloy, Si-Am-Kap)	163	43
1997	Smales[242]	5 10 15	II	Amalgam (alloys not specified)	160	
1998	Kreulen[118]	15	II	New True Dentalloy, Tytin, Cavex	1,117	183
1998	Mair[144]	10	II	New True Dentalloy, Solila Nova	35	
1998	Plasmans[204]	8	II	Cavex (non–gamma-2)	266	130
1999	Burke[24]		I II	Amalgam (alloys not specified)	268 1,142	
1999	Cichon[29]	8	1-surface 2-surface 3-surface	Amalgam (alloys not specified)	820	
1999	Kamann[104]	6	I II	Luxalloy	62 21	

Method	Study design	Survival rate (%)	Annual failure rate (%)	Median survival time (y)	Remarks
	Meta-analysis	25 70 70 85	5.8 2.3 2.3 1.2		Zinc and copper content of the alloy contributed to the corrosion resistance of the amalgams; main failure reasons: fractures, marginal ditching, recurrent caries
Defined criteria for clinical failure	Cross-sectional			9	Main reasons for replacement: secondary caries (50%) and fracture (29%)
Modified USPHS criteria	Cross-sectional	87.5	2.1		Kaplan-Meier method; main reason for replacement: fracture
Defined criteria for clinical failure	Cross-sectional	77.6 66.7 47.8	4.5 3.3 3.5	14.6	Extensive amalgam restorations with cusp replacement
Defined criteria for clinical failure	Longitudinal	83	1.1		Replacement risk for MOD restorations is significantly higher than for MO/OD restorations
Modified USPHS criteria	Longitudinal	94.3	0.6		
Defined criteria for clinical failure	Longitudinal	88	1.5		Large amalgam restorations in molars with cusp replacement
	Cross-sectional			7.4 6.6	
Defined criteria for clinical failure	Cross-sectional	80 73.2 71.1	2.5 3.4 3.6		Patients had severe mental and/or physical handicaps
	Longitudinal	83.9 66.7	2.7 5.6		Main reason for replacement: secondary caries

amalgam in the United Kingdom. As a result of large cross-sectional studies, a median longevity of 9.5 years for Class I and 8 years for Class II amalgam restorations in a patient population in Denmark were described.[208,210] Bjertness and Sonju[17] reported a survival rate of 81% for amalgam restorations after 17 years in service. The median survival time for the failed restorations was five years. Smales and Hawthorne[241] found a survival rate of 66.7% after 10 years and 47.8% after 15 years for large cuspal-replacement amalgam restorations in Australia. An interesting study that compared the longevity of dental restorations in a developing country (Pakistan) with data from Australian patients exhibited an almost equal median survival time for amalgam restorations—8 and 9 years respectively.[143] The median longevity of 4.7 years recorded for amalgam restorations in Italy is low in comparison to other studies.[173]

Wilson et al[273] evaluated 172 Class I and Class II amalgam restorations and found a survival rate of 94.8% after 5 years. The results indicated a tendency for more deterioration in large restorations than in moderate-sized restorations and in molar teeth compared to premolars. Plasmans et al[204] investigated extensive amalgam restorations, ie, restorations that replaced at least one cusp, in molars and found a retention rate of 88% after 8 years. Different operators had no statistical significant influence on the treatment outcome, whereas an age effect was apparent. Extensive amalgam restorations performed significantly better for a young age group of patients (≤ 30 years of age) than for an older patient population (> 30 years of age).

Cichon and Kerschbaum[29] studied the longevity of amalgam restorations in a patient population comprising patients with severe mental and/or physical handicaps treated under general anesthesia. The findings indicate an annual failure rate of 2.5% for one-surface, 3.4% for two-surface, and 3.6% for multi-surface restorations—figures that are comparable to the annual failure rates for all patients. These results indicate that a physical or mental handicap per se is not a high risk factor affecting the longevity of amalgam restorations.[29]

Letzel et al[133] analyzed the survival rate of 3,119 amalgam restorations with respect to four different alloy groups. After 13 years, conventional zinc-free alloys exhibited a survival rate of only 25%, while conventional zinc-containing alloys and high-copper zinc-free alloys had 70% survival. High-copper, zinc-containing alloys had the highest survival rate, 85%. The zinc and copper content of the alloys contributed to the corrosion resistance of the amalgams and influenced the survival rate.

Given that most of the long-term clinical studies on amalgam were conducted during a time of high caries incidence[223,224] and knowing that the clinical diagnosis of secondary caries was recorded to be the main reason for the failure of amalgam restorations,[24,34,74,170,180,218] the overall findings in respect of state-of-the-art dental amalgam must be considered excellent.

Direct Composite Restorations

There is now widespread use of composite resins for the restoration of posterior teeth, even in stress-bearing areas. The results of selected clinical studies are summarized in Table 16-2. Annual failure rates of posterior composite restorations range from 0% to 9%.[7,53,75,138,139,167,178,182,188,236]

Mjör[180] reported a median longevity of 6 years for 537 composite restorations placed by general practitioners in Sweden. In addition to secondary caries (38%), bulk fracture (16%), marginal fracture (4%), discoloration (12%), poor anatomic form (9%), and fracture of the tooth (13%) accounted for the failure of the restorations. Discoloration as a reason for replacement of restorations is limited to tooth-colored dental materials.

Moffa,[182] in 1989, described a survival rate of 80% for Class I and 55% for Class II composite restorations after 5 years. In another patient population, a survival rate of 41.7% after 12 years of clinical service was reported with recurrent caries (40.6%), fracture (20.7%), and wear (13.4%) being the main reasons for failure.

Letzel[130] described in the results of a multicenter clinical trial of 711 Class I and Class II restorations of Occlusin (ICI Dental, Macclesfield, UK) a 4-year survival rate of 94%. Loss of material due to insufficient wear resistance and recurrent caries accounted for the failure of 35 Class I and 13 Class II restorations respectively.

The results of a cross-sectional survey in Scandinavia indicated a median survival time of 4 years for Class I and 4 to 7 years for Class II posterior composite restorations.[102] Secondary caries (> 65%) was stated as the main reason for restoration failure, followed by bulk fracture (> 20%).

Interestingly, Burke et al[24] found recently a higher mean longevity for Class II composite restorations (4.6 years) compared with Class I restorations (3.3 years). Scheibenbogen-Fuchsbrunner et al[227] re-

ported a 90% survival rate for composite restorations in Class I and Class II cavities after 2 years. Qvist et al,[210] in 1990, reported only 3 years as the median longevity for Class I and Class II composite restorations in Denmark. El-Mowafy et al,[45] in 1994, published the results of a comprehensive statistical meta-analysis. They observed a 89.5% survival rate after 5 years of clinical service for posterior composite restorations. A cross-sectional survey in Sweden exhibited a mean age of 8 years for 2,609 failed resin composite restorations with approximately 33% having secondary caries as diagnosis for replacement.[179]

Mjör[175] stated a median longevity of 7 years for Class I composite restorations and 4 years for Class II, mesio-occluso-distal (MOD) restorations. Wilson et al found in a 5-year prospective clinical trial with yearly follow-up intervals a success rate of 84%[268-272] with 75% of the failed restorations having been inserted in Class II cavities, while the remaining 25% were simple occlusal restorations. Wassell et al[262] reported a survival rate of 96% after 3 years of clinical service for 71 Class I and Class II incrementally placed direct composite restorations. No case of recurrent caries could be detected.

Smales et al[236] indicated in a 3-year survey of Class I restorations a perfect survival rate for P-30 (3M, St. Paul, MN) composite restorations and 93.9% for Visio-Molar (ESPE, Seefeld, Germany) restorations. Geurtsen and Schoeler[63] described a clinical survival rate of 87% for 1,209 Class I and Class II Herculite XR (Kerr, Orange, CA) restorations. Statistical analysis revealed significantly more Alpha ratings in premolars (82%) than in molars (77%). No difference was found for Class I

Table 16-2 Longevity of direct composite restorations in posterior teeth

Year of publication	First author	Observation period (y)	Black class	Restorative materials	Restorations (n)	Patients (n)
1988	Wilson[272]	5	I and II	Occlusin	67	
1989	Letzel[130]	4	I and II	Occlusin	711	
1989	Lundin[139]	4	I and II	Occlusin and PC4502	137	65
1989	Moffa[182]	5	I II	Composite resins (not specified)	356	
1990	Mjör[171]		II	Composite resins (not specified)		
1990	Qvist[210]		I II	Composite resins (not specified)		
1990	Smales[236]	3	I	Visio-Molar P-30	42 251	
1990	Welbury[263]	5	I	Prisma-Fil and Prisma-Shield	150	103
1991	Barnes[7]	5 8	I and II	Ful-Fil	33	12
1992	Freilich[53]	3	I and II	Heliomolar, Marathon, P-30, Experimental composite	105	46
1993	Mjör[178]	5	II	P-10	91	
1994	el-Mowafi[45]	5	I and II	Composite resins (not specified)	191	
1994	Jokstad[102]	> 10	I II	Composite resins (not specified)	22 79	
1995	Wassell[262]	3	I and II	Brilliant	71	54
1996	Lösche[138]	2	II	Herculite and P-50 + glass ceramic inserts	24	

Method	Study design	Survival rate (%)	Annual failure rate (%)	Median survival time (y)	Remarks
Modified USPHS criteria	Longitudinal	86	2.8		Large and moderately sized restorations; higher failure rate in Class II than in Class I
Defined criteria for clinical failure	Longitudinal	94	1.5		Multicenter clinical trial; main reason for replacement: wear and recurrent caries
Modified USPHS criteria	Longitudinal	84	4		142 μm average wear after 4 years; most of the failed restorations were classified as large
Modified USPHS criteria		80 55	4 9		Interproximal gingival area of Class II restoartions was found to be an area of early failure
				4	MOD composite restorations in Scandinavia
Defined criteria for clinical failure	Cross-sectional			3 3	
Defined criteria for clinical failure	Longitudinal	93.9 100	2 0		Small restorations
Modified USPHS criteria	Longitudinal	94.7	1.1		Minimal composite restorations combined with a fissure sealant
Modified USPHS criteria	Longitudinal	90 77	2 2.9		Main reason for replacement: recurrent caries
Modified USPHS criteria	Longitudinal	99	0.3		
Modified USPHS criteria	Longitudinal	85	3		Estimated survival function; small Class II cavities
Meta-analysis		89.5	2.1		
	Cross-sectional			4 4–7	Main reason for replacement: recurrent caries (> 65%) and fracture (> 20%)
Modified USPHS criteria	Longitudinal	96	1.3		61% Class II restorations; no secondary caries
Modified USPHS criteria and SEM	Longitudinal	100	0		Only premolars in the maxilla

Table 16-2 (continued)

Year of publication	First author	Observation period (y)	Black class	Restorative materials	Restorations (n)	Patients (n)
1997	Geurtsen[63]	4	I	Herculite XR	109	412
			II		1,100	
1997	Mjör[180]	> 25		Composite resins (not specified)	537	
1998	Helbig[75]	5	I and II	P-50	27	22
1998	Kiremitci[108]	2	I and II	Charisma + Beta-quartz inserts	22	
1998	Mair[144]	10	II	P-30, Occlusin, Cleartil Posterior	56	
1998	Mertz-Fairhurst[167]	10	I	Miradapt + Delton sealant	85	
1998	Nordbo[188]	7	II	Occlusin	34	37
				Ful-Fil	17	
1999	Burke[24]		I	Composite resins	27	
			II	(not specified)	71	
1999	Raskin[212]	10	I and II	Occlusin	100	36
1999	Rosin[221]	0.5	I	Definite (ormocer)	17	
			II		30	
1999	Scheibenbogen-Fuchsbrunner[228]	2	I and II	Tetric, Pertac-Hybrid Unifil, Blend-a-lux	43	
1999	Wilder[266]	17	I and II	Estilux, Nuva-Fil, Nuva-Fil PA, Uvio-Fil	85	33
2000	Sjögren[235]	3	I	Heliomolar +	9	16
			II	Beta-quartz inserts	30	

Method	Study design	Survival rate (%)	Annual failure rate (%)	Median survival time (y)	Remarks
Modified USPHS criteria	Cross-sectional	87	3.3	9	More Alpha ratings in premolars than in molars; no difference between Class I and II cavities
Defined criteria for clinical failure	Cross-sectional			6	Main reasons for replacement: secondary caries (38%) and fracture (20%)
Modified USPHS criteria	Longitudinal	88.9	2.2		Marginal integrity and surface texture significantly deteriorated after 5 years
Modified USPHS criteria and SEM	Longitudinal	95.5	2.3		
Modified USPHS criteria	Longitudinal	92.9	0.7		P-30 and Occlusin showed approximately 400 µm wear, Clearfil Posterior 300 µm after 10 years
Modified USPHS criteria	Longitudinal	80	2		Ultraconservative restorations
Modified USPHS criteria	Longitudinal	88	1.7		Main reason for replacement: recurrent caries
		59	5.9		
	Cross-sectional			3.3	
				4.6	
Modified USPHS criteria	Longitudinal	50–60	4–5		Main reason for replacement: loss of anatomic form and approximal contacts
Modified USPHS criteria	Longitudinal	100			Resin-based restorative material with modified matrix: inorganic-organic copolymer matrix
		96.7			
Modified USPHS criteria	Longitudinal	90	5		Main reason for replacement: recurrent caries
Modified USPHS criteria	Longitudinal	76	1.4		264 µm wear after 17 years; most wear occured in the first 5 years
CDA criteria	Longitudinal	69	10.3		4 restorations lost the insert

and II restorations. The 50% survival time was calculated by extrapolation of the clinical data with a Weibull analysis and determined a life expectancy of 9 years. Barnes et al[7] reported a survival rate of 90% for posterior Ful-Fil (Dentsply, Milford, DE) restorations after 5 years and a survival rate of 77% after 8 years of clinical service. Reasons for the replacement of restorations were predominated by secondary caries and excessive wear. Similar results with a survival rate of 88.9% for bonded P-50 (3M) restorations after 5 years were reported by Helbig et al.[75] Raskin et al[212] reported an estimated 10-year failure rate between 40% and 50% for Class I and Class II restorations of Occlusin. Loss of occlusal anatomic form during the first 5 years and loss of approximal contacts near the end of the study accounted for most of the failures. Recurrent caries and bulk fracture were recorded only infrequently. In contrast to other studies, location, class, and size of the restorations were not found to significantly influence the treatment outcome.

A 17-year study of ultraviolet-cured posterior composites by Wilder et al[266] demonstrated an excellent success rate of 76%. Color matching (94% Alpha), marginal discoloration (100% Alpha), marginal integrity (100% Alpha), secondary caries (92% Alpha), surface texture (72% Alpha), anatomic form (22% Alpha), and a mean occlusal wear of 264 µm were recorded after 17 years. Most of the wear (75%) occurred in the first 5 years, confirming the findings of Raskin et al.[212] Mair[144] indicated a survival rate of 92.9% for three posterior composite resins after 10 years with mean wear rates between 300 µm and 400 µm.

For the new composite restorative materials based on the ormocer (organ-ically modified ceramics) technology, only preliminary 6-month data of one clinical trial are available, indicating 100% survival for 17 Class I and a 96.7% survival rate for 30 Class II restorations.[221] Ormocers were introduced in the European market in 1998 and are characterized by a novel inorganic-organic copolymer matrix. [83,154–156,278]

Only a very limited number of clinical studies reporting the performance of direct composite restorations in combination with prefabricated glass-ceramic inserts are available. Lösche[138] restored 24 Class II cavities in premolars with composites and glass-ceramic inserts and observed a 100% success rate after 2 years. Kiremitci et al[108] observed after 2 years a survival rate of 95.5% for Class II composite restorations reinforced with Beta-quartz glass-ceramic inserts (Lee Pharmaceuticals, South El Monte, CA). However, Sjögren et al[235] rated only 69% of 39 Heliomolar Beta-quartz insert restorations in Class I and Class II cavities satisfactory after 3 years in clinical service. Four restorations lost their inserts, seven restorations fractured or exhibited flaking surfaces, and one restoration failed because of recurrent caries.

Glass-Ionomer Cements and Compomers

Annual failure rates for posterior glass ionomer, resin-modified glass ionomer, and compomer restorations range within 1.4% to 14.4%.[56,70,71,78,146,236,249] The results of selected clinical studies are summarized in Table 16-3. Mjör[180] reported a median longevity of 3 years for 155 glass-ionomer restorations, comprising all cavity classes, placed by general practitioners in Sweden. For glass-ionomer restorations, fracture of restorations (18%), including bulk fracture (12%) and marginal fracture (6%), together with poor anatomic form as a result of low wear resistance, were the main reasons for failure.[180] In another study that included 790 restorations, Mjör revealed a mean age of 5 years for failed glass-ionomer cement restorations.[179] Reasons for replacement were predominantly secondary caries (50%), anatomic form (12%), bulk fracture (11%), and marginal fracture (5%).

Smales et al[237] reported a median survival time of 2.2 years for glass-ionomer restorations, and 6.2 years and 0.8 years for the 25% and 75% quartiles, respectively. In a further study, Smales et al[236] assessed 132 Class I Ketac-Silver (ESPE) cermet restorations and found a 56.8% survival rate after 3 years, corresponding to an annual failure rate of 14.4%. Of the cermet restorations, 11.4% failed as a result of surface cracking or crazing, sometimes within the first 6 months of placement.

Mount[184] reported no failures after 10 to 12 years for eight Class I glass-ionomer restorations placed in a private practice. From the results of the 5-year clinical observation of metal-modified glass-ionomer restorations (Ketac-Silver) in small Class II cavities, Mjör and Jokstad[178] described an estimated survival rate of 55%. Failures were mainly attributed to fracture phenomena. Krämer et al[112] reported a Kaplan-Meier survival rate of approximately 90% for Class I and 72% for Class II cermet restorations as part of the findings of a 4-year clinical investigation. For Class II cavities, in particular, many fracture-related failures were observed. Hickel et al[78] re-ported a survival rate of 88.5%, 50%, and 80.8% after 2.5 to 3.5 years of observation for cermet restorations (Ketac-Silver) in Class I, Class II, and small Class II cavities, respectively.

Tunnel restorations

Hasselrot[71] placed 232 Class I tunnel (partial tunnel) restorations with an unbroken enamel wall and 35 Class II tunnel (total tunnel) restorations with perforated approximal enamel and observed an annual failure rate of 7% for both restoration types after 7 years. The main reasons for failure included fracture of the marginal ridge (41%), secondary caries (40%), and progressive enamel cavitation and/or degradation of the glass-ionomer restorations (19%). No performance difference could be revealed between molars and premolars or between maxillary and mandibular teeth. A comparable annual failure rate of 7.6% was observed in a study examining the survival of glass-ionomer tunnel restorations after 3.5 years.[70] Svanberg[249] found an appreciably higher survival rate with 94.4% success and 1.9% annual failure rate after 3 years for 18 cermet (Ketac-Silver) Class II tunnel restorations in a population of 18 caries-active Swedish adolescents. Strand et al[246] reported a success rate of 70% for 161 cermet tunnel restorations after 3 years. Marginal ridge fracture accounted for 14% and caries formation for 16% of the failures.

ART restorations

Ho et al[85] reported the 2-year findings for two glass-ionomer cements (ChemFil Superior, Dentsply, and Fuji IX, GC, Tokyo, Japan) that were placed according to an

Table 16-3 Longevity of glass-ionomer and compomer restorations in posterior teeth

Year of publication	First author	Observation period (y)	Black class	Restorative materials	Restorations (n)	Patients (n)
1988	Hickel[78]	3.5	I II II (small)	Ketac-Silver (cermet)	87 104 52	
1990	Smales[236]	3	I	Ketac-Silver (cermet)	132	
1991	Smales[237]	9	All	Aaps, Fuji II, Ketac	465	
1992	Svanberg[249]	3	II	Ketac-Silver	18	18
1993	Hasselrot[70]	3.5	I and II	Base Line and Ketac-Silver	282	
1993	Mjör[178]	5	II	Ketac-Silver (cermet)	95	
1994	Krämer[112]	4	I II	Ketac Silver (cermet)	49 39	50
1995	Mallow[145]	0.5	I	Fuji GC MAGIC		102
1996	Frencken[55]	1	I	ChemFil Superior	213	
1996	Phantum-vanit[201]	1 2 3	I	Glass-ionomer cement	241	144
1996	Strand[246]	3	I and II	Ketac-Silver (cermet)	161	85
1997	Benz[13]	0.5	II	Fuji IX, Ketac Molar Dyract, Compoglass	28, 19 37, 50	

Method	Study design	Survival rate (%)	Annual failure rate (%)	Median survival time (y)	Remarks
Defined criteria for clinical failure	Longitudinal	88.5 50 80.8	3.3 14.3 5.5		Small (modified) Class II restorations showed better results than regular Class II cavities
Defined criteria for clinical failure	Longitudinal	56.8	14.4		Main reasons for replacement: surface cracking and crazing
Defined criteria for clinical failure	Cross-sectional			2.2	
Defined criteria for clinical failure	Longitudinal	94.4	1.9		Caries-active individuals; tunnel restorations
Defined criteria for clinical failure	Longitudinal	73.5	7.6		Tunnel restorations
Modified USPHS criteria	Longitudinal	55	9		Estimated survival function; small Class II cavities
Modified USPHS criteria	Longitudinal	89.8 71.8	2.6 7.1		Main reasons for replacement: bulk fracture
Defined criteria for clinical failure	Longitudinal	87.1 58.8			ART technique in Cambodia; placed by dental nurse students
Defined criteria for clinical failure	Longitudinal	93.4	6.6		ART technique in Zimbabwe; no secondary caries
Defined criteria for clinical failure	Longitudinal	93 83 71	7 8.5 9.7		ART technique in Thailand
Defined criteria for clinical failure	Longitudinal	70	10		Tunnel restorations; main failure reasons: caries 16%, marginal ridge fracture 14%
Modified USPHS criteria	Longitudinal	91 97			Significantly better wear and marginal integrity for compomers

Table 16-3 (continued)

Year of publication	First author	Observation period (y)	Black class	Restorative materials	Restorations (n)	Patients (n)
1997	Mjör[180]	> 25	All	Glass ionomers (not specified)	155	
1997	Mount[184]	10–12	I	Glass ionomers (not specified)	8	
1998	Benz[14]	0.5	II	Dyract AP	40	
1998	Frencken[56]	1 2 3	I	Fuji IX	297	142
1998	Hasselrot[71]	7	I II	Base Line Ketac-Silver (cermet)	232 35	193
1998	Mallow[146]	1 3	I	Fuji II	89	53
1999	Ho[85]	2	I	Fuji IX ChemFil Superior	55 45	21
1999	Huth[95]	0.5	I and II	Hytac (compomer)	88	24
1999	Kontou[111]	1	I and II	Hytac, Dyract AP (compomers)	71	31
1999	Manhart[153]	0.5	I	Hytac (compomer)	40	25

Method	Study design	Survival rate (%)	Annual failure rate (%)	Median survival time (y)	Remarks
Defined criteria for clinical failure	Cross-sectional			3	Main reasons for replacement: secondary caries (50%), fracture (18%)
Defined criteria for clinical failure	Cross-sectional	100	0		Very small number of restorations
Modified USPHS criteria	Longitudinal	100	0		
Defined criteria for clinical failure	Longitudinal	98.6 93.8 88.3	1.4 3.1 3.9		ART technique in Zimbabwe
Defined criteria for clinical failure	Longitudinal	7 7	6 6		Tunnel restorations; no difference in failure rates between Class I and II
Defined criteria for clinical failure	Longitudinal	76.3 57.9	14		ART technique in Cambodia; placed by dental nurse students
Defined criteria for clinical failure	Longitudinal	93	3.5		ART technique in Asia; small Class I cavities in molar teeth; main failure reasons: wear, fracture, recurrent caries
Modified USPHS criteria	Longitudinal	91			Main reasons for replacement: wear and secondary caries
Modified USPHS criteria	Longitudinal	96	4		
Modified USPHS criteria	Longitudinal	100			

atraumatic treatment (ART) regimen. Ninety-three percent of the restorations survived. The remaining restorations failed because of wear, fracture, and recurrent caries. Mean cumulative wear was 83.1 μm for Fuji IX and 104 μm for ChemFil Superior.

The ART technique is based on removing tooth decay using hand instruments only, after which the cavity is filled with a glass-ionomer cement.[55] This technique was established to facilitate the provision of dental care in rural areas of developing countries, where no electricity-driven dental equipment can be used and there is a minimum of dental health care. Frencken et al[55] reported after 1 year a survival rate of 93.4% for one-surface ART restorations in an oral health program in Zimbabwe. These results are comparable to the treatment outcome of 93% success rate after 1 year for ART glass-ionomer restorations in Thailand.[54] Phantumvanit et al[201] indicated 93%, 83%, and 71% success rates for ART restorations in a rural village in Thailand after 1, 2, and 3 years, respectively. The use of the highly viscous glass-ionomer cement Fuji IX yielded slightly better results with a survival rate of 98.6%, 93.8%, and 88.3% after 1, 2, and 3 years, respectively.[56] A somewhat low survival rate after 6 months was found for ART restorations placed by dental nurse students under field conditions in rural Cambodia: 87.1% of the Fuji-GC (GC) restorations and only 58.8% of MAGIC (Nulite, Hornsby, Austrailia) glass-ionomer restorations survived.[145] A further study by the same author reported a success rate of 76.3% after 1 year for ART Fuji II (GC) Class I restorations placed by student dental nurses in Cambodia and only 57.9% survival rate after 3 years of service.

Compomer Restorations

Clinical trials are ongoing to determine the clinical performance of compomers in stress-bearing Class I and Class II cavities in the permanent dentition. Survival rates of between 91% and 100% were reported for the 6-month clinical behavior of several compomer materials.[13,14,95,153] Kontou et al[111] described a 4% failure rate for compomers in Class I and Class II cavities after 1 year. These short-term results must, however, be viewed as having relatively limited value. It will be of specific interest to monitor the further performance of these restorations. The ease of handling of compomer materials is probably the main reason for their widespread acceptance by practitioners, especially in European countries,[82,91,150,152] although they exhibited significantly inferior wear rates compared with hybrid composites.[83,205]

Longevity of Indirect Posterior Restorations (Class I and II)

Composite Inlays and Onlays

Composite inlays are indicated for the restoration of large defects. The major advantage is that most of the composite is formed by the precured composite inlay, which is inserted in the cavity using a minimum of resin cement, offering good control of anatomic form and proximal contacts.[16,23,40,191,224,228] The mechanical properties of composite inlays can be enhanced by postcuring the inlay in a light oven or by heat and pressure curing, resulting in a higher degree of conversion. There have been few in vivo studies of the long-term behavior of indirect posterior composite restorations. The results of selected clinical studies are summarized in Table 16-4.

Annual failure rates for posterior composite inlays and onlays range from 0% to 10%.[16,62,67,110,113,117] Wendt and Leinfelder[264] reported a failure of two heat-treated Occlusin inlays after 3 years of clinical service, which corresponds to a 96.7% success rate. Füllemann et al[62] found a 100% survival rate for 24 Brilliant (Coltène, Altstätten, Switzerland) inlays after 1 year and Krejci et al[117] described a success rate of 100% for APH (Dentsply) inlays for the same duration of service.

Wassell et al[262] restored Class I and Class II cavities and reported an 8% failure rate for 71 Brilliant composite inlays. A cause for concern was the fact that four restorations had to be removed because of postoperative sensitivity. The other restorations failed because of fracture of the inlay or tooth. Thordrup et al[251] assessed 15 direct Brilliant inlays and 14 indirect Estilux (Kulzer, Wehrheim, Germany) composite inlays and found an overall survival rate of 96.6% after 1 year, with one Brilliant inlay having failed because of recurrent caries formation. The Brilliant inlays showed a smooth surface texture, whereas the Estilux inlays exhibited a rough texture.

Krämer et al[113] assessed 118 Visio-Gem (ESPE) inlays over a 6-year period and found a survival rate of only 41% using the Kaplan-Meier estimator. After 4 years, 56% of the inlays were at risk. The main reason for failure during the first 2 years of the study was postoperative sensitivity, while after 2 years material-related effects of the microfilled composite (inlay fracture, loss of retention, marginal openings, and secondary caries) prevailed. A similarly high failure rate was described by a study of Isosit (Ivoclar, Schaan, Liechtenstein) inlays.[16] Donly et al[40] reported a survival rate of 75% for 36 Concept (Ivoclar) composite inlays and onlays after 7 years. Failures due to secondary caries and fracture were predominantly observed for restorations in molars.

Wiedmer et al[265] studied the longevity of 24 composite inlays in Class I and Class II cavities over a 5-year period and found 100% success. No differences in performance were found between molars and premolars or between direct and indirect inlays. These results were confirmed in a study by Frederickson and Setcos,[52] reporting a 100% survival rate for 31 Concept composite inlays and onlays after 5 years. Hannig[69] reported a success rate of 92.5% for 40 Isosit inlays in Class I and Class II cavities after 5 years. Scanning electron microscopic (SEM) analysis indicated 50% marginal imperfections for Class I and 60% for Class II inlays. Three inlays failed because of extensive marginal fractures related to bruxism by the patients. Similar results with a survival rate of 88% after 5 to 6 years were found for 100 Brilliant inlays in Class II cavities.[256] In a recent study, Klimm et al[110] found a 100% survival rate for 13 Herculite XRV (Kerr) Class II composite inlays after 2 years of clinical service.

Ceramic Inlays and Onlays

Ceramic inlays can be made of feldspathic ceramic materials by sintering or by milling. Glass-ceramic inlays can be cast or pressed using the lost wax technique or by milling.[81,224,247] CAD/CAM technology is used in the Cerec system, which mills ceramic inlays from blocks of ceramic

Table 16-4 Longevity of composite inlays and onlays

Year of publication	First author	Observation period (y)	Black class	Restorative materials	Restorations (n)	Patients (n)
1991	Bessing[16]	1		Isosit	34	19
1992	Füllemann[62]	1	I and II	Brilliant	24	
1992	Haas[67]	2	Inlays	Coltene-composite	30	
				Kulzer-composite	30	
1992	Wendt[264]	3	I and II	Occlusin	60	
1994	Frederickson[52]	3	Inlays and onlays	Concept	31	23
1994	Krejci[117]	1	Inlays	APH	21	24
			Onlays		9	
1994	Thordrup[251]	1	I and II	Estilux, Brilliant	29	
1994	van Dijken[256]	5	II	Brilliant	100	
1995	Wassell[262]	3	I and II	Brilliant	71	54
1996	Hannig[69]	5	I	Isosit	20	
			II		20	
1996	Krämer[113]	6	I and II	Visio-Gem	118	28
1997	Wiedmer[265]	5	I and II	Brilliant, APH	24	
1999	Donly[40]	7	Inlays	Concept	32	18
			Onlays		4	
1999	Klimm[110]	2	II	Herculite XRV	13	
1999	Scheibenbogen-Fuchsbrunner[228]	2	I and II	Tetric, Pertac-Hybrid Unifil, Blend-a-lux	45	

Method	Study design	Survival rate (%)	Annual failure rate (%)	Median survival time (y)	Remarks
CDA criteria	Longitudinal	88.2	11.8		
Modified USPHS criteria and SEM		100	0		
Defined criteria for clinical failure	Longitudinal	80 80	10 10		No difference between molars and premolars
Modified USPHS criteria		96.7	1.1		
Modified USPHS criteria		100	0		All restorations moderate to large in size
Modified USPHS criteria and SEM	Longitudinal	100 100	0 0		Excellent marginal integrity after 1 year
CDA criteria	Longitudinal	96.6	3.4		1 inlay: secondary caries
Modified USPHS criteria	Longitudinal	88	2.4		
Modified USPHS criteria	Longitudinal	92	2.7		66% Class II restorations; main failure reasons: fracture, postoperative sensitivity
Defined criteria for clinical failure and SEM	Longitudinal	92.5	1.5		Marginal imperfections: 60% in Class II and 50% in Class I
Modified USPHS criteria	Longitudinal	41	9.8		Kaplan-Meier estimator; main failure reasons: fracture, marginal opening, postoperative sensitivity
Modified USPHS criteria and SEM	Longitudinal	100	0		No differences between molars and premolars and between direct and indirect inlays
Modified USPHS criteria	Longitudinal	75 75	3.6 3.6		Main failure reasons: secondary caries, fracture
Modified USPHS criteria	Longitudinal	100	0		
Modified USPHS criteria	Longitudinal	93	3.5		

material that are formed under optimum, controlled conditions.[159] In this way, it is possible to obtain a high quality inlay without the inevitable variations seen in a manually produced restoration.[185,232] The Celay system (Mikrona Technologie AG, Spreitenbach, Switzerland) is designed as a high-precision copy milling machine using a composite "pro-inlay" as guidance to mill the ceramic inlay out of a ceramic block.[44,77,81]

The results of selected clinical studies investigating ceramic inlays and onlays are summarized in Table 16-5. Annual failure rates of ceramic inlay restorations range from 0% to 7.5%.[46,51,57,58,61,67,73,89,114,207,227] Isidor and Brondum[97] reported a 52% survival rate for sintered ceramic inlays after 2 to 4.5 years of clinical service. The average length of clinical service before failure of the restorations was 15.7 months. Jensen[99] described a success rate of 95.8% for 310 Mirage (Miron Int, Kansas City, KS) inlays and onlays in 59 patients after 2 years.

Scheibenbogen et al[227] and Manhart et al[157,158] found a 100% survival rate for heat-pressed Empress (Vivadent, Schaan, Liechtenstein) glass ceramic inlays inserted by students in a German dental school after 1, 2, and 3 years. These results are confirmed by the findings of Krejci et al,[116] who reported a 100% survival rate of 10 Empress inlays after 1.5 years. Krejci et al, however, revealed a significant deterioration of marginal quality over time using SEM analysis. Identical results were published by Thonemann et al.[250] Tidehag and Gunne[252] observed only one fractured Empress onlay after 2 years (failure rate, 1.6%). All other restorations received 82% excellent ratings for anatomic form and 84% for marginal integrity.

Thordrup et al[251] exhibited a survival rate of 92.9% for 14 Vitadur N (Vita Zahnfabrik, Bad Säckingen, Germany) inlays after 1 year. One inlay had to be replaced because of bulk fracture. Roulet[225] evaluated 123 Dicor (Dentsply) inlays up to 6 years in service and found a 76% success rate using the Kaplan-Meier method. Twelve inlays failed, seven because of fractures and four because of endodontic problems. All fractures could be traced back to case selection errors (bruxing patients, replacing cusps, over-extension). Studer et al[247] reported 97.5% success for leucite-reinforced Empress glass-ceramic inlays and onlays after 2 years. Three restorations had to be replaced within the observation period because of fracture-related failures. After 4 years of clinical service, 93% of extensive Empress inlays and onlays survived, with 79% of the remaining restorations exhibiting marginal deficiencies.[114]

Höglund et al[89] studied the effect of the luting agent on the clinical performance of 118 fired Mirage inlays in Class II cavities. Half of the restorations were luted with either a dual-cured composite cement or a glass-ionomer cement. The assessment after 2 years exhibited a 2% failure rate for resin-cemented inlays while 15% of the restorations cemented with the glass-ionomer luting agent failed. The 3-year follow-up examination confirmed these observations.[90] At the 6-year follow-up examination, a significantly higher failure rate could be revealed for the ceramic inlays placed with a glass-ionomer cement (74% survival) compared with resin cement-bonded restorations (88% survival).[258] Similar failure rates were observed for Dicor inlays inserted with a glass-ionomer luting cement, showing 8% failure after 2 years.[244]

Haas et al[67] observed Dicor, Optec (Jeneric/Pentron, Wallingford, CT), Hi-Ceram (Vita Zahnfabrik), and Du-Ceram (Ducera Dental, Rosbach, Germany) inlays (n = 30 of each) over a 3-year period and found 93.3%, 80%, 80%, and 90% survival rates, respectively. Secondary caries and fracture were recorded as the main causes for restoration failure.

Hayashi et al[73] reported a 6-year study of 49 fired ceramic inlays (G-Cera Cosmotech II, GC) that demonstrated a survival rate of 92%. The results of the different examinations at baseline, 6 months, and 1, 2, 4, and 6 years showed a decrease of Alpha ratings and an increase of Bravo ratings (modified USPHS system) for the clinical criteria "marginal adaptation" and "marginal discoloration." Additional SEM analysis revealed marginal microfractures in 49% of the restorations, wear of the restorative material (15%), and wear of the resin cement (36%).

Fuzzi and Rapelli[61] studied the longevity of 183 fired ceramic inlays over a 10-year observation period and estimated with Kaplan-Meier curves a 97% overall survival rate—99% for inlays in premolars and 95% in molars. A perfect survival rate (100%) was reported for 50 fired Mirage II (Miron Int) ceramic inlays in Class II cavities after 2 years.[57] Further SEM investigation revealed a marginal deterioration from baseline to the 1-year and 2-year follow-up assessment. The 4-year follow-up of the same restorations indicated continued 100% survival of the 50 ceramic inlays. Marginal deterioration of the restorations still increased from 2 years up to 4 years, albeit at a slower rate.[58]

Felden et al[46] conducted a cross-sectional survey on different systems of 232 ceramic inlays and 55 partial ceramic crowns and found that 94.2% of all restorations survived more than 7 years. Seventeen restorations failed during the observation period, consisting of fourteen partial crowns and three inlays. Kaplan-Meier survival probability for 7 years was 98% for ceramic inlays and only 56% for partial ceramic crowns. Qualtrough and Wilson[207] reported the 3-year findings of 50 fired Mirage porcelain inlays and found a survival rate of 82%. Five of nine lost inlays failed within the first month after placement because of fracture. More inlays in molars (n = 6) had to be replaced than restorations inserted in premolars (n = 3).

Computer-Generated Ceramic Inlays and Onlays (CAD/CAM)

The results of selected clinical studies examining the longevity of computer-generated ceramic inlays are summarized in Table 16-6. Annual failure rates for CAD/CAM-ceramic restorations have ranged between 0% and 4.4%.[15,67,186,195, 251,261,279]

Thordrup et al[251] revealed after 1 year no failure of 15 Cerec inlays in a selected patient population. These results are confirmed by the findings of Mörmann and Krejci,[186] who reported a 100% survival rate for Vita Mark I (Vita Zahnfabrik) Cerec restorations after 5 years of clinical service. Sjögren et al[232] found in an assessment of 205 Cerec inlays up to 24 months of age a survival rate of 98%. Four inlays fractured and 14% of the 72 patients suffered from postoperative hypersensitivity. Excellent ratings, using the California Dental Association (CDA) quality evaluation system, were scored with 26% for surface, 57% for color match, 55% for anatomic surface, and 83% for marginal integrity.

Table 16-5 Longevity of ceramic inlays and onlays

Year of publication	First author	Observation period (y)	Black class	Restorative materials	Restorations (n)	Patients (n)
1988	Jensen[99]	2	I and II	Mirage	310	59
1992	Haas[67]	3	Inlays	Dicor	30	
				Optec	30	
				Hi-Ceram	30	
				Du-Ceram	30	
1992	Höglund[89]	2	II	Mirage (resin cement)	59	50
				Mirage (GI cement)	59	
1992	Krejci[116]	1.5	II	Empress	10	10
1993	Stenberg[244]	2	II	Dicor (GI cement)	25	20
1994	Höglund[90]	3	II	Mirage (resin cement)	59	50
				Mirage (GI cement)	59	
1994	Thordrup[251]	1	I and II	Vita Dur N	14	
1995	Isidor[97]	2–4.5	II	Mirage	25	
1995	Tidehag[252]	2	II	Empress	62	18
1996	Friedl[57]	2	II	Mirage II	50	20
1996	Qualtrough[207]	3	I and II	Mirage	50	27
1996	Studer[247]	2	I and II	Empress	130	36
1997	Fradeani[51]	4.5	Inlays and onlays	Empress	125	29

Method	Study design	Survival rate (%)	Annual failure rate (%)	Median survival time (y)	Remarks
Modified USPHS criteria		95.8	2.1		
Defined criteria for clinical failure	Longitudinal	93.3 80 80 90	2.2 6.7 6.7 3.3		Main reasons for replacement: fracture of the inlays, secondary caries
Modified USPHS criteria		98 85	1 7.5		Comparison of a resin cement and a glass-ionomer cement as luting agent
Modified USPHS criteria and SEM	Longitudinal	100	0		Only inlays in premolars; significant deterioration of marginal quality over time
Modified USPHS criteria		92	4		Glass-ionomer cement as luting agent
Modified USPHS criteria		96.6 84.7	1.3 5.1		Comparison of a resin cement and a glass-ionomer cement as luting agent
CDA criteria	Longitudinal	92.9	7.1		Fracture of one inlay
Defined criteria for clinical failure	Longitudinal	52			Main reasons for replacement: fracture of the inlay
CDA criteria	Longitudinal	98.4	0.8		Fracture of one onlay
Modified USPHS criteria and SEM	Longitudinal	100	0		
Modified USPHS criteria and SEM	Longitudinal	82	6		Main failure reasons: inlay fracture; more failures in molars (n = 6) than in premolars (n = 3)
Modified USPHS criteria	Longitudinal	97.5	1.3		Kaplan-Meier method; main reasons for replacement: fracture of the inlays
Modified USPHS criteria	Longitudinal	95.6	1		Kaplan-Meier method; main failure reason: inlay fracture

Table 16-5 (continued)

Year of publication	First author	Observation period (y)	Black class	Restorative materials	Restorations (n)	Patients (n)
1997	Friedl[58]	4	II	Mirage II	50	20
1997	Roulet[225]	6	I and II	Dicor	123	29
1997	Thonemann[250]	2	I II	Empress	14 37	11
1998	Felden[46]	7	Inlays and onlays	Dicor, Empress, Mirage II, Cerec Vita Mark I, Duceram LFC	287	106
1998	Fuzzi[61]	10	I and II	Microbond Natural Ceramic and Fortune Ceramic	183	67
1998	Hayashi[73]	6	I and II	G-Cera Cosmotech II	49	29
1998	Lehner[127]	6	Inlays Onlays	Empress	138 17	43
1998	Scheibenbogen[227]	1	I and II	Empress	24	
1998	van Dijken[258]	6	II	Mirage (resin cement) Mirage (GI cement)	58 57	50
1999	Krämer[114]	4	Inlays and onlays	Empress	96	34

Method	Study design	Survival rate (%)	Annual failure rate (%)	Median survival time (y)	Remarks
Modified USPHS criteria and SEM	Longitudinal	100	0		64% of the margins were perceptible clinically after 4 years
Modified USPHS criteria	Cross-sectional	76	4		Kaplan-Meier method; main reason for replacement: fracture of the inlays
Modified USPHS criteria and SEM		100	0		All margins located within enamel; significant deterioration of marginal quality over time
Modified USPHS criteria	Cross-sectional	94.2	0.8		Kaplan-Meier method; 17 restorations failed (3 inlays, 14 onlays)
Defined criteria for clinical failure	Longitudinal	97	0.3		Kaplan-Meier method; premolars better than molars (99% vs 95%)
Modified USPHS criteria and SEM	Longitudinal	92	1.3		SEM showed marginal microfractures in 49% of the inlays
Modified USPHS criteria	Longitudinal	94.9	0.9		Kaplan-Meier method; no Class I inlay failed
Modified USPHS criteria	Longitudinal	100	0		Student operators
Modified USPHS criteria	Longitudinal	88 74	2 4.3		Higher failure rate in inlay group luted with a glass-ionomer (GI) cement rather than a resin cement
Modified USPHS criteria and SEM	Longitudinal	93	1.8		Kaplan-Meier method; main failure reasons: bulk fractures, need for endodontic therapy

Table 16-6 Longevity of computer-generated ceramic inlays and onlays (CAD/CAM)

Year of publication	First author	Observation period (y)	Black class	Restorative materials	Restorations (n)	Patients (n)
1991	Reiss[214]	3	I and II	Cerec	426	142
1992	Haas[67]	3	Inlays	Cerec	30	
1992	Mörmann[186]	5	II	Cerec; Vita Cerec Mark I	8	8
1992	Sjögren[232]	1–2	I and II	Cerec; Vita Cerec Mark I and II	205	72
1994	Thordrup[251]	1	I and II	Cerec; Vita-Blocks	15	
1994	Walther[261]	5	I and II	Cerec	1,011	299
1995	Otto[195]	5	II	Cerec; Vita-Blocks	100	62
1996	Heymann[77]	4	I	Cerec; Dicor MGC	19	28
			II		31	
1997	Berg[15]	5	II	Cerec I	51	46
1998	Reiss[215]	7.5	I and II	Cerec	1,011	299
1998	Zuellig-Singer[279]	3	II	Cerec; Vita Mark II (RC)	28	18
				Cerec; Vita Mark II (GIC)	9	
2000	Reiss[216]	10 12	I and II	Cerec	1,010	299

Method	Study design	Survival rate (%)	Annual failure rate (%)	Median survival time (y)	Remarks
Modified USPHS criteria	Longitudinal	95	1.7		Kaplan-Meier method; main reasons for replacement: fracture, postoperative symptoms
Defined criteria for clinical failure	Longitudinal	86.7	4.4		
Modified USPHS criteria and SEM		100	0		73.6% to 86% perfect margins in the SEM
CDA criteria		98			4 inlays fractured; 14% postoperative sensitivity
CDA criteria	Longitudinal	100	0		
Defined criteria for clinical failure	Longitudinal	95	1		Kaplan-Meier method; main reasons for replacement: inlay fracture, tooth fracture, caries
Defined criteria for clinical failure	Longitudinal	98	0.4		2 restored teeth required endodontic therapy
Modified USPHS criteria and SEM	Longitudinal	100	0		
Defined criteria for clinical failure and SEM	Longitudinal	94.1	1.2		All inlays showed marginal defects after 5 years
Defined criteria for clinical failure	Longitudinal	91.6	1.1		Kaplan-Meier method; premolars exhibited a better performance than molars
SEM	Longitudinal	96.4 100	1.2 0		Quantitative margin analysis; RC = resin cement; GIC = glass-ionomer cement (Ketac-Cem)
Defined criteria for clinical failure	Longitudinal	90 84.9	1 1.3		Kaplan-Meier method; premolars exhibited a better performance than molars

The assessment of 426 Cerec restorations in 142 patients showed a 95% survival rate in a 3-year observation period.[214] Six restorations showed fracture-related failures and four restorations exhibited symptoms of postoperative sensitivity, which made it necessary to replace the restorations. The failure rates between restorations in molars and premolars were not statistically significant, however the ratios (10 failures in 228 molars vs two failures in 198 premolars) indicated a slightly better trend for premolars.

Walther et al[261] reported the findings of a large longitudinal clinical trial in general practice with 1,011 Cerec inlays. Kaplan-Meier estimator revealed a 95% survival probability after 5 years of clinical service. Thirty-nine restorations failed during the observed time period, twenty-one of them because of fracture (fourteen inlay fractures; seven tooth fractures), five because of postoperative sensitivity, seven because of caries formation, and six because of other reasons. While fractures as a cause for failure could be observed equally distributed throughout the observation period, hypersensitivity was limited to the first 24 months. Comparable results with a 94.1% survival rate of Class II Cerec inlays were found in a population of 51 Swedish patients after 5 years.[15]

Reiss and Walther[215] reported an estimated survival probability of 91.6% after a clinical observation period of 7.5 years. Premolars showed better results than molars and vital teeth exhibited significantly less failures than endodontically treated teeth. Ceramic fractures and tooth fractures accounted for most of the failures. These results were confirmed by the 10- and 12-year findings that exhibited a survival rate of 90% and 84.9%,

respectively.[216] Otto[195] published in 1995 the results of a further survey of 100 Cerec restorations made in a general practice in Switzerland and found a survival rate of 98%. Two restored teeth required endodontic treatment and 27% of the involved patients suffered from postoperative sensitivity, which disappeared in most cases after a few weeks.

Zuellig-Singer and Bryant[279] compared Cerec-Vita Mark II (Vita Zahnfabrik) restorations in Class II cavities luted with either three different resin cements or a glass-ionomer cement. After 3 years of service, 100% of the latter were still intact, while one inlay (3.6%) inserted with a composite cement fractured. Heymann et al[77] found a 100% survival of 50 Cerec restorations in 28 patients after 4 years of clinical service. Average cement loss up to 61 μm was detected in the luting gap.

Cast Gold Inlays and Onlays

Limited data are available on the longevity of gold restorations. Usually cast gold restorations tend to be used on patients with excellent oral hygiene, which influences the results of clinical studies significantly.[172] The results of selected clinical studies examining the longevity of cast gold inlays are summarized in Table 16-7. Annual failure rates of cast gold restorations range within 0 to 5.9%.[31,59,67,125,245]

The survival analysis of cast gold inlays in Class II cavities inserted by undergraduate dental students and faculty members in a teaching hospital yielded a mean survival time of 7 years.[31] This result must be considered in light of the varying levels of treatment skills among the operators. Mjör[172] reported in a review article a median survival time of 22 years for small (one-surface) gold restorations and 14 years for large (two- or three-surface) restorations. Bentley and Drake[11] indicated that 95% of cast gold inlays and onlays in an American dental school survived 10 years. A median survival time of 13 years is described for functional gold restorations,[171] which corresponds to the findings of Maryniuk and Kaplan.[161]

Data from selected practices in the US show a median age of 15 years for cast gold restorations.[175] Jokstad et al[102] reported a median age ranging from 15 to 17 years for Class II gold restorations resulting from a comprehensive cross-sectional survey in Scandinavia. These results are comparable to the mean longevity of 18.5 years reported by Burke et al.[24] Smales and Hawthorne[241] indicated a 91% survival rate for cast gold restorations at 10 years and 78% at 15 years of clinical service in an Australian population. Cast gold restorations in Australia (10.6 years) exhibited a much higher survival result than restorations in a Pakistan group (5 years).[143] This may reflect different individual patient factors in developing countries such as poor oral hygiene, a lack of adequate clinical and laboratory facilities, and the general unavailability of fluorides. Stoll et al[245] reported the results of a comprehensive survey of 890 patients with more than 3,000 cast gold restorations at a German dental school and found a 10-year survival rate of 76.1% for Class I restorations, 88.3% for mesio-occlusal (MO), 83.4% for occlusodistal (OD), 87.5% for mesio-occlusodistal (MOD) restorations, and 86.1% for partial crowns. In total, 111 restorations failed because of caries (n = 38), insufficient retention (n = 36), endodontic treatment (n = 33), insufficient mar-

ginal adaptation (n = 3), and tooth extraction (n =1). Statistical analysis revealed no significant difference in longevity between MO and DO inlays, inlays in molars and premolars, and inlays in the maxilla or mandible. However, Stoll et al[245] detected a significantly lower survival rate for occlusal inlays compared with Class II gold restorations and attributed this finding to a higher risk of approximal caries when the inlay is confined to the occlusal surface. Schlösser et al[230] published a very similar survival rate (87.3%) for partial crowns after 9 years, while the findings of Leempoel et al[125] indicated a slightly superior clinical performance with a 96% survival rate after 5 years and 91% after 11 years. Fritz et al[59] found distinctly lower 10-year survival rates: 65% for one-surface, 60% for two-surface, and 68% for three-surface cast gold inlays and 70% for partial crowns. Class I inlays failed significantly more frequently because of formation of caries than all other inlays.

Mjör and Medina[177] reported a median age of 15 to 16 years for 1,689 cast gold restorations. The main reasons for replacement were fracture of tooth (36%) and the formation of secondary caries (22%). Mjör and Medina[177] further reported a median age of 18.5 years for 111 failed cast and compacted gold restorations. Nordbo and Lyngstadaas[189] described a median longevity of 16.5 years for Class II cast gold inlays placed by clinicians with limited experience and 34 years for inlays inserted in a selected practice. These results are comparable to a study in Australia, indicating a mean survival time of 13.8 years for gold castings and 8.3 years for the 75th quartile.[72]

As a result of a 7-year controlled clinical trial, Donly et al[40] described a failure rate

271

Table 16-7 Longevity of cast gold inlays and onlays

Year of publication	First author	Observation period (y)	Black class	Restorative materials	Restorations (n)	Patients (n)
1981	Crabb[31]	10	II	Gold	146	
1985	Leempoel[125]	5	Partial crown	Gold	895	
		11	Partial crown			
		5	Crown		785	
		11	Crown			
1986	Bentley[11]	10	I and II	Gold	173	
			Crown		295	
1992	Fritz[59]	10	I	Gold	2,717	548
			II (2-surface)			
			II (3-surface)			
			Partial crown			
1992	Haas[67]	5	Inlays	Gold (RC)	30	
				Gold (CC)	30	
1993	Mjör[177]		Cast gold restorations	Gold	1,689	
1993	Schlösser[230]	9	Partial crown	Gold	725	
			Crown		390	
1994	Jokstad[102]	> 10	II	Gold	> 250	
1994	Mahmood[143]	> 12		Gold	120 (P)	
					80 (A)	
1996	Pelka[198]	> 10	Inlays and onlays	Gold	520	56
1996	Smales[241]	15	I and II	Gold	96	
1997	Hawthorne[72]		I and II	Gold	49	
1999	Donly[40]	7	Inlays	Gold	11	18
			Onlays		7	
1999	Stoll[245]	10	I	Gold	171	890
			II (MO)		294	
			II (OD)		427	
			II (MOD)		862	
			Partial crown		1,679	

Method	Study design	Survival rate (%)	Annual failure rate (%)	Median survival time (y)	Remarks
Defined criteria for clinical failure	Cross-sectional	41.1	5.9	7	
		96	0.8		Kaplan-Meier-estimator
		91	0.8		
		99	0.2		
		97	0.3		
	Cross-sectional	95	0.5		Life table method
		89	1.1		
	Cross-sectional	65	3.5		Kaplan-Meier estimator; main reason for failure: caries (42%), need for endodontic therapy (18%)
		60	4		
		68	3.2		
		70	3		
Defined criteria for clinical failure	Longitudinal	100	0		No difference between adhesively inserted (RC) inlays and conventionally cemented (CC) inlays
		100	0		
	Cross-sectional			15–16	Main reasons for failure: tooth fracture, recurrent caries
	Cross-sectional	87.3	1.3		Life-table method
		92.1	0.9		
	Cross-sectional			15–17	
Defined criteria for clinical failure	Cross-sectional			5	Study conducted in Pakistan (P) and Australia (A)
				10.6	
Modified USPHS criteria	Cross-sectional	94.6			Premolars performed better than molars and small restorations better than large restorations
	Cross-sectional	78	1.5		
Defined criteria for clinical failure	Cross-sectional			13.8	Life-table method
Modified USPHS criteria	Longitudinal	81.8	2.6		Main failure reasons: secondary caries and fracture
		85.7	2		
Defined criteria for clinical failure	Cross-sectional	76.1	2.4		Kaplan-Meier estimator; main reasons for failure: caries, insufficient retention, endodontic treatment
		88.3	1.2		
		83.4	1.7		
		87.5	1.3		
		86.1	1.4		

of 18.2% and 14.3% for cast gold inlays and onlays, respectively. Haas et al[67] compared two modes of cementation on the clinical performance of 60 cast gold inlays. Half of the inlays were conventionally cemented with zinc oxide phosphate cement, the other 30 restorations were treated with the Silicoater system and subsequently adhesively inserted with a resin cement. After 5 years of clinical service, both groups showed 100% survival rates with no differences between the cementation modes. Pelka et al[198] evaluated the quality of 520 gold inlays and onlays in 56 patients and described a success rate of 94.6%. Restorations with more than three surfaces involved and molars showed distinctly lower ratings.

Longevity of Anterior Restorations (Class III and IV)

Despite the nearly universal use of composite resins as a restorative material for anterior teeth, there is only a limited number of investigations on the long-term clinical performance in such situations available.[103] The results of selected clinical studies are summarized in Table 16-8. Annual failure rates of anterior composite restorations range within 0% to 11.6%.[36,103,168,203,217,240,257]

Paterson[197] reported in 1984 a 50% survival time of 4.5 years for Adaptic (Johnson & Johnson Dental Products Ltd, East Windsor, NJ) and Prisma-Fil (Dentsply) composite restorations in Class III and IV cavities. Qvist et al[210] found a 7-year median survival time of Class III composite restorations in Denmark. Jokstad et al[102]

reported a median age of 9 years for Class III composite restorations and 7 years for Class IV defects as a result of a cross-sectional survey of dental practitioners in Scandinavia. However, the results of Burke et al[24] indicated a mean longevity of only 5 years for Class III and 3.9 years for Class IV composite restorations in the United Kingdom. The results of an 11-year assessment of 104 Class III composite restorations showed a survival rate of 84%.[211] Earlier follow-up assessments of these restorations showed a gradual deterioration of the clinical quality over time, with 100% optimal ratings at baseline, 60% at 2 years, 55% at 4 years, 40% at 6 years, and approximately 20% optimal scores at the 11-year recall. Smales and Hawthorne[241] reported a survival rate of 72% after 10 years and 54.6% after 15 years for Class III composite restorations in Australia. In an earlier study, Smales et al[237] reported a median survival time of 7.9 years for anterior composite restorations, and 16.2 years and 3.4 years for the 25% and 75% quartile, respectively. The comparison of the median longevity of anterior composite restorations in Pakistan (8 years) with those assessed in Australia (6 to 7 years) showed a slightly better performance for the restorations in Pakistan.[143]

Jokstad et al[103] reported the 10-year clinical performance of the microfilled composite Silar (3M) and of the macrofiller Concise (3M) in anterior restorations and found a survival rate of 80% and 95%, respectively. A higher number of microfilled composite restorations were replaced because of recurrent caries compared with macrofilled restorations. The increased proportion of organic matrix in Silar results in a lower modulus of elasticity and a higher coefficient of thermal expansion.

These material properties are related to increased potential for microleakage and secondary caries.[202] A 5-year study of four types of anterior composites reported a survival rate of 87% for Class III restorations and only 42% for high-stress Class IV restorations, a statistically significant difference.[240] The restorations of all four composite materials deteriorated at slightly different rates for different clinical criteria with time, but most of the changes were slight. Hawthorne and Smales[72] reported composite restoration survival times derived from life-table estimates being 34.4 years for the 25th quartile, 16.7 years for the 50th quartile, and 7.9 years for the 75th quartile for three private dental practices in Australia. Pieper et al[203] investigated 239 Class III and Class IV composite restorations and found a failure rate of 7.1% after 2 to 4 years, 10.8% after 5 to 8 years, and 10.5% after 9 to 11 years of service.

Reusens et al[217] compared the clinical performance of a microfilled composite (Silux Plus, 3M) and a hybrid composite (Herculite XRV) over a 2-year period and found a 100% survival rate for both materials with a significantly higher rate of marginal discoloration for the microfiller (48% vs 78% Alpha ratings). De Araujo et al[36] confirmed the excellent clinical behavior of Herculite XRV and reported a survival rate of 100% for the composite and also 100% for a glass-ionomer cement in Class III cavities after 2 years. However, the composite exhibited significantly more Alpha ratings in terms of color match and esthetic appearance. Van Djiken[259] compared a resin-modified glass ionomer (Fuji II LC, GC), a compomer (Dyract, Dentsply), and a composite resin (Pekafill, Bayer, Dormagen, Germany) after 5 years in Class III cavities and found a significantly better clinical performance for the two latter materials.

Short-term results for compomer materials in Class III cavities are encouraging with 98% to 100% survival rate for up to 3 years.[12,206,257] However, these results need to be confirmed by further observations over a longer time period.

Longevity of Cervical Restorations (Class V)

The results of selected clinical studies reporting the long-term behavior of restorations in cervical lesions are summarized in Table 16-9. Annual failure rates for Class V restorations are reported in a wide range, from 0% to 26%.[1,2,21,22,25,66,183,187,206,231]

Crabb[31] reported in 1981 a median survival time of 9 years for amalgam in Class V lesions. The results of a comprehensive cross-sectional survey conducted by Jokstad et al[102] indicated a median age of 11 years for amalgam and 6 years for composite restorations in Class V defects. Qvist et al[210] reported an 8-year median survival time for amalgam and 5 years for composite in Class V restorations. These results are completed by the observations of Burke et al,[24] who found for amalgam, composite, and glass ionomer a mean survival time of 7.0, 4.6, and 3.2 years, respectively. This trend toward a higher survival rate for amalgam (73.2%) compared with composite (57.1%) in cervical lesions could be confirmed by a 6-year longitudinal study by Kamann and Gängler.[104]

A substantial number of Class V restorations are inserted in noncarious,

Table 16-8 Longevity of anterior restorations (Class III and IV) (GI = glass-ionomer cement; RMGI = resin-modified glass ionomer)

Year of publication	First author	Observation period (y)	Black class	Restorative materials	Restorations (n)	Patients (n)
1984	Paterson[197]	6	III and IV	Adaptic, Prisma-Fil (composites)	130	
1990	Qvist[210]		III	Composite resins (not specified)		
1991	Pieper[203]	9–11	III and IV	Composite resins (not specified)	239	
1991	Smales[237]	15	III and IV	Adaptic, Concise, Nuva-Fil, Silar (composites)	1,770	
1992	Smales[240]	5	III IV	Concise, Silar, Estic Miradapt (composites)	340 38	86
1993	Qvist[211]	11	III	Silar (composite)	104	35
1994	Jokstad[102]	> 10	III IV	Composite resins (not specified)	1,461 72	
1994	Jokstad[103]	10	III and IV	Concise (composite) Silar (composite)	118	57
1994	Mahmood[143]	12	III and IV	Composite resins (not specified)	109 (P) 200 (A)	
1996	Smales[241]	15	III	Composite resins (not specified)	284	
1996	van Dijken[257]	3	III	Pekafill (composite) Dyract (compomer) Fuji II LC (RMGI)	56 52 44	
1997	Benz[13]	0.5	III	Tetric (composite) Compoglass (compomer) Dyract (compomer)	26 16 15	
1997	Hawthorne[72]		III and IV	Composite resins (not specified)	341	
1997	Millar[168]	8	III and IV	Opalux (composite)	28	24
1998	de Araujo[36]	2	III	Chelon-Fil (GI) Herculite XRV (composite)	21 21	21
1998	Prati[206]	3	III	Dyract (compomer)	23	
1999	Burke[24]		III IV	Composite resins (not specified)	243 151	
1999	Reusens[217]	2	III	Silux Plus (composite) Herculite XRV (composite)	28 28	28

Method	Study design	Survival rate (%)	Annual failure rate (%)	Median survival time (y)	Remarks
Defined criteria for clinical failure	Cross-sectional			4.5	
Defined criteria for clinical failure	Cross-sectional			7	
Modified USPHS criteria	Cross-sectional	89.5	1–1.2		
Defined criteria for clinical failure	Cross-sectional			7.9	
Defined criteria for clinical failure	Longitudinal	87 42	2.6 11.6		Higher failure rate for Class IV restorations; no significant difference among the materials
Modified USPHS criteria	Longitudinal	84	1.5		Main reasons for replacement: secondary caries, marginal discrepancies, discoloration
	Cross-sectional			9 7	
USPHS criteria	Longitudinal	95 80	0.5 2		The macrofilled composite Concise showed a better performance than the microfilled Silar
Defined criteria for clinical failure	Cross-sectional			7.9 6.6	Study conducted in Pakistan (P) and Australia (A)
	Cross-sectional	54.6	3		
Modified USPHS criteria	Longitudinal	100 98 98	0 0.7 0.7		
Modified USPHS criteria	Longitudinal	100 100 100			
Defined criteria for clinical failure	Cross-sectional			16.7	Life-table method
Modified USPHS criteria	Longitudinal	73	3.4		
Modified USPHS criteria	Longitudinal	100 100	0 0		Composite exhibited significantly more Alpha ratings for color match than the GI
Modified USPHS criteria	Longitudinal	100	0		
	Cross-sectional			5.0 3.9	
Modified USPHS criteria	Longitudinal	100 100	0 0		Significantly more marginal discoloration for Silux Plus

Table 16-9 Longevity of cervical restorations (Class V). GI = glass ionomer cement; RMGI = resin-modified glass ionomer

Year of publication	First author	Observation period (y)	Black class	Restorative materials	Restorations (n)	Patients (n)
1981	Crabb[31]	10	V	Amalgam (alloys not specified, gamma-2 alloys)	219	
1986	Mount[183]	7	V	ASPA (GI)	306	
				Fuji II (GI)	191	
				Ketac-Fil (GI)	421	
1986	Ngo[187]	1	V	Ketac-Fil (GI)	30	
1990	Qvist[210]		V	Amalgam		
				Composite		
1994	Jokstad[101]	> 10	V	Amalgam	1,045	
				Composite	580	
1995	Barnes[8]	1	V	Variglass (RMGI) nret	75	31
				Variglass (RMGI) ret	31	17
				Prisma APH (composite) nret	32	25
1996	Matis[162]	10	V	Ketac-Fil (GI) fi	18	18
				Ketac-Fil (GI) fd	18	
				Chelon-Fil (GI)	18	
				Cervident (composite)	18	
1996	Smales[241]	10	V	Amalgam, posterior	270	
				Composite, anterior	96	
				Glass ionomer, anterior	69	
				Glass ionomer, posterior	117	
1997	Abdalla[2]	2	V	Compoglass (compomer)	28	
				Dyract (compomer)	29	
				Fuji II LC (RMGI)	28	
				Vitremer (RMGI)	29	
1997	Abdalla[1]	2	V	Dyract (compomer)	18	
				Fuji II LC (RMGI)	20	
				Photac-Fil (RMGI)	17	
				Vitremer (RMGI)	18	
1997	Jedynakiewicz[98]	3	V	Dyract (compomer)	54	

Method	Study design	Survival rate (%)	Annual failure rate (%)	Median survival time (y)	Remarks
Defined criteria for clinical failure	Cross-sectional	41.1	5.9	9	
Defined criteria for clinical failure	Longitudinal	85.3	2.1		
		95.8	0.6		
		97.9	0.3		
Defined criteria for clinical failure		86.7	13.3		Erosion/abrasion lesions; main reason for failure: loss of retention
Defined criteria for clinical failure	Cross-sectional			8	
				5	
	Cross-sectional			11	
				6	
Modified USPHS criteria	Longitudinal	97.1	2.9		nret = nonretentive erosive lesions; ret = retentive Class V cavities
		100	0		
		96.4	3.6		
Modified USPHS criteria	Longitudinal	83	1.7		Erosion/abrasion lesions; no tooth preparations; each patient received 4 restorations; fi = finished immediately; fd = finished after delay
		78	2.2		
		67	3.3		
		17	8.3		
	Cross-sectional	70.2	3		
		69.9	3		
		84.1	1.6		
		78.7	2.1		
Modified USPHS criteria		100	0		
		100	0		
		100	0		
		100	0		
Modified USPHS criteria		100	0		
		100	0		
		94	3		
		100	0		
		98	0.7		

Table 16-9 (continued)

Year of publication	First author	Observation period (y)	Black class	Restorative materials	Restorations (n)	Patients (n)
1997	Loher[137]	1.3	V	Tetric (composite)	33	37
				Dyract (compomer)	83	
				Fuji II LC (RMGI)	51	
				Photac-Fil (RMGI)	31	
1997	Schuster[231]	1	V	Compoglass (compomer)	24	
				Dyract (compomer)	46	
1998	Burrow[25]	1	V	Composite and RMGI	95	
1998	Folwaczny[49]	3	V	Tetric (composite)	33	37
				Dyract (compomer)	83	
				Fuji II LC (RMGI)	51	
				Photac-Fil (RMGI)	31	
1998	Gladys[66]	1.5	V	HiFi Master (GI)	33	86
				Fuji II LC (RMGI)	30	
				Vitremer (RMGI)	30	
				Experimental (RMGI))	62	
				Dyract (compomer)	32	
1998	Prati[206]	3	V	Dyract (compomer)	57	
1998	Tyas[255]	1	V	Dyract (compomer)	36	
1999	Brackett[22]	1	V	Fuji II LC (RMGI)	31	
				Compoglass (compomer)	31	
1999	Brackett[21]	2	V	Ketac-Fil (GI)	29	
				Photac-Fil (RMGI)	29	
1999	Burke[24]		V	Amalgam	115	
				Composite	101	
				Glass ionomer	130	
1999	Kamann[104]	6	V	Luxalloy (amalgam)	56	
				Durafill (composite)	56	
1999	Oberländer[191]	1	V	Dyract (compomer)	40	20
				Hytac (compomer)	40	

Method	Study design	Survival rate (%)	Annual failure rate (%)	Median survival time (y)	Remarks
Modified USPHS criteria	Longitudinal	100	0		Mixed Class V cavities
		94	4.6		
		93	5.4		
		90	7.7		
Modified USPHS criteria		92	8		Marginal discoloration:
		74	26		Dyract 23%, Compoglass 14%
Modified USPHS criteria	Longitudinal	98	2		
Modified USPHS criteria	Longitudinal	93	2.3		Mixed Class V cavities
		83.3	5.6		
		66.7	11.1		
		60	13.3		
Modified USPHS criteria and SEM	Longitudinal	97	2		Unprepared cavities;
		100	0		all materials showed
		100	0		microleakage over time
		96	2.7		
		89	7.3		
Modified USPHS criteria	Longitudinal	100	0		
		97	3		22% marginal discoloration
Modified USPHS criteria		100	0		Main reasons for failure: loss of
		74	26		retention, recurrent caries
Modified USPHS criteria	Longitudinal	93	3.5		
		93	3.5		
	Cross-sectional			7.0	
				4.6	
				3.2	
Defined criteria for clinical failure	Longitudinal	73.2	4.5		Main reason for composite
		57.1	7.2		replacement: loss of retention
Modified USPHS criteria and SEM	Longitudinal	100	0		Softstart polymerization;
		100	0		no significant differences in
					marginal integrity between
					Hytac and Dyract

nonretentive cavities, which favors the use of composite and glass-ionomer materials because no macromechanical retention is required with the use of these materials. Smales and Hawthorne[241] differentiated between anterior and posterior Class V restorations in a large cross-sectional study in Australia. They found for glass-ionomer materials after 10 years a 84.1% survival rate for anterior restorations and 78.7% for posterior Class V cavities. Anterior composite restorations exhibited a 69.9% survival rate after 10 years and 59.2% after 15 years, while posterior amalgam restorations had survival rates of 70.2% and 62.1%, respectively. However, Ngo and Mount[187] stated a much worse performance for Ketac-Fil (ESPE) glass-ionomer restorations in erosion/abrasion lesions. They reported a 13.7% failure after 1 year mainly because of loss of retention.

Brackett et al[22] and Schuster et al[231] reported after 1 year of clinical service a 26% failure of compomer restorations in cervical lesions. Adverse storage conditions for the material and nonuse of rubber dam were discussed as possible causes for this catastrophic failure rate. Other investigators found in studies of up to 3 years survival rates for compomers between 97% and 100%.[1,2,98,255]

Barnes et al[8] compared the clinical performance of composite restorations in nonretentive, noncarious Class V lesions with a resin-modified glass ionomer (RMGI) and the same RMGI in retentively prepared Class V cavities. After 1 year, survival rates of 96.4%, 97.1%, and 100%, respectively, were recorded. No significant difference existed among the retention rates of the different types of restorations.

Matis et al[162] described the findings of a 10-year study investigating the success of a composite and glass-ionomer cement in erosive/abrasive Class V cavities without tooth preparation. Patients with at least four cervical lesions received one restoration of each of the following: Ketac-Fil, finished immediately after placement; Ketac-Fil, finished after a 24-hour delay; Chelon-Fil (ESPE), finished immediately; and Cervident composite (SS White, Lakewood, NJ). The recorded survival rates were 83%, 78%, 67%, and 17%, respectively. All the glass-ionomer restorations exhibited a significantly greater retention than Cervident.

Oberländer et al[191] compared the clinical performance of two compomer materials in both erosive/abrasive Class V lesions and Class V cavities after caries excavation with and without softstart polymerization.[165] After 1 year, all restorations were in function with no significant differences between the different treatment modes having been found. Hawthorne and Smales[72] reported a survival time of 11.3 years for the 75th quartile for glass ionomers in cervical defects in three private dental practices in Australia. Gladys et al[66] investigated the clinical performance and marginal adaptation of a conventional glass-ionomer cement (HiFi Master, Shofu), three resin-modified glass ionomers (Fuji II LC; Vitremer, 3M; exp. Material), and one compomer (Dyract) over a period of 18 months. The survival rates of the glass ionomer–derived materials were 97%, 100%, 100%, and 96% respectively. Dyract was applied using a non-etch procedure and realized an 89% survival rate only. Similar results were reported by Loher et al[137] who, 15 months after placement, found a success rate of 100% for Tetric composite restorations, 94% for Dyract, 93% for Fuji II LC, and 90% for the resin-modified glass ionomer Photac-Fil (ESPE) in mixed Class V cavities. The restorations exhibited a slight deterioration at the 2-year follow-up assessment.[137] At the 3-year recall, these restorations demonstrated survival rates of 93%, 83.3%, 66.7%, and 60%, respectively.[49] The resin-modified glass-ionomer restorative materials (Fuji II LC, Photac-Fil) exhibited a distinct deterioration during the period of clinical service. In contrast, Prati et al[206] found a 100% survival rate after 3 years for Class V restorations of Dyract in nonretentive cavities.

Discussion

Amalgam Restorations

Amalgam is considered to be a restorative material with low technique sensitivity, favorable mechanical properties, and good clinical performance over time.[171] Secondary caries, a high incidence of bulk and tooth fracture, cervical overhang, and marginal degradation have been reported as the main problems limiting the survival of amalgam restorations.[24,34,74,101,102,131,132,169,170,176,178,180,237,274]

However, the assessment of secondary caries at the margins of a restoration, an important aspect of quality evaluation, is a more complex procedure than generally assumed. The rating system is simple in that it has only two ratings: "caries" or "no caries." But in order to obtain consistency in the rating of secondary caries, it is crucial that a thorough calibration of the examiners precedes the clinical study.[226] The necessity of this calibration is obvious on reviewing the findings of a study published by Merrett and Elderton[166] in which nine dentists examined 228 teeth. One

dentist scored "caries" in 11 teeth, while another diagnosed "caries" in 54 teeth.

The zinc and copper content of the alloy has been found to have a strong impact on the survival rates of amalgam restorations because it influences the corrosion resistance of the amalgam.[133] High-copper amalgams have higher survival rates than conventional amalgams.[132,133]

In contrast to the adhesive capabilities with modern composite systems, the lack of adhesive stabilization of the hard tooth tissues in combination with amalgam frequently results in the fracture of restored teeth. Large amalgam restorations exhibit more deterioration than moderate- and small-sized restorations.[273] Several authors have emphasized that, despite the low technique sensitivity of amalgam, the majority of amalgam failures result from the poor technical skill of the dentist combined with faulty cavity preparation, rather than from failure of the amalgam itself.[42,74,124,275]

Direct Posterior Composite Restorations

The reasons for the limited periods of clinical service of direct composite restorations have changed significantly.[199] Insufficient wear characteristics resulting in loss of anatomic form and interproximal contacts with general degradation were the main problems in the 1970s and early 1980s.[128] Improvements in the filler technology and construction of composite materials have resulted in changes in reasons for restoration replacement, as well as the increasing trend to insert composite restorations in stress-bearing areas of posterior teeth.[227] Wear, fracture of the

283

restorations, marginal deterioration, discoloration, and secondary caries are now the principal modes of failure and reasons for limitations in the longevity of resin-based composites.[63,40,174,178,180,188,228,237,274] Microfilled composites showed more fracture-related failures, especially in high-stress Class II cavities, compared with hybrid composites because of their inferior mechanical properties. The relatively high incidence of secondary caries associated with the composite resin restorations may be explained on the basis of microbiologic studies that indicate a significantly higher proportion of *Streptococcus mutans* at the cavity margins of composites compared with amalgam and glass-ionomer restorations.[178,248] Furthermore, the efficacy of older generation dentin bonding agents limited the marginal quality of composite restorations, in particular when cavity finish lines were within dentin. Despite the dramatic improvements in the formulation of newer generation bonding agents with enhanced marginal adaptation and bond strengths, a perfect marginal seal is still not achievable. Premolars generally offer more favorable conditions for composite restorations than do molars.[63,226,228] Cavities are tending to become smaller and, as a consequence, the effect of the chewing forces is less intense. In addition, the knowledge and understanding of newer materials, notably adhesive systems, which are very susceptible to variations in handling and application, has improved. The possibility of effective tooth care in this area of the mouth is also better. Daily cleaning procedures by the patient, as well as professional care executed by dentists and dental hygienists, can be performed and controlled more efficiently and effectively.

Negative effects of polymerization shrinkage have often been cited, in addition to wear, as being common causes of failure of direct posterior composite restorations.[10,123,128,141,222] An inherent weakness of composite resin restorations has been attributed to the organic matrix component.[108] In the past 30 years there have been no fundamental changes in the monomer systems since the introduction of dimethacrylates (Bis-GMA) by Bowen in 1962.[156] With the introduction of the first ormocer-based composite restorative material in 1998, a novel inorganic-organic copolymer matrix emerged in dentistry. Photochemically curable methacrylate groups are linked to an inorganic Si-O-Si network by covalent atomic bonds.[154,276-278] Following incorporation of filler particles, the ormocer composites can be manipulated like a hybrid composite. Currently only two ormocer systems are available (Definite, Degussa, Hanau, Germany and Admira, Voco, Cuxhaven, Germany). Laboratory trials exhibited excellent wear rates and a promising marginal quality for the ormocer materials.[9,120,147,154,156] Ongoing clinical trials are needed to determine the in vivo performance of the ormocer-based restorative materials, together with the clinical behavior of the recently introduced group of high-viscosity packable composites. A comprehensive assessment of these materials is not possible at present, given the limited data available.

The use of beta-quartz glass-ceramic inserts in combination with direct composite restorations was intended to reduce the clinical problems related to the resin matrix component of composite materials.[235] The placement of large volumes of composite is avoided by the insertion of inorganic megafiller inserts.[18,19,43] The maximum advantage with this approach can be achieved when a composite restoration contains the largest volume of insert possible, reducing polymerization contraction stresses and lowering the effects of thermal expansion.[23,119,121] The literature, however, includes conflicting views on the effects that prefabricated inserts have on the general wear of composite restorations. While Kawai and Leinfelder[107] reported that inserts have only limited influence on the wear of the surrounding composite but may be helpful to maintain functional occlusion, Ishikawa et al[96] suggested that glass-ceramic inserts are effective in reducing the wear of composites. Flessa et al[48] observed a trend for lower wear in direct composite restorations with beta-quartz glass-ceramic inserts compared to restorations without inserts; the results, however, were not statistically significant. Little information is available to date on the clinical performance of direct composite restorations reinforced with megafiller inserts. Two clinical studies provided promising results,[108,138] while a 3-year follow-up study[235] reported only 69% satisfactory insert-reinforced composite restorations. The latter study reported the loss of several inserts while the composite restorative material still covered the cavity walls, indicating a bond failure between the insert and the composite. Care has to be taken to avoid contamination of the presilaned surfaces of the inserts. It is also recommended that "try-in" inserts be employed when determining the size of the insert to be used.[121] These clinical data are based on a very limited number of investigations and more detailed information on the long-term clinical performance of insert restorations is required.

Glass-Ionomer Cements as Posterior Restorative Materials

Glass-ionomer cements have certain advantageous properties,[85] such as sustained fluoride release, chemical bonding to tooth substance, and biocompatibility. These materials are not, however, considered to possess adequate mechanical properties for general use as definitive restorations in stress-bearing situations in posterior teeth.[82,83,171,175,178,184,267] Many glass-ionomer restorations failed because of bulk fractures due to their low mechanical strength.[84,112,150,178] Silver particles sintered into the glass-ionomer powder particles increase the strength and radiopacity[163]; however, metal-reinforced glass-ionomer cements (cermet) are not suitable as a long-term restorative material for use in Class II cavities.[32,78,112,178]

In contrast to expectations and despite the release of fluoride ions, secondary caries surprisingly has been found to be the main reason for the clinical failure of glass-ionomer restorations.[24,71,179,180,274] The release of fluoride ions has been anticipated to reduce the incidence of secondary caries,[187,267] although the fluoride concentration required to establish a long-term anticariogenic effect has not been established. The longevity of glass-ionomer restorations is furthermore dependent on the use of appropriate clinical techniques because these materials tend to be rather technique sensitive, especially with respect to water adsorption and dehydration.[84,249]

For patients with small approximal lesions and intact marginal ridges free of cracks and opacities, glass-ionomer cements have been suggested as suitable for the restoration of Class I and Class II tunnel preparations.[70,71,249] The tunnel preparation technique is a conservative approach to the treatment of approximal lesions. Caries is removed via the occlusal surface through an occlusal tunnel preparation.[92,93,196] Unless the approximal surface is cavitated, it is considered better to preserve the demineralized enamel wall because fluoride leaching from a glass-ionomer restorative material may contribute to remineralization.[50,267] However, a high failure rate has been recorded for such an approach when treating patients with high caries activity, large initial lesions, and tunnel restorations that do not reach the approximal surface.[246]

Composite Inlays and Onlays

Many of the problems associated with the direct placement of large posterior composite restorations can be overcome by the use of an indirect composite inlay technique. It has been concluded that composite inlays are a favorable, longer-lasting alternative to direct plastic composite restorations in large Class II situations.[256] Indications for esthetic inlays include teeth in which strengthening of the remaining structure is indicated, the cavity is free from marked undercuts, and the patients are regular attenders requesting tooth-colored restorations in posterior teeth.[23,81] Strict patient and case selection, ie, frequent attenders with a good standard of oral hygiene and cavities that allow adequate moisture control, will increase the longevity of adhesive inlays.

The indirect technique allows the production of restorations in the laboratory with appropriate proximal contours and contacts and control of anatomic form.

Polymerization shrinkage is limited to the width of the lute space. Post-curing the inlay with heat, pressure, and/or light increases the degree of conversion through an annealing process, improving the mechanical properties of the composite and resulting in a better wear resistance.[23,37,47,52,192,213,262,264] Several authors have indicated that premolars offer more favorable conditions for indirect composite restorations than do molars.[40,226,228] A premolar restoration is subjected to much less occlusal stress than a molar restoration, the access for dental treatment is easier, and oral hygiene measures are more easily controlled by the patient.

Ceramic Inlays and Onlays

The use of all-ceramic restorations was mainly limited to anterior teeth until high-strength reinforced ceramic materials and new processing techniques were introduced approximately two decades ago.[233] Bulk fracture is a relatively frequent cause of failure of ceramic inlays.[97,176,207,233,234,247,261] The risk of fracture of a ceramic inlay depends, among other factors, on the strength of the material. The fracture properties of the ceramic are important for the longevity of the restoration. Ceramic materials are brittle and are susceptible to failure in tensile mode while their resistance to compressive stresses is high. Flaws at internal or external surfaces are in many cases the origin of cracks that can propagate and lead to catastrophic failure.[26,159] Other important factors, such as the design of the cavity preparation, the shape of the restoration, a minimum thickness of 1.5 mm, and internal fit, influence the strength of the ceramic restoration.[227,233] Strict case selection, avoiding the placement of ceramic inlays in bruxists and situations that require crowns, increases the probability for ceramic inlay success.[28,69]

The fit of ceramic restorations, especially the fit of CAD/CAM-manufactured ceramic inlays, has been controversial.[106,129,233] Laboratory studies have indicated that indirect ceramic inlays have a better marginal fit than direct Cerec inlays.[251] After adhesive cementation of Cerec restorations, however, a clinically acceptable marginal adaptation has been observed in several in vivo studies.[86,87,195,251] A major problem associated with the Cerec system is the high frequency of rough surfaces in the restorations.[232] In the improved Cerec 2 system, the operating software provides for the milling of a central groove in the occlusal section of the restoration. This facility has been enhanced in the Cerec 3 system launched in January 2000. However, adjustment and shaping of the occlusal anatomy after adhesive cementation is still the most time-consuming element of the CAD/CAM restorative procedure. Rough ceramic surfaces following occlusal adjustment require meticulous finishing that is often difficult to carry out with appropriate accuracy in the mouth.[232]

Cerec cavity preparations, especially for the Cerec 1 system, are different from preparations necessary for laboratory-made ceramic inlays. This difference may affect the clinical outcome.[225] In general, preparation dimensions have an important influence on the fracture resistance of all-ceramic restorations.[159,250,261] Failure to achieve necessary cavity dimensions may contribute more to failure by fracture than does the nature of the ceramic system.[88]

Hypersensitivity is a complication frequently encountered after the luting of an adhesive inlay.[60,79,195,232,251] The risk of postplacement hypersensitivity has been attributed to the method of luting and could be significantly reduced by improved dentin bonding agents and resin cements, as well as the meticulous use of recommended techniques and avoidance of tooth desiccation.[116,195,250]

Cast Gold Inlays and Onlays

Compared with other restorations for posterior teeth, cast gold restorations are considered to be costly but long-lasting.[245] The relative cost factor of gold restorations has been calculated to be 3.8 to 6.3 times that of amalgam restorations.[172,241] Gold restorations are, however, considered to be the most durable restorations for posterior teeth.[27] Tooth fracture, marginal defects, insufficient retention, and secondary caries are main reasons for the failure of cast gold inlays.[176,177,245] If the size of a lesion requires the replacement of one or more cusps, gold onlays or partial crowns are still an excellent method to achieve tooth restoration, despite the possibilities offered by adhesively bonded all-ceramic restorations. Smales and Hawthorne[241] found that posterior cast gold restorations had significantly greater longevity than cuspal replacement amalgam restorations.

Anterior Restorations (Class III and IV)

Qvist et al[210] reported secondary caries as the most frequent reason for the replacement of tooth-colored Class III restorations. Loose or lost and fractured restorations were frequent reasons for the failure of Class IV restorations in addition to the formation of recurrent caries. More Class IV restorations were observed to have failed than Class III restorations.[168,240] Class IV defects present a high tensile and flexural stress situation that challenges the physical properties of the restorative material, as well as the bond strength to the underlying enamel and dentin. Microfilled materials were, in particular, reported to be unsuitable for the restoration of Class IV lesions, despite their excellent esthetics. Cohesive chip fractures were observed by several authors.[39,122,240,253]

Short-term results indicate good clinical performance for glass ionomers and compomers in Class III cavities, however, resin-based composites were still superior when compared with glass ionomers in terms of color stability and esthetics.[36] Composite materials exhibit a smoother surface than do glass ionomers as a consequence of small porosities and larger filler particles within the glass-ionomer cement. In addition, composites have a better translucency when compared with glass ionomers.[20,164]

Cervical Restorations (Class V)

Glass ionomers, hybrid ionomers, compomers, and composite resins are widely used to restore Class V defects.[2,134,260] Amalgam and gold restorations have been used in such situations in the past but are now rarely seen because of alleged adverse health effects related to the release of mercury from amalgam restorations and, more importantly, esthetic shortcomings.[84] Composite resins and compomers in combination with the acid-etch technique and adhesive systems have

already replaced glass ionomers and hybrid ionomers to a great extent for the restoration of cervical lesions because of their excellent esthetics, superior mechanical and physical properties, significantly reduced susceptibility to bulk fracture, and higher bond strengths to enamel and dentin.[2,65,83,135,150,152,191] The various bonding systems have a crucial impact on the retention rate and marginal adaptation of restorations of composite and compomer materials.[206] Retention, marginal integrity, and marginal discoloration are closely related to the adhesion of the material along dentinal and enamel margins. Although the formulation of compomers is very similar to that of composite resins,[83] it was initially claimed that etching of enamel was unnecessary for compomers.[206] The use of acidic modified monomers and the addition of mild organic acids to the formulation of compomer bonding agents should assure sufficient adhesion to tooth substrates. Meanwhile, many studies have shown that etching of enamel and dentin results in considerably better adhesion with higher bond strengths and less gap formation.[30,68,148,149,152,220]

The complex morphology of Class V defects with margins in enamel as well as in root dentin presents a challenge for the restorative material. When a noninvasive procedure is indicated, glass-ionomer cements have an excellent clinical performance, notably in noncarious lesions, given their long-term retention values.[162] However, they do not possess either convenient handling properties or esthetic qualities to satisfy the current demands of patients and dentists.[21,192] Since their introduction in 1993, compomers have grown in importance as a substitute for glass-ionomer cements. The ease of handling of compomers is probably the main reason for their wide acceptance by practitioners.[152,153]

Loss of retention is a frequent cause for the failure of nonretentive Class V restorations.[183,187] Other restorations tend to be in preparations with mechanical undercuts in sound tooth structure and are therefore less likely to fail. Tooth flexure as a result of occlusal stresses may rupture the bond between tooth and restorative material,[255] especially if the restoration does not flex in the same way as the tooth. Thus, it has been suggested that the elastic modulus of a cervical restorative material should be similar to that of dentin.[76] Normally, the strength of the bond between glass-ionomer cements and clean tooth surfaces is sufficient to withstand typical clinical stress if the restoration is not under direct occlusal load. However, sclerotic dentin, which is often associated with abrasion lesions, presents unfavorable conditions for the adhesion of restorative materials.[8] Conditioning the surfaces of the cavity with polyacrylic acid prior to the placement of a glass-ionomer restoration increases the bond strengths. In such situations, cohesive failures, rather than adhesive failures, have been observed more frequently.[184]

The high incidence of marginal discoloration in Class V compomer restorations has been attributed in several studies to the lack of use of the acid-etch technique.[6,136,231,255]

Clinical Trials: Design, Variables, and Statistical Analysis

Clinical trials of restorative materials are major investigations in terms of time commitment, numbers of investigators involved, and associated research costs.[45] For these reasons, clinical trials tend to be time-limited and long-term observations are relatively rare. Although controlled longitudinal, prospective studies are best when the longevity of restorations is to be studied, it is unrealistic to expect such investigations to exceed 10 years.[171] Cross-sectional, retrospective studies based on records in dental practices present a suitable alternative approach to determining the survival of a large number of restorations.

Studies on the longevity of dental restorations are subjective and based on the individual clinician's opinion as to what is acceptable or unacceptable.[170] Handling of a dental restorative material under ideal circumstances produces a restoration that can last for many years. However, the longevity of the restoration is dependent upon many factors,[80] some of which are related to the practitioner, including level of expertise, experience, manual skills, time for restoration placement, and strict observation of the recommended directions for use.[3,23,56,64,72,198,226,238] Other factors are patient related, including the quality of the tooth tissues, the size of the defect following caries excavation, patient age, and the inherent properties of the material.[94] Furthermore, dietary habits, interest in oral hygiene, and treatment compliance are patient-related factors that are only subject to limited influence by the dental team. All these and other factors contribute to the time a dental restoration may survive in the oral cavity.

The longevity of restorations has been investigated in different ways in survival analysis studies, eg, percentage of restorations remaining after a specified number of years in clinical service, by recording the mean or median age, by determining the 95% survival time, and by determining the cumulative survival rate.[102,172,175,245] Actuarial life table methods and the Kaplan-Meier method have been employed as statistical survival functions in several longevity studies to estimate the survival probabilities for dental restorations.[245] Leempoel et al[126] indicated that the Kaplan-Meier method provides more accurate estimates for survival probabilities than the life table method. The latter subdivides the period of time under observation into intervals. For each interval, the probability of an event is calculated and combined to estimate cumulative probabilities.[33] The method suggested by Kaplan and Meier[105] does not use fixed intervals but calculates the probability of an event each time an event is observed.

A direct comparison of the longevity of different types of restorations in different studies reported by different authors is problematic for various reasons.[41,45,100] The variables in the study designs are often poorly described or omitted, or differences in clinical procedures, materials used, and variations in study characteristics make direct comparisons impossible.[160] The annual failure rates from different studies investigating the same type of restorations vary widely (Table 16-10). The influence of factors such as the intraoral location of the restoration, the dental and hygiene status of the patients, the availability of fluoride, the frequency of dental visits, and other clinical factors prevent valid comparisons of the results from the different reports. Furthermore, improvements in the qualities of restorative materials over time may have more effect on one group of materials than on

another.[180] Irrespective of these limitations, however, certain trends are apparent from comparisons of the results of different clinical studies. Cross-sectional surveys differ from controlled longitudinal studies in which the clinicians operate under ideal conditions for the materials investigated. However, results from controlled clinical studies do not reflect the situation in general dental practice[243,254] and may be of limited significance to general dental practice.[180] Results from longitudinal clinical studies may not be generalized and are difficult to compare with retrospective cross-sectional investigations because the outcome is highly dependent on the individual skills of the dentist and the care taken in placing the restoration.[118,224]

One study compared restoration longevity in Pakistan and Australia, indicating a significantly greater longevity for restorations in female than in male patients, with the differences being most evident in the developing country (Pakistan), possibly reflecting different levels of compliance with oral hygiene measures.[143] Furthermore, in both patient groups, the median survival time for the restorations was significantly greater in those patients who were classified as infrequent attenders (> 1 year), indicating a tendency for frequent attenders (≤ 1 year) to receive more dental treatment.[190] These findings were confirmed by Hawthorne and Smales,[72] who reported that less frequent attenders had higher survival rates for gold castings and glass ionomers than frequent attenders. However, in another study by Dawson and Smales,[35] no significant differences in restoration longevity between frequent and less frequent attenders was shown. Lundin and Koch[139] reported a high inci-

Table 16-10 Annual failure rates of the different types of direct and indirect restorations in clinical studies as determined by the present review of the dental literature

Restoration type	Annual failure rate (%)			
	All studies	Studies > 3 y	Longitudinal studies	Cross-sectional studies
Amalgam restorations	0–7	0–7	0–7	1–6.3
Direct posterior composite restorations	0.7–9	0.7–9	0.7–5.9	3.3–9
Glass-ionomer restorations	0–14.4	0–14.3	0–14.4	–
Composite inlays and onlays	0–10	1.5–9.8	0–10	–
Ceramic inlays and onlays	0–7.1	0–4.3	0–7.1	0.8–4
CAD/CAM inlays and onlays	0–4.4	0–1.3	0–4.4	–
Cast gold inlays and onlays	0–5.9	0–5.9	0–2.6	0.5–5.9
Anterior restorations (Class III and IV)	0–11.6	0.5–11.6	0–11.6	1–3
Cervical restorations (Class V)	0–26	0.3–7.2	0–26	1.6–5.9

dence of posterior composite restoration failures in cavities classified as large. There was a tendency for large restorations with a long cavosurface margin to show greater deterioration than smaller restorations. The findings of several studies supported the view that single-surface restorations show a greater longevity than do multi-surface restorations.[4,11,31,104,112,127,161,175,273] However, restorations limited to the occlusal surface may be found to suffer significantly more failures due to caries than do Class II restorations.[59,219,245] The development of new caries lesions on unprotected approximal surfaces during the lifetime of the Class I restorations was considered to account for this phenomenon. Furthermore, premolars rather than molars were found to offer significantly more favorable conditions for the long-term survival of adhesive inlays,[61,63,207,215,226,228] gold castings,[198] and amalgam restorations.[273] Several authors observed that the age of the patient had an important influence on the treatment outcome.[11,72,94,100,204,238] Smales et al[238] mentioned an age effect, but found no statistical evidence, whereas Plasmans et al[204] and Bentley and Drake[11] found a superior survival rate for restorations placed in younger patients compared with older patients. Differences in the quality of oral hygiene measures, fluoride availability, dietary habits, and periodontal problems may be associated with these findings.

Conclusions

The importance and use of esthetic tooth-colored restorative materials is still increasing. Amalgam and even cast gold restorations are being replaced because of alleged adverse health effects and inferior esthetic appearance. However, all restorative materials and procedures have certain limitations. Direct and indirect composite res-torations and ceramic restorations are time-consuming, costly treatment procedures and are only indicated for patients with excellent oral hygiene. Glass ionomers, resin-modified glass ionomers, and compomers can only be considered as long-term provisional restorations in stress-bearing posterior situations. However, these materials, together with composites, more than satisfy requirements for the restoration of Class V defects. Composite resin is the material of choice for the restoration of Class III and Class IV defects.

The quality of dental restorations is difficult to define and longevity is only one aspect of quality. The longevity of restorations is dependent upon many factors including material-, dentist-, and patient-related factors. For posterior stress-bearing restorations, cast gold inlays, CAD/CAM ceramic restorations, and amalgam restorations exhibit the lowest annual failure rates. Main reasons for the failure of restorations are secondary caries, bulk fracture of the restoration or fracture of the tooth, marginal defects, and for cervical restorations, loss of retention.

References

1. Abdalla AI, Alhadainy HA. Clinical evaluation of hybrid ionomer restoratives in Class V abrasion lesions: Two year results. Quintessence Int 1997; 28:255–258.

2. Abdalla AI, Alhadainy HA, Garcia-Godoy F. Clinical evaluation of glass ionomers and compomers in Class V carious lesions. Am J Dent 1997;10:18–20.

3. Akerboom HB, Advokaat JG, van Amerongen WE, Borgmeijer PJ. Long-term evaluation and rerestoration of amalgam restorations. Community Dent Oral Epidemiol 1993;21:45–48.

4. Allan DN. The durability of conservative restorations. Br Dent J 1969;126:172–177.

5. Allan DN. A longitudinal study of dental restorations. Br Dent J 1977;143:87–89.

6. Attin T, Buchalla W. Werkstoffkundliche und klinische Bewertung von Kompomeren. Dtsch Zahnärztl Z 1998;53:766–774.

7. Barnes DM, Blank LW, Thompson VP, Holston AM, Gingell JC. A 5- and 8-year clinical evaluation of a posterior composite resin. Quintessence Int 1991;22:143–151.

8. Barnes DM, Blank LW, Gingell JC, Gilner PP. A clinical evaluation of a resin-modified glass ionomer restorative material. J Am Dent Assoc 1995; 126:1245–1253.

9. Bauer CM, Kunzelmann KH, Hickel R. Simulierter Nahrungsabrieb von Kompositen und Ormoceren. Dtsch Zahnärztl Z 1995;50: 635–638.

10. Bayne SC, Taylor DF, Roberson TM, et al. Long term clinical failures in posterior composites [abstract 32]. J Dent Res 1989;68(special issue): 185.

11. Bentley C, Drake CW. Longevity of restorations in a dental school clinic. J Dent Educ 1986; 50:594–600.

12. Benz C, Landenhammer H, Hickel R. Die Qualität von Klasse-III-Kompomerfüllungen nach 6 Monaten. Dtsch Zahnärztl Z 1997;52:804–805.

13. Benz C, Stabel W, Mehl A, Hickel R. Clinical evaluation of modified glass ionomers in Class II restorations [abstract 1209]. J Dent Res 1997;76(special issue):165.

14. Benz C, Gust C, Folwaczny M, Benz B, Hickel R. Clinical evaluation of a compomer material in Class II restorations [abstract 103]. J Dent Res 1998;77(special issue A):118.

15. Berg NG, Derand T. A 5-year evaluation of ceramic inlays (Cerec). Swed Dent J 1997;21: 121–127.

16. Bessing C, Lundqvist P. A 1-year clinical examination of indirect composite resin inlays: a preliminary report. Quintessence Int 1991; 22:153–157.

17. Bjertness E, Sonju T. Survival analysis of amalgam restorations in long-term recall patients. Acta Odontol Scand 1990;48:93–97.

18. Bowen RL, Eichmiller FC, Marjenhoff WA. Glass-ceramic inserts anticipated for 'megafilled' composite restorations. Research moves into the office. J Am Dent Assoc 1991;122: 71–75.

19. Bowen RL, Eichmiller FC, Misra DN. Beta quartz microcrystalline glass as megafillers for composites [abstract 534]. J Dent Res 1991; 68(special issue):248.

20. Bowen RL, Eichmiller FC, Marjenhoff WA. Gazing into the future of esthetic restorative materials. J Am Dent Assoc 1992;123:32–39.

21. Brackett WW, Gilpatrick RO, Browning WD, Gregory PN. Two-year clinical performance of a resin-modified glass-ionomer restorative material. Oper Dent 1999;24:9–13.

22. Brackett WW, Browning WD, Ross JA, Gregory PN, Owens BM. 1-year clinical evaluation of Compoglass and Fuji II LC in cervical erosion/abfraction lesions. Am J Dent 1999;12:119–122.

23. Burke EJ, Qualtrough AJ. Aesthetic inlays: Composite or ceramic? Br Dent J 1994;176:53–60.

24. Burke FJT, Cheung SW, Mjör IA, Wilson NHF. Restoration longevity and analysis of reasons for the placement and replacement of restorations provided by vocational dental practitioners and their trainers in the United Kingdom. Quintessence Int 1999;30:234–242.

25. Burrow MF, Tyas MJ. Clinical evaluation of a resin-modified glass ionomer adhesive system. Oper Dent 1998;23:290–293.

26. Chen HY, Hickel R, Setcos JC, Kunzelmann KH. Effects of surface finish and fatigue testing on the fracture strength of CAD/CAM and pressed ceramic crowns. J Prosthet Dent 1999; 82:468–475.

27. Christensen GJ. The coming demise of the cast gold restoration? J Am Dent Assoc 1996; 127:1233–1236.

28. Christensen GJ. Longevity vs. esthetics in restorative dentistry. J Am Dent Assoc 1998; 129:1023–1024.

29. Cichon P, Kerschbaum T. Verweildauer zahnärztlicher Restaurationen bei Behinderten. Dtsch Zahnärztl Z 1999;54:96–102.

30. Cortes O, Garcia-Godoy F, Boj JR. Bond strength of resin-reinforced glass ionomer cements after enamel etching. Am J Dent 1993;6:299–301.

31. Crabb HSM. The survival of dental restorations in a teaching hospital. Br Dent J 1981; 150:315–318.

32. Croll TP, Phillips RW. Six years' experience with glass-ionomer-silver cermet cement. Quintessence Int 1991;22:783–793.

33. Cutler SJ, Ederer F. Maximum utilization of the life table method in analyzing survival. J Chronic Dis 1958;8:699–712.

34. Dahl JE, Eriksen HM. Reasons for replacement of amalgam dental restorations. Scand J Dent Res 1978;86:404–407.

35. Dawson AS, Smales RJ. Restoration longevity in an Australian Defence Force population. Aust Dent J 1992;37:196–200.

36. de Araujo MAM, Araujo RM, Marsilio AL. A retrospective look at esthetic resin composite and glass-ionomer Class III restorations: A 2-year clinical evaluation. Quintessence Int 1998;29: 87–93.

37. de Gee AJ, Pallav P, Werner A, Davidson CL. Annealing as a mechanism of increasing wear resistance of composites. Dent Mater 1990; 6:266–270.

38. Doglia R, Herr P, Holz J, Baume LJ. Clinical evaluation of four amalgam alloys: A five-year report. J Prosthet Dent 1986;56:406–415.

39. Dogon IL, Murray L, Van Leeuwen M, Norris D, Sobel M. The clinical evaluation of a new anterior restorative material with improved edge strength [abstract 484]. J Dent Res 1987;66(special issue):167.

40. Donly KJ, Jensen ME, Triolo P, Chan D. A clinical comparison of resin composite inlay and onlay posterior restorations and cast-gold restorations at 7 years. Quintessence Int 1999;30:163–168.

41. Downer MC, Azli NA, Bedi R, Moles DR, Setchell DJ. How long do routine dental restorations last? A systematic review. Br Dent J 1999;187:432–439.

42. Easton GS. Causes and prevention of amalgam failures. J Am Dent Assoc 1941;28:392–400.

43. Eichmiller FC. Clinical use of beta-quartz glass-ceramic inserts. Compend Contin Educ Dent 1992;13:568–574.

44. Eidenbenz S, Lehner CR, Scharer P. Copy milling ceramic inlays from resin analogs: A practicable approach with the CELAY system. Int J Prosthodont 1994;7:134–142.

45. el-Mowafy OM, Lewis DW, Benmergui C, Levinton C. Meta-analysis on long-term clinical performance of posterior composite restorations. J Dent 1994;22:33–43.

46. Felden A, Schmalz G, Federlin M, Hiller KA. Retrospective clinical investigation and survival analysis on ceramic inlays and partial ceramic crowns: Results up to 7 years. Clin Oral Investig 1998;2:161–167.

47. Flessa HP, Kunzelmann KH, Mehl A, Hickel R. 3D-Verschleissanalyse von Kompositfüllungen. Kompositinlays und Keramikinlays in vivo. [Proceedings of the Annual Meeting of the German Scientific Dental Association (DGZMK), 3–6 Oct 1996, Düsseldorf]. Düsseldorf: DGZMK, 1996:37.

48. Flessa HP, Kunzelmann KH, Mehl A, Hickel R. Quantitative 3D wear analysis of composite fillings with and without inserts [abstract 1629]. J Dent Res 1999;78(special issue):309.

49. Folwaczny M, Loher C, Mehl A, Benz C, Hickel R. Class V fillings with four different light-curing materials: Three-year results [abstract 673]. J Dent Res 1998;77(special issue A):190.

50. Forsten L, Mount GJ, Knight G. Observations in Australia of the use of glass ionomer cement restorative material. Aust Dent J 1994;39: 339–343.

51. Fradeani M, Aquilano A, Bassein L. Longitudinal study of pressed glass-ceramic inlays for four and a half years. J Prosthet Dent 1997; 78:346–353.

52. Frederickson D, Setcos J. Clinical evaluation of indirect posterior composite restorations over three years [abstract 2232]. J Dent Res 1994;73(special issue):381.

53. Freilich MA, Goldberg AJ, Gilpatrick RO, Simonsen RJ. Direct and indirect evaluation of posterior composite restorations at three years. Dent Mater 1992;8:60–64.

54. Frencken JE, Songpaisan Y, Phantumvanit P, Pilot T. An atraumatic restorative treatment (ART) technique: Evaluation after one year. Int Dent J 1994;44:460–464.

55. Frencken JE, Makoni F, Sithole WD. Atraumatic restorative treatment and glass ionomer sealants in a school oral health programme in Zimbabwe: Evaluation after 1 year. Caries Res 1996;30:428–433.

56. Frencken JE, Makoni F, Sithole WD. ART restorations and glass ionomer sealants in Zimbabwe: Survival after 3 years. Community Dent Oral Epidemiol 1998;26:372–381.

57. Friedl KH, Schmalz G, Hiller KA, Saller A. In-vivo evaluation of a feldspathic ceramic system: 2-year results. J Dent 1996;24:25–31.

58. Friedl KH, Hiller KA, Schmalz G, Bey B. Clinical and quantitative marginal analysis of feldspathic ceramic inlays at 4 years. Clin Oral Investig 1997;1:163–168.

59. Fritz U, Fischbach H, Harke I. Langzeitverweildauer von Goldgußfüllungen. Dtsch Zahnärztl Z 1992;47:714–716.

60. Fuzzi M, Bonfiglioli R, Di Febo G, Marin C, Caldari R, Tonelli PM. Posterior porcelain inlay: Clinical procedures and laboratory technique. Int J Periodontics Restorative Dent 1989;9: 275–287.

61. Fuzzi M, Rappelli G. Survival rate of ceramic inlays. J Dent 1998;26:623–626.

62. Füllemann J, Krejci I, Lutz F. Kompositinlays: Klinische und rasterelektronenmikroskopische Untersuchung nach einjähriger Funktionszeit. Schweiz Monatsschr Zahnmed 1992;102: 292–298.

63. Geurtsen W, Schoeler U. A 4-year retrospective clinical study of Class I and Class II composite restorations. J Dent 1997;25:229–232.

64. Gjerdet NR, Hegdahl T. Porosity, strength and mercury content of amalgam made by different dentists in their own practice. Dent Mater 1985; 1:150–153.

65. Gladys S, Van Meerbeek B, Braem M, Lambrechts P, Vanherle G. Comparative physico-mechanical characterization of new hybrid restorative materials with conventional glass-ionomer and resin composite restorative materials. J Dent Res 1997;76:883–894.

66. Gladys S, Van Meerbeek B, Lambrechts P, Vanherle G. Marginal adaptation and retention of a glass-ionomer, resin-modified glass-ionomers and a polyacid-modified resin composite in cervical Class V lesions. Dent Mater 1998;14:294–306.

67. Haas M, Arnetzl G, Wegscheider WA, Konig K, Bratschko RO. Klinische und werkstoffkundliche Erfahrungen mit Komposit-, Keramik- und Goldinlays. Dtsch Zahnärztl Z 1992;47:18–22.

68. Haller B, Moll K, Hofmann N, Klaiber B. Initiale Scherhaftfestigkeit von Glasionomer-Komposit-Hybridmaterialien an konditioniertem und unkonditioniertem Schmelz. Dtsch Zahnärztl Z 1997;52:680–684.

69. Hannig M. Five-year clinical evaluation of a heat- and pressure-cured composite resin inlay system [abstract 1908]. J Dent Res 1996;75(special issue):256.

295

70. Hasselrot L. Tunnel restorations. A 3 1/2-year follow up study of Class I and II tunnel restorations in permanent and primary teeth. Swed Dent J 1993;17:173–182.

71. Hasselrot L. Tunnel restorations in permanent teeth. A 7 year follow up study. Swed Dent J 1998;22:1–7.

72. Hawthorne WS, Smales RJ. Factors influencing long-term restoration survival in three private dental practices in Adelaide. Aust Dent J 1997;42:59–63.

73. Hayashi M, Tsuchitani Y, Miura M, Takeshige F, Ebisu S. 6-year clinical evaluation of fired ceramic inlays. Oper Dent 1998;23:318–326.

74. Healey HJ, Phillips RW. A clinical study of amalgam failures. J Dent Res 1949;28:439–446.

75. Helbig EB, Klimm W, Haufe E, Richter G. Klinische Fünfjahresstudie zum Feinpartikelhybrid P-50 in Kombination mit Scotchbond 2. Acta Med Dent Helv 1998;3:171–177.

76. Heymann HO, Sturdevant JR, Bayne SC, Wilder AD, Sluder TB, Brunson WD. Examining tooth flexure effects on cervical restorations: A two-year clinical study. J Am Dent Assoc 1991;122: 41–47.

77. Heymann HO, Bayne SC, Sturdevant JR, Wilder-AD J, Roberson TM. The clinical performance of CAD-CAM-generated ceramic inlays: A four-year study. J Am Dent Assoc 1996;127: 1171–1181.

78. Hickel R, Petschelt A, Maier J, Voß A, Sauter M. Nachuntersuchung von Füllungen mit Cermet-Zement (Ketac-Silver). Dtsch Zahnärztl Z 1988; 43:851–853.

79. Hickel R. Zur Problematik hypersensibler Zähne nach Eingliederung von Adhäsivinlays. Dtsch Zahnärztl Z 1990;45:740–742.

80. Hickel R. Glass Ionomers, cermets, hybrid ionomers and compomers–(long-term) clinical evaluation. Trans Acad Dent Mater 1996;9:105–129.

81. Hickel R, Kunzelmann KH. Keramikinlays und Veneers. Munich: Hanser, 1997.

82. Hickel R. Moderne Füllungswerkstoffe. Dtsch Zahnärztl Z 1997;52:572–585.

83. Hickel R, Dasch W, Janda R, Tyas M, Anusavice K. New direct restorative materials. Int Dent J 1998;48:3–16.

84. Hickel R, Manhart J. Glass-ionomers and compomers in pediatric dentistry. In: Davidson CL, Mjör IA (eds). Advances in Glass-Ionomer Cements. Berlin: Quintessence, 1999:201–226.

85. Ho TFT, Smales RJ, Fang DTS. A 2-year clinical study of two glass ionomer cements used in the atraumatic restorative treatment (ART) technique. Community Dent Oral Epidemiol 1999;27: 195–201.

86. Hofmann N, Klaiber B, Heners M. Okklusale Randschlussqualität von Cerec-Inlays nach mehrmonatiger Tragedauer. Dtsch Zahnärztl Z 1990;45:289–292.

87. Hofmann N. Die Herstellung und Eingliederung von computergefrästen Keramikinlays. ZWR 1990;99:530–537.

88. Hofmann N, Popp M, Klaiber B. Klinische und rasterelektronenmikroskopische Nachuntersuchung von Cerec-Inlays nach fünf Jahren Liegedauer. Dtsch Zahnärztl Z 1995;50: 835–839.

89. Höglund CH, van Dijken JW, Olofsson AL. A clinical evaluation of adhesively luted ceramic inlays. A two year follow-up study. Swed Dent J 1992;16:169–171.

90. Höglund CH, van Dijken JW, Olofsson AL. Three-year comparison of fired ceramic inlays cemented with composite resin or glass ionomer cement. Acta Odontol Scand 1994;52: 140–149.

91. Höhnk HD, Hannig M. Dentalmaterialien mit Potential: Compomere & Co. Phillip J 1998; 15:264–269.

92. Hunt PR. A modified Class II cavity preparation for glass ionomer restorative materials. Quintessence Int 1984;10:1011–1018.

93. Hunt PR. Microconservative restorations for approximal carious lesions. J Am Dent Assoc 1990;120:37–40.

94. Hunter B. Survival of dental restorations in young patients. Community Dent Oral Epidemiol 1985;13:285–287.

95. Huth K, Selbertinger S, Kunzelmann KH, Hickel R. Compomer for Class I/II restorations—Results after 6 months [abstract 1439]. J Dent Res 1999;78(special issue):285.

96. Ishikawa A, Katsuyama S, Tani Y. Wear resistance of composite resins inserted with glass-ceramic inserts [abstract 1795]. J Dent Res 1994;73(special issue):326.

97. Isidor F, Brondum K. A clinical evaluation of porcelain inlays. J Prosthet Dent 1995;74: 140–144.

98. Jedynakiewicz NM, Martin N, Fletcher JM. A three year clinical evaluation of a compomer restorative [abstract 1189]. J Dent Res 1997; 76(special issue):162.

99. Jensen ME. A two-year clinical study of posterior etched-porcelain resin-bonded restorations. Am J Dent 1988;1:27–33.

100. Jokstad A, Mjör IA. Analyses of long-term clinical behavior of Class-II amalgam restorations. Acta Odontol Scand 1991;49:47–63.

101. Jokstad A, Mjör IA. Replacement reasons and service time of Class II amalgam restorations in relation to cavity design. Acta Odontol Scand 1991;49:109–126.

102. Jokstad A, Mjör IA, Qvist V. The age of restorations in situ. Acta Odontol Scand 1994; 52:234–248.

103. Jokstad A, Mjör IA, Nilner K, Kaping S. Clinical performance of three anterior restorative materials over 10 years. Quintessence Int 1994; 25:101–108.

104. Kamann WK, Gängler P. Zur Funktionszeit von Amalgam-, Komposite- und Goldhämmerfüllungen. ZWR 1999;108:270–273.

105. Kaplan EL, Meier P. Nonparametric estimation from incomplete observations. J Am Stat Assoc 1958;53:457–481.

106. Kawai K, Isenberg BP, Leinfelder KF. Effect of gap dimension on composite resin cement wear. Quintessence Int 1994;25:53–58.

107. Kawai K, Leinfelder KF. Effect of glass inserts on resin composite wear. Am J Dent 1995; 8:249–252.

108. Kiremitci A, Bolay S, Gurgan S. Two-year performance of glass-ceramic insert-resin composite restorations: Clinical and scanning electron microscopic evaluation. Quintessence Int 1998; 29:417–421.

109. Klausner LH, Charbeneau GT. Amalgam restorations: A cross-sectional survey of placement and replacement. J Mich Dent Assoc 1985; 67:249–252.

110. Klimm W, Wolff U, Natusch I. Evaluation of Class II composite and ceramic restorations in vivo and in vitro [abstract 1620]. J Dent Res 1999;78(special issue):308.

111. Kontou E, Frankenberger R, Krämer N. Posterior performance of two compomer materials after 12 months [abstract 303]. [Proceedings of the Continental European Division, 1999, Montpellier, France] 1999:120.

112. Krämer N, Kunzelmann KH, Pollety T, Pelka M, Hickel R. Langzeiterfahrungen mit Cermet-Zementfüllungen in Klasse-I/II-Kavitäten. Dtsch Zahnärztl Z 1994;49:905–909.

113. Krämer N, Kunzelmann KH, Mumesohn M, Pelka M, Hickel R. Langzeiterfahrungen mit einem mikrogefüllten Komposit als Inlaysystem. Dtsch Zahnärztl Z 1996;51:342–344.

114. Krämer N, Frankenberger R, Pelka M, Petschelt A. IPS Empress inlays and onlays after four years—A clinical study. J Dent 1999; 27:325–331.

115. Krejci I, Lutz F. Marginal adaptation of Class V restorations using different restorative techniques. J Dent 1991;19:24–32.

116. Krejci I, Krejci D, Lutz F. Clinical evaluation of a new pressed glass ceramic inlay material over 1.5 years. Quintessence Int 1992;23:181–186.

117. Krejci I, Guntert A, Lutz F. Scanning electron microscopic and clinical examination of composite resin inlays/onlays up to 12 months in situ. Quintessence Int 1994;25:403–409.

118. Kreulen CM, Tobi H, Gruythuysen RJM, van Amerongen WE, Borgmeijer PJ. Replacement risk of amalgam treatment modalities: 15-year results. J Dent 1998;26:627–632.

119. Kunzelmann KH, Obermeier T, Mehl A, Hickel R. Finite element analysis of megafillers/inserts to optimize shape and material properties [abstract 1402]. J Dent Res 1995;74(special issue):187.

120. Kunzelmann KH, Mehl A, Hickel R. Sliding-wear of an experimental ormocer and 15 commercial composites [abstract 965]. J Dent Res 1998;77(special issue A):226.

121. Kunzelmann KH, Manhart J. Plastische Kompositfüllungen mit Sonicsys-Approx-Inserts. Ästhet Zahnmed 2000;3:34–39.

122. Lambrechts P, Vanherle G. Structural evidences of the microfilled composites. J Biomed Mater Res 1983;17:249–260.

123. Lambrechts P, Braem M, Vanherle G. Klinische Erfahrungen mit Composites und Dentin-Adhäsiven im Seitenzahnbereich I: Klinische Beurteilung von Composites. Phillip J 1988;1:12–28.

124. Lavelle CLB. A cross-sectional survey into the durability of amalgam restorations. J Dent 1976;4:139–143.

125. Leempoel PJB, Eschen S, De Haan AF, van't Hof MA. An evaluation of crowns and bridges in general dental practice. J Oral Rehabil 1985;12:515–528.

126. Leempoel PJB, van't Hof MA, De Haan AF. Survival analysis studies of dental restorations: Criteria, methods and an analysis. J Oral Rehabil 1989;16:387–394.

127. Lehner C, Studer S, Brodbeck U, Schärer P. Six-year clinical results of leucite-reinforced glass ceramic inlays and onlays. Acta Med Dent Helv 1998;3:137–146.

128. Leinfelder KF, Sluder TB, Santos JFF, Wall JT. Five-year clinical evaluation of anterior and posterior restorations of composite resins. Oper Dent 1980;5:57–65.

129. Leinfelder KF, Isenberg BP, Essig ME. A new method for generating ceramic restorations: A CAD/CAM system. J Am Dent Assoc 1989;118:703–707.

130. Letzel H. Survival rates and reasons for failure of posterior composite restorations in multicentre clinical trial. J Dent 1989;17:10–17.

131. Letzel H, van't Hof MA, Vrijhoef MMA, Marshall GW, Marshall SJ. Failure, survival, and reasons for replacement of amalgam restorations. In: Anusavice K (ed). Quality Evaluation of Dental Restorations. Chicago: Quintessence, 1989:83–94.

132. Letzel H, van't Hof MA, Vrijhoef MM, Marshall GW J, Marshall SJ. A controlled clinical study of amalgam restorations: survival, failures, and causes of failure. Dent Mater 1989;5:115–121.

133. Letzel H, van't Hof MA, Marshall GW, Marshall SJ. The influence of the amalgam alloy on the survival of amalgam restorations: A secondary analysis of multiple controlled clinical trials. J Dent Res 1997;76:1787–1798.

134. Levitch LC, Bader JD, Shugars DA, Heymann HO. Non-carious cervical lesions. J Dent 1994;22:195–207.

135. Li D, Manhart J, Fay RM, Hickel R, Powers JM. Color stability of composites, compomers and ormocer by staining [abstract P33]. Trans Acad Dent Mater 1998;12:235.

136. Loher C, Kunzelmann KH, Hickel R. Klinische Studie mit Hybridglasionomerzement-, Kompomer- und Kompositfüllungen in Klasse-V-Kavitäten. Dtsch Zahnärztl Z 1997;52:525–529.

137. Loher C, Kunzelmann KH, Hickel R. Clinical evaluation of glass ionomer cements (LC), compomer and composite restorations in Class V cavities—Two-year results [abstract 1190]. J Dent Res 1997;76(special issue):162.

138. Lösche GM. Klasse-II-Kompositfüllungen mit und ohne konfektionierte Glaskeramik-Inserts. Eine In-vivo-Studie. Dtsch Zahnärztl Z 1996;51:389–394.

139. Lundin SA, Koch G. Class I and II composite restorations: A 4-year clinical follow up. Swed Dent J 1989;13:217–227.

140. Lussi A, Schaffner M, Suter P, Hotz P. Toxikologie der Amalgame. Schweiz Monatsschr Zahnmed 1989;99:55–59.

141. Lutz F, Phillips RW, Roulet JF, Setcos JC. In vivo and in vitro wear of potential posterior composites. J Dent Res 1984;63:914–920.

142. Mackert JR. Dental amalgam and mercury. J Am Dent Assoc 1991;122:54–61.

143. Mahmood S, Smales RJ. Longevity of dental restorations in selected patients from different practice environments. Aust Dent J 1994; 39:15–17.

144. Mair LH. Ten-year clinical assessment of three posterior resin composites and two amalgams. Quintessence Int 1998;29:483–490.

145. Mallow P, Durward C, Klaipo M. Comparison of two glass ionomer cements using the ART technique [abstract 33]. J Dent Res 1995;74:405.

146. Mallow PK, Durward CS, Klaipo M. Restoration of permanent teeth in young rural children in Cambodia using the atraumatic restorative treatment (ART) technique and Fuji II glass ionomer cement. Int J Paediatr Dent 1998;8:35–40.

147. Manhart J, Hollwich B, Mehl A, Kunzelmann KH, Hickel R. Marginal adaptation of ormocer- and composite-fillings in Class II cavities [abstract 223]. J Dent Res 1997;76:1122.

148. Manhart J, Li D, Powers JM, Hickel R. Bond strength of VLC GICs, compomers, and composites [abstract P34]. Trans Acad Dent Mater 1998;12:236.

149. Manhart J, Li D, Powers JM, Hickel R. Bonding of compomers to deep dentin under various surface conditions [abstract 1246]. J Dent Res 1998;77(special issue):787.

150. Manhart J, Hickel R. Esthetic compomer restorations in posterior teeth using a new all-in-one adhesive: case presentation. J Esthet Dent 1999;11:250–258.

151. Manhart J, Mehl A, Schroeter R, Obster B, Hickel R. Bond strength of composite to dentin treated by air abrasion. Oper Dent 1999;24:223–232.

152. Manhart J, Chen HY, Kunzelmann KH, Hickel R. Bond strength of a compomer to dentin under various surface conditions. Clin Oral Investig 1999;3:175–180.

153. Manhart J, Hickel R. Klinische Studie zum Einsatz eines All-in-one-Adhäsivs. Erste Ergebnisse nach 6 Monaten. Quintessenz 1999;50: 1277–1288.

154. Manhart J, Hollwich B, Mehl A, Kunzelmann KH, Hickel R. Randqualität von Ormocer- und Kompositfüllungen in Klasse-II-Kavitäten nach künstlicher Alterung. Dtsch Zahnärztl Z 1999; 54:89–95.

155. Manhart J, Chen HY, Kunzelmann KH, Hickel R. Werkstoffkundliche Charakterisierung eines Füllungsmateriales auf Ormocer-Basis im Vergleich zu einem Komposit und einem Kompomer. ZMK 1999;15:807–812.

156. Manhart J, Kunzelmann KH, Chen HY, Hickel R. Mechanical properties and wear behavior of light-cured packable composite resins. Dent Mater 2000;16:33–40.

157. Manhart J, Scheibenbogen-Fuchsbrunner A, Chen HY, Hickel R. 2-year clinical study of composite and ceramic inlays. Clin Oral Investig 2000;4:192–198.

158. Manhart J, Chen HY, Neuerer P, Scheibenbogen-Fuchsbrunner A, Hickel R. Composite and ceramic inlays after 3 years of clinical service. Am J Dent (in press).

159. Martin N, Jedynakiewicz NM. Clinical performance of Cerec ceramic inlays: A systematic review. Dent Mater 1999;15:54–61.

160. Maryniuk GA. In search of treatment longevity: A 30-year perspective. J Am Dent Assoc 1984;109:739–744.

161. Maryniuk GA, Kaplan SH. Longevity of restorations: Survey results of dentists' estimates and attitudes. J Am Dent Assoc 1986;112:39–45.

162. Matis BA, Cochran M, Carlson T. Longevity of glass-ionomer restorative materials: Results of a 10-year evaluation. Quintessence Int 1996; 27:373–382.

163. McLean JW, Gasser O. Glass-cermet cements. Quintessence Int 1985;16:333–343.

164. McLean JW. Clinical applications of glass ionomer cements. Oper Dent 1992;17:184–190.

165. Mehl A, Hickel R, Kunzelmann KH. Physical properties and gap formation of light-cured composites with and without softstart-polymerization. J Dent 1997;25:321–330.

166. Merrett MCW, Elderton RJ. An in vitro study of restorative dental treatment decisions and dental caries. Br Dent J 1984;157:128–133.

167. Mertz-Fairhurst EJ, Curtis JW Jr, Ergle JW, Rueggeberg FA, Adair SM. Ultraconservative and cariostatic sealed restorations: Results at year 10. J Am Dent Assoc 1998;129:55–66.

168. Millar BJ, Robinson PB, Inglis AT. Clinical evaluation of an anterior hybrid composite resin over 8 years. Br Dent J 1997;182:26–30.

169. Mjör IA. Placement and replacement of restorations. Oper Dent 1981;6:49–54.

170. Mjör IA. Amalgam and composite resin restorations: Longevity and reasons for replacement. In: Anusavice K (ed). Quality Evaluation of Dental Restorations. Chicago: Quintessence, 1989:61–80.

171. Mjör IA, Jokstad A, Qvist V. Longevity of posterior restorations. Int Dent J 1990;40:11–17.

172. Mjör IA. Long term cost of restorative therapy using different materials. Scand J Dent Res 1992;100:60–65.

173. Mjör IA, Toffenetti F. Placement and replacement of amalgam restorations in Italy. Oper Dent 1992;17:70–73.

174. Mjör IA, Toffenetti F. Placement and replacement of resin-based composite restorations in Italy. Oper Dent 1992;17:82–85.

175. Mjör IA. Problems and benefits associated with restorative materials: Side-effects and long-term cost. Adv Dent Res 1992;6:7–16.

176. Mjör IA. Repair versus replacement of failed restorations. Int Dent J 1993;43:466–472.

177. Mjör IA, Medina JE. Reasons for placement, replacement, and age of gold restorations in selected practices. Oper Dent 1993;18:82–87.

178. Mjör IA, Jokstad A. Five-year study of Class II restorations in permanent teeth using amalgam, glass polyalkenoate (ionomer) cerment and resin-based composite materials. J Dent 1993;21:338–343.

179. Mjör IA. Glass ionomer restorations and secondary caries. A preliminary report. Quintessence Int 1996;27:171–174.

180. Mjör IA. The reasons for replacement and the age of failed restorations in general dental practice. Acta Odontol Scand 1997;55:58–63.

181. Mjör IA. Selection of restorative materials in general dental practice in Sweden. Acta Odontol Scand 1997;55:53–57.

182. Moffa JP. Comparative performance of amalgam and composite resin restorations and criteria for their use. In: Anusavice K (ed). Quality evaluation of dental restorations. Chicago: Quintessence, 1989:125–133.

183. Mount GJ. Longevity of glass ionomer cements. J Prosthet Dent 1986;55:682–685.

184. Mount GJ. Longevity in glass-ionomer restorations: Review of a successful technique. Quintessence Int 1997;28:643–650.

185. Mörmann W, Brandestini M. Die Cerec Computer Rekonstruktion. Inlays, Onlays und Veneers. Berlin: Quintessenz, 1989.

186. Mörmann W, Krejci I. Computer-designed inlays after 5 years in situ: Clinical performance and scanning electron microscopic evaluation. Quintessence Int 1992;23:109–115.

187. Ngo H, Mount GJ. Glass-ionomer cements: A 12-month evaluation. J Prosthet Dent 1986;55:203–205.

188. Nordbo H, Leirskar J, von der Fehr FR. Schüsselförmige Kavitätenpräparation für approximale Kompositrestaurationen im Seitenzahnbereich – Beobachtungen bis zu 10 Jahren. Quintessenz 1988;49:773–779.

189. Nordbo H, Lyngstadaas SP. The clinical performance of two groups of functioning Class II cast gold inlays. Acta Odontol Scand 1992;50:189–192.

190. Nuttal NM. General dental service treatment received by frequent and infrequent dental attendees in Scotland. Br Dent J 1984;156:363–366.

191. Oberländer H, Friedl K-H, Schmalz G, Hiller K-A, Kopp A. Clinical performance of polyacid-modified resin restorations using "softstart-polymerization". Clin Oral Investig 1999;3:55–61.

192. O'Neal SJ, Miracle RL, Leinfelder KF. Evaluating interfacial gaps for esthetic inlays. J Am Dent Assoc 1993;124:48–54.

193. Osborne JW, Binon PP, Gale EN. Dental amalgam: Clinical behavior up to eight years. Oper Dent 1980;5:24–28.

194. Osborne JW, Normann RD, Gale EN. A 14-year clinical assessment of 12 amalgam alloys. Quintessence Int 1991;22:857–864.

195. Otto T. Cerec-Restaurationen. Schweiz Monatsschr Zahnmed 1999;105:1039–1044.

196. Papa J, Wilson PR, Tyas MJ. Tunnel restorations: A review. J Esthet Dent 1992;4:4–9.

197. Paterson N. The longevity of restorations. Br Dent J 1984;157:23–25.

198. Pelka M, Schmidt G, Petschelt A. Klinische Qualitätsbeurteilung von gegossenen Metallinlays und -onlays. Dtsch Zahnärztl Z 1996;51:268–272.

199. Pelka M. Haltbarkeit von Füllungen aus verschiedenen Materialien. Zahnärztl Mitt 1998;88:42–47.

200. Peters MCRB, Roeters JJM, Frankenmolen FWA. Clinical evaluation of Dyract in primary molars: 1-year results. Am J Dent 1996;9:83–87.

201. Phantumvanit P, Songpaisan Y, Pilot T, Frencken JE. Atraumatic restorative treatment (ART): A three-year community field trial in Thailand–Survival of one-surface restorations in the permanent dentition. J Public Health Dent 1996;56:141–145.

202. Phillips RW. Past, present and future composite resin systems. Dent Clin North Am 1981;25:209–218.

203. Pieper K, Meyer G, Marienhagen B, Motsch A. Eine Langzeitstudie an Amalgam- und Kunststoff-Füllungen. Dtsch Zahnärztl Z 1991;46:222–225.

204. Plasmans PJJM, Creugers NHJ, Mulder J. Long-term survival of extensive amalgam restorations. J Dent Res 1998;77:453–460.

205. Powers JM, Farah JW. Compomers. The Dental Advisor 1998;15:1–5.

206. Prati C, Chersoni S, Cretti L, Montanari G. Retention and marginal adaptation of a compomer placed in non-stress-bearing areas used with the total-etch technique: A 3-year retrospective study. Clin Oral Investig 1998;2:168–173.

207. Qualtrough AJE, Wilson NHF. A 3-year clinical evaluation of a porcelain inlay system. J Dent 1996;24:317–323.

208. Qvist J, Qvist V, Mjör IA. Placement and longevity of amalgam restorations in Denmark. Acta Odontol Scand 1990;48:297–303.

209. Qvist V, Thylstrup A, Mjör IA. Restorative treatment pattern and longevity of amalgam restorations in Denmark. Acta Odontol Scand 1986;44:343–349.

210. Qvist V, Qvist J, Mjör IA. Placement and longevity of tooth-colored restorations in Denmark. Acta Odontol Scand 1990;48:305–311.

211. Qvist V, Strom C. 11-year assessment of Class-III resin restorations completed with two restorative procedures. Acta Odontol Scand 1993;51:253–262.

212. Raskin A, Michotte-Theall B, Vreven J, Wilson NHF. Clinical evaluation of a posterior composite: 10-year report. J Dent 1999;27:13–19.

213. Reinhardt KJ. Vorteil und Risiko des Kunststoffinlays. Dtsch Zahnärztl Z 1989;44:769–773.

214. Reiss B, Walther W. Überlebensanalyse und klinische Nachuntersuchungen von zahnfarbenen Einlagefüllungen nach dem CEREC-Verfahren. ZWR 1991;100:329–332.

215. Reiss B, Walther W. Ereignisanalyse und klinische Langzeitergebnisse mit Cerec-Keramikinlays. Dtsch Zahnärztl Z 1998;53:65–68.

216. Reiss B, Walther W. Clinical long-term results and 10-year Kaplan-Meier analysis of Cerec restorations. Int J Comput Dent 2000;3:9–23.

217. Reusens B, D`Hoore W, Vreven J. In vivo comparison of a microfilled and a hybrid minifilled composite resin in Class III restorations: 2-year follow-up. Clin Oral Investig 1999;3:62–69.

218. Richardson AS, Boyde MA. Replacement of silver amalgam restorations by 50 dentists during 246 working days. Can Dent Assoc J 1973;39:556–559.

219. Robinson AD. The life of a filling. Br Dent J 1971;130:206–208.

220. Roeder LB, Kim HB, Powers JM. Bond strength of bonding agents/compomers to dentin [abstract 498]. J Dent Res 1998;77(special issue A):168.

221. Rosin M, Hartmann A, Konschake C, Greese U, Schwahn B, Meyer G. A clinical evaluation of a new ormocer restorative at 6 months [abstract 1438]. J Dent Res 1999;78(special issue):285.

222. Roulet JF. The problems associated with substituting composite resins for amalgam: A status report on posterior composites. J Dent 1988;16:101 113.

223. Roulet JF. Esthetic posterior restorations. In: dall'Orologia GD, Fuzzi M, Prati C (eds). Adhesion in Restorative Dentistry. [Proceedings of the International Symposium, 18 Nov 1995, Bologna]. 1995:27–47.

224. Roulet JF. Benefits and disadvantages of tooth-coloured alternatives to amalgam. J Dent 1997;25:459–473.

225. Roulet JF. Longevity of glass ceramic inlays and amalgam–Results up to 6 years. Clin Oral Investig 1997;1:40–46.

226. Rykke M. Dental materials for posterior restorations. Endod Dent Traumatol 1992;8:139–148.

227. Scheibenbogen A, Manhart J, Kunzelmann KH, Hickel R. One-year clinical evaluation of composite and ceramic inlays in posterior teeth. J Prosthet Dent 1998;80:410–416.

228. Scheibenbogen-Fuchsbrunner A, Manhart J, Kremers L, Kunzelmann KH, Hickel R. Two-year clinical evaluation of direct and indirect composite restorations in posterior teeth. J Prosthet Dent 1999;82:391–397.

229. Schiele R. Die Amalgamfüllung – Verträglichkeit. Dtsch Zahnärztl Z 1991;46:515–518.

230. Schlösser R, Kerschbaum T, Ahrens FJ, Cramer M. Überlebensrate von Teil- und Vollgußkronen. Dtsch Zahnärztl Z 1993;48:696–698.

231. Schuster S, Schreger E, Klimm W, Koch R. Klinische Untersuchungen von Klasse-V-Kompomerfüllungen. Dtsch Zahnärztl Z 1997;52:828–832.

232. Sjögren G, Bergman M, Molin M, Bessing C. A clinical examination of ceramic (Cerec) inlays. Acta Odontol Scand 1992;50:171–178.

233. Sjögren G. Dental ceramics and ceramic restorations. An in vitro and in vivo study. Swed Dent J Suppl 1996;111:3–50.

234. Sjögren G, Lantto R, Granberg A, Sundström BO, Tillberg A. Clinical examination of leucite-reinforced glass-ceramic crowns (Empress) in general practice: A retrospective study. Int J Prosthodont 1999;12:122–128.

235. Sjögren G, Hedlund SO, Jonsson C, Sandström A. A 3-year follow-up study of preformed beta-quartz glass-ceramic insert restorations. Quintessence Int 2000;31:25–31.

236. Smales RJ, Gerke DC, White IL. Clinical evaluation of occlusal glass ionomer, resin, and amalgam restorations. J Dent 1990;18:243–249.

237. Smales RJ, Webster DA, Leppard PI. Survival predictions of four types of dental restorative materials. J Dent 1991;19:278–282.

238. Smales RJ, Webster DA, Leppard PI. Survival predictions of amalgam restorations. J Dent 1991;19:272–277.

239. Smales RJ. Longevity of cusp-covered amalgams: Survivals after 15 years. Oper Dent 1991;16:17–20.

240. Smales RJ, Gerke DC. Clinical evaluation of four anterior composite resins over 5 years. Dent Mater 1992;8:246–251.

241. Smales RJ, Hawthorne WS. Long-term survival and cost-effectiveness of five dental restorative materials used in various Classes of cavity preparations. Int Dent J 1996;46:126–130.

242. Smales RJ, Hawthorne WS. Long-term survival of extensive amalgams and posterior crowns. J Dent 1997;25:225–227.

243. Stanford JW. Future of materials and materials research. Adv Dent Res 1988;2:187–192.

244. Stenberg R, Matsson L. Clinical evaluation of glass ceramic inlays (Dicor). Acta Odontol Scand 1993;51:91–97.

245. Stoll R, Sieweke M, Pieper K, Stachniss V, Schulte A. Longevity of cast gold inlays and partial crowns—A retrospective study at a dental school clinic. Clin Oral Investig 1999;3:100–104.

246. Strand GV, Nordbo H, Tveit AB, Espelid I, Wikstrand K, Eide GE. A 3-year clinical study of tunnel restorations. Eur J Oral Sci 1996;104:384–389.

247. Studer S, Lehner C, Brodbeck U, Scharer P. Short-term results of IPS-Empress inlays and onlays. J Prosthodont 1996;5:277–287.

248. Svanberg M, Mjör IA, Orstavik D. Mutans streptococci in plaque from margins in amalgam, composite and glass ionomer restorations. J Dent Res 1990;69:861–864.

249. Svanberg M. Class II amalgam restorations, glass-ionomer tunnel restorations, and caries development on adjacent tooth surfaces: a 3-year clinical study. Caries Res 1992;26:315–318.

250. Thonemann B, Federlin M, Schmalz G, Schams A. Clinical evaluation of heat-pressed glass-ceramic inlays in vivo: 2-year results. Clin Oral Investig 1997;1:27–34.

251. Thordrup M, Isidor F, Hörsted-Bindslev P. A one-year clinical study of indirect and direct composite and ceramic inlays. Scand J Dent Res 1994;102:186–192.

252. Tidehag P, Gunne J. A 2-year clinical follow-up study of IPS Empress ceramic inlays. Int J Prosthodont 1995;8:456–460.

253. Tyas MJ. Correlation between fracture properties and clinical performance of composite resins in Class IV cavities. Aust Dent J 1990;35:46–49.

254. Tyas MJ. Dental materials science—The maintenance of standards. J Oral Rehabil 1992;18:105–110.

255. Tyas MJ. Clinical evaluation of a polyacid-modified resin composite (compomer). Oper Dent 1998;23:77–80.

256. van Dijken JW. 5-6 year evaluation of direct composite inlays [abstract 1801]. J Dent Res 1994;73(special issue):327.

257. van Dijken JW. 3-year clinical evaluation of a compomer, a resin-modified glass ionomer and a resin composite in Class III restorations. Am J Dent 1996;9:195–198.

258. van Dijken JW, Höglund-Aberg C, Olofsson AL. Fired ceramic inlays: A 6-year follow up. J Dent 1998;26:219–225.

259. van Dijken JW. Longevity of new hybrid restorative materials in Class III cavities. Eur J Oral Sci 1999;107:215–219.

260. Van Meerbeek B, Peumans M, Gladys S, Braem M, Lambrechts P, Vanherle G. Three-year clinical effectiveness of four total-etch dentinal adhesive systems in cervical lesions. Quintessence Int 1996;27:775–784.

261. Walther W, Reiss B, Toutenburg H. Longitudinale Ereignisanalyse von Cerec-Einlagefüllungen. Dtsch Zahnärztl Z 1994;49:914–917.

262. Wassell RW, Walls AWG, McCabe JF. Direct composite inlays versus conventional composite restorations: Three-year clinical results. Br Dent J 1995;179:343–349.

263. Welbury RR, Walls AW, Murray JJ, McCabe JF. The management of occlusal caries in permanent molars. A 5-year clinical trial comparing a minimal composite with an amalgam restoration. Br Dent J 1990;169:361–366.

264. Wendt SL, Leinfelder KF. Clinical evaluation of a heat-treated resin composite inlay: 3-year results. Am J Dent 1992;5:258–262.

265. Wiedmer CS, Krejci I, Lutz F. Klinische, röntgenologische und rasterelektronenoptische Untersuchung von Kompositinlays nach fünfjähriger Funktionszeit. Acta Med Dent Helv 1997;2:301–307.

266. Wilder AD, May KN, Bayne SC, Taylor DF, Leinfelder KF. Seventeen-year clinical study of ultraviolet-cured posterior composite Class I and II restorations. J Esthet Dent 1999;11: 135–142.

267. Wilson AD, McLean JW. Glass-Ionomer Cement. Chicago: Quintessence, 1988.

268. Wilson MA, Wilson NHF, Smith GA. A clinical trial of a visible light-cured posterior composite resin restorative: Two-year results. Quintessence Int 1986;17:151–155.

269. Wilson NHF, Wilson MA, Smith GA. A clinical trial of a new visible light-cured posterior composite restorative—Initial findings and one-year results. Quintessence Int 1985;16:281–290.

270. Wilson NHF, Smith GA, Wilson MA. A clinical trial of a visible light cured posterior composite resin restorative material: Three-year results. Quintessence Int 1986;17:643–652.

271. Wilson NHF, Wilson MA, Smith GA. A clinical trial of a visible light-cured posterior composite resin restorative material: Four-year results. Quintessence Int 1987;19:133–139.

272. Wilson NHF, Wilson MA, Wastell DG, Smith GA. A clinical trial of a visible light cured posterior composite resin restorative material: Five-year results. Quintessence Int 1988;19: 675–681.

273. Wilson NHF, Wastell DG, Norman RD. Five-year performance of high-copper content amalgam restorations in a multiclinical trial of a posterior composite. J Dent 1996;24:203–210.

274. Wilson NHF, Burke FJT, Mjör IA. Reasons for placement and replacement of restorations of direct restorative materials by a selected group of practitioners in the United Kingdom. Quintessence Int 1997;28:245–248.

275. Wolcott RB. Failures in dental amalgam. J Am Dent Assoc 1958;56:479–491.

276. Wolter H, Storch W. Urethane (meth)acrylate alkoxysilanes, a new type of reactive compounds for the preparation of inorganic-organic copolymers (ORMOCERs). [Proceedings of the Polymer & Materials Research Symposium, 1993, Bayreuth]. 1993:14–17.

277. Wolter H, Storch W, Ott H. Dental filling materials (posterior composites) based on inorganic/organic copolymers (ORMOCERs). In: Percec V, Lando J (eds). Proceedings of the 35th International Union of Pure and Applied Chemistry International Symposium on Macromolecules [11–15 July 1994, Akron, Ohio]. Heidelberg, Germany, 1995:503.

278. Wolter H, Storch W, Ott H. New inorganic/organic copolymers (ORMOCERs) for dental applications. Mater Res Soc Symp Proc 1994; 346:143–149.

279. Zuellig-Singer R, Bryant RW. Three-year evaluation of computer-machined ceramic inlays: Influence of luting agent. Quintessence Int 1998;29:573–582.

Chapter 17

Quality Guidelines of Operative Dentistry: The Swiss Approach

Felix Lutz and Ivo Krejci

Introduction

The belief that all oral health care is appropriate and proper is considered naive.[24] Only about 25% of dental procedures have been shown to have a sound scientific basis.[17] Questions have recently been raised in operative dentistry, and with good reason, as to who actually benefits from restorative procedures.[11,12] Consequently, the dental profession should address the reasons to continue as it currently does.[6]

In health policy, the future of dentistry can be secured by defining clear, generally accepted goals, and by achieving patient satisfaction with the dental care offered and practiced. This approach has been followed in Switzerland:

Goals

Dentistry in Switzerland is based on the officially accepted opinion that caries and tooth loss caused by periodontitis can be prevented in healthy individuals solely through self-care.[1,22] Therefore, the main-

tenance of primary oral health (defined as the absence of disease of the teeth, the periodontium, and the oral mucosa, as well as the ability to maintain dental function) must be the primary goal in dental care. In secondary oral health, the aim is to rectify at an early stage any damage that has occurred, thereby restoring functional ability. Placing restorations to achieve unclear goals that are not patient-centered is therefore unacceptable. A targeted approach to the restoration of oral health is imperative.[11,12]

Satisfaction

The patients (in "need dentistry") and the consumers (in "want dentistry") must be satisfied with their dental care. This satisfaction should also extend to the relatives of the patients and consumers and to society at large. The key to this satisfaction is quality. The relevant types of qualities must be set at a sufficiently high level and include: access quality (access to dental care[14]), structural quality (practice team, equipment, structure, and organization), indication quality (treatment decision-making[9]), process quality (applied clinical concept and performance), and result quality (quality of the dental service rendered[15]). Subjectively, however, two issues are eminently important from the patient's point of view. First, the access to quality dental care must be unhampered and, second, the quality of the dental service must meet the patient's requirements and expectations.[3,4,10,13] In Europe the amounts paid by patients for dental care are continually increasing, especially in Switzerland, where there is no third-party insurance.

Defining quality seeks to ensure the patient's satisfaction and the pursuit of specific professional goals. By establishing quality standards, a time-based, quality-compatible, fee-per-item system can be secured. Service reductions and service rationing can be avoided and thus the demise of the profession prevented.[7] Demands for information and transparency can be simultaneously fulfilled by making the various types of dental service better known, by clearly defining the range of services, and by warranting the services offered.[10]

In operative dentistry, quality guidelines must not be confined to assessing restorations only. Preventive care must be well-defined and structured in the context of maintaining and enhancing both primary and secondary oral health.[9,21] With the restoration of secondary oral health, therapeutic decision making is of primary concern. This process includes:

1. Diagnosis of caries
2. Monitoring of caries
3. Assessment of individual caries risk
4. Caries-reducing measures

5. Tooth surface–specific preventive and therapeutic procedures in terms of the depth and progress of any lesion relative to an individual's risk of caries
6. Sophisticated patient-handling according to a decision tree or flow chart, which guarantees optimal individual care[9]

Thus, the question, "to drill or not to drill," should be readily answerable. Also, the extremes of patient-damaging care, ie, "supervised neglect" and "aggressive overtreatment," are avoidable.

Operative Goals of Restorations

According to the "Swiss Guidance to Dentists on Professional and Personal Conduct," the maintenance of primary oral health must be given priority.[22] Operative dentistry forms part of the restoration of oral health. Consequently, the targets to be defined for restorations must focus on secondary oral health and solely on the patient. Interestingly, the definition of secondary oral health fails to mention esthetics. It is correctly confined to "need dentistry," thus respecting the luxury aspect of esthetics. Goals within "want dentistry" can also be envisaged with restorations if, additionally or exclusively, the fulfillment of esthetic demands is of primary concern. Thus, the targets must be differentiated according to the patient's request for care.

Based on these considerations, a definition of restoration grades was developed (Table 17-1)[11,12] and accepted as the basis of the quality guidelines in operative dentistry, as edited by the Swiss Dental Society in January 2000.[21] In these

Table 17-1 Operative goals of restorations

Goal	Restoration type	Restoration grade
Pulp protection, preservation of enamel and dentin	• Atraumatic restorative technique* (ART) • Nonfunctional provisional restorations • Sealing of caries[†]	Grade 1 (Preservation)
Preservation + restoration of tooth form (contour, proximal contacts and occlusion) and tooth function	• Functional provisional restorations[‡] • Restorations in primary teeth • Amalgam restorations • Restorations placed with amalgam substitutes[§] • Gold, non–tooth-colored, nonadhesive restorations • Functional anterior and cervical restorations[‡]	Grade 2 (Preservation + Form and Function)
Preservation + form and function + imperceptible restitution/esthetics	• Esthetic restorations placed with amalgam alternatives[‖] • Adhesive anterior and cervical restorations[¶]	Grade 3 (Preservation + Form and Function + Imperceptible Restitution)

*Caries excavation with hand instruments; simply placed glass-ionomer restorations in compliance with restoration grade 1; restorative concept developed for underdeveloped countries.

[†]Currently experimental with dentinal caries.

[‡]According to the current clinical potential of glass-ionomer cements, resin-reinforced glass-ionomer cements, and compomers.

[§]Potentially compomers, simply-worked composites, and resin-based amalgam substitutes.

[‖]Direct composite fillings comprising preventive resin restorations, adhesive restorations, ball- and U-shaped Class I and II fillings, box-shaped Class I and II fillings, and indirect restorations made of resin-based composites, or ceramics comprising inlays, onlays, partial-coverage crowns, and inlay/onlay fixed partial dentures fabricated according to the principles of operative dentistry; envisaged quality warranty: 8 years for direct restorations, 10 years for indirect restorations.

[¶]Direct composite fillings, direct or indirect laboratory-made additions, and composite and ceramic veneers; envisaged quality warranty: 8 years for direct restorations, 10 years for indirect restorations.

guidelines, the terms amalgam substitutes and amalgam alternatives are unambiguously defined. According to these quality guidelines, the requirements must be fulfilled both on completing the restoration and by each individual restoration for a minimum service time. This has been defined as 8 and 10 years, respectively, for tooth-colored direct and indirect restorations. Currently, it is apparent that not only do various goals exist in operative dentistry, but various classes of dentistry. Class 1 dentistry, corresponding to restoration grade 1, is the dentistry appropriate for developing countries, emergencies, or for the "have-nots." Class 2 dentistry, corresponding to restoration grade 2, is worldwide standard dentistry, conforming with the amalgam age. This is dentistry for patients of limited means, for practitioners with modest or conventional dental training, for patients with mediocre dental awareness, and for National Health Service dentistry as generally offered to the public. Class 3 dentistry, corresponding to restoration grade 3, is, at least for the time being, luxury dentistry outside the realm of procedures covered by health insurance, high-end dentistry, and dentistry for the dentally-aware "haves."

It is remarkable that the three classes of dentistry are not identically distributed within the population of different countries. In Switzerland, for example, two thirds of the population fits into class 3 dentistry. Consequently, dentistry in Switzerland is both demanding and rewarding, because increasing numbers of clients are consumers asking for "want dentistry," rather than patients requesting "need dentistry."

Evaluation Criteria for Restorations

Defining goals for restorations according to the restoration grade or class of dentistry is insufficient. The goals described in Table 17-1 must be defined not only qualitatively, but also quantitatively using evaluation criteria. Furthermore, a distinction has to be made between initial quality and performance quality.

Initial quality is highly influenced by the dental practice (equipment, facilities, and ancillary staff), the individual dentist (training, ability, skills, and knowledge), the patient (cooperativeness during treatment), the operative technique, and the materials used (simplicity and sensitivity of technique). The restoration grade chosen and how well it has been achieved determine the performance quality. Furthermore, the following factors play an important role: the restorative material (physical properties and durability), the patient (dental awareness, self-care, dietary habits, and saliva quality and quantity), and restoration maintenance (recall frequency and nondestructive professional tooth cleaning and refinishing).

Both of the above qualities need to be defined, but not just semiquantitatively as has been done by the United States Public Health Service, the Royal College of Surgeons of England, and the American Academy of Pediatric Dentistry.[2,8,20] In contrast, the evaluation criteria must be defined quantitatively, according to the following four levels:

- A+: Excellent or perfect
- A: Good, but with minor shortcomings; not damaging and improvement easily possible

- B: Major shortcomings or prospectively damaging
- C: Irreversible damage or prospectively severely damaging

The selected evaluation criteria include:

1. Caries
2. Postoperative sensitivity
3. Pulp vitality
4. Anatomic form and wear
5. Occlusion
6. Marginal quality
7. Marginal discoloration
8. Color match
9. Restoration surface
10. Restoration esthetics (imperceptible restitution according to restoration grade 3 in Table 17-1)
11. Preventive and maintenance care
12. Patient self-care
13. Patient satisfaction

In contrast to other quality guidelines, the current scheme includes self-care and patient satisfaction. These two criteria must not be used when restorations are assessed. However, if the warranty pertaining to each restoration is not adequately fulfilled, these two criteria may be helpful when trying to explain the failure and assigning responsibility. The detailed descriptions of each criterion for levels A+, A, B, and C are presented in Table 17-2 and are considered the clinical centerpiece of the quality guidelines.

Assessment Tables for Restorations

Table 17-2 defines each criterion for levels A+, A, B, and C. Although this does not set the standards in restorative dentistry, it is a prerequisite to assessing restorations. In fact, the quality standards are then set by the assessment tables for restorations. Restorations are rated as follows:

- E: Excellent, meets the highest rating levels
- G: Good, fulfils the restorative goals
- I: Insufficient, to be corrected or replaced for damage prevention
- U: Unacceptable, unbearable, to be replaced compulsorily and urgently for damage control

As there are three different classes of dentistry, the requirements that must be fulfilled for various restoratives are different. Consequently, there is more than just one quality standard based on one assessment table.

Categories

The currently available restoratives can be grouped in four categories, as follows.

Category I
- Tooth-colored restoratives: Adhesive Class III and IV restorations, direct and indirect additions, and veneers
- Amalgam alternatives: Direct Class V restorations, fissure sealing, extended fissure sealing, and adhesive Class I restorations

Category II
- Amalgam alternatives: Adhesive Class II restorations, ball-, U-, and box-shaped restorations, and in general stress-bearing direct and indirect restorations

Table 17-2 Definition of the evaluation criteria according to levels A+, A, B, and C

Level	Caries	Postoperative sensitivity	Pulp vitality
A+	No signs of caries at the tooth-restoration interface	No sensitivity to various stimuli or occlusal load	Pulp free of symptoms; adequate pulp protection
A	Marginal discolorations and marginal imperfections indicate an increased caries risk at the tooth-restoration interface; no catching of the probe; no caries detectable	Sensitivity to various stimuli or occlusal load that cannot be attributed to preexistent pulp damage (caries, trauma) or to inadequate treatment, arising shortly after restoration placement; a spontaneous abatement can be expected, possibly after refinements	Pulp free of symptoms; questionable sufficiency of pulp protection; shortcoming can be readily eliminated through refinements
B	Suspected caries at the tooth restoration interface; catching of the probe	Sensitivity to various stimuli or occlusal load that can be attributed objectively to inadequate treatment; duration and prognosis is uncertain, even after refinements	Symptoms of a pulpitis; inadequate pulp protection; problems can be attributed to inadequate treatment; unclear prognosis
C	Caries at the tooth-restoration interface threatening pulp and/or preservation of hard tooth tissue; caries is detectable with a probe and/or is visible radiographically	Pain on various stimuli or occlusal load that can be attributed objectively to inadequate treatment; pain therapy is urgent	Irreversible pulpitis and/or necrosis; undiagnosed nonvital tooth; problems can be attributed to inadequate treatment; treatment is usually urgent

*Centric = habitual, maximum intercuspation.

Anatomic form and wear	Occlusion*
Smooth transition between tooth and restoration; no signs of structural defects in the occlusal contact point area; normal proximal contacts; the contour of the restoration is harmoniously adapted to the extant anatomic form; cusps, cusp slopes, fissures, pits, marginal ridges, and the characteristic tooth form, including the texture, are ideally and harmoniously restored	Individually correct centric and functional contacts; supporting cusps are restored and fossae hold a Shimstock foil in centric occlusion; the restoration harmonizes with the existing occlusion; there are neither lateral glides in centric occlusion nor functional interferences
Slightly under- or overcontoured restoration; no signs of structural defects in the occlusal contact point area; vertical loss of substance noticeable; light or inadequate proximal contact; proximal surface is slightly undercontoured; the contour of the restoration is adapted to the existing anatomic form; cusps, cusp slopes, fissures, pits, marginal ridges, and the characteristic tooth form, including the texture, are restored, but with some shortcomings	Occlusal contact is too heavy or too light; occlusion is satisfactory in centric, however there exist slight functional interferences; pathologic findings or symptoms are missing; adjustment of occlusion can be readily achieved
Markedly under- or overcontoured restoration; signs of structural defects in the occlusal contact point area with clear vertical loss of substance; dentin or base material is partly exposed; too light proximal contact; contour of proximal surface results in gingival harm; the contour of the restoration is insufficiently adapted to the existing anatomic form; cusps, cusp slopes, fissures, pits, marginal ridges, and the characteristic tooth form, including the texture, are partly unrestored	Missing or reversibly traumatic occlusal and/or functional contacts
Missing restoration or parts of restoration; clear structural defects in the occlusal contact point area with significant vertical loss of substance; dentin or base material is exposed; missing proximal contact; proximal overhangs; the contour of the restoration is not adapted to the existing anatomic form; cusps, cusp slopes, fissures, pits, marginal ridges, and the characteristic tooth form, including the texture, are mostly unrestored; the restoration causes tooth or pulpal pain	Missing or irreversibly traumatic occlusal and/or functional contacts; masticatory dysfunctions and/or speech impediment

311

Table 17-2 (continued)

Level	Marginal quality	Marginal discoloration[†]	Color match
A+	Even with meticulous inspection, imperceptible transition from restoration to hard tooth substance throughout the whole marginal length; smooth, continuous transition	Even with meticulous inspection, no marginal discoloration perceptible	Color, opacity, and/or translucency match harmoniously with surrounding hard tooth substance; the restoration is barely perceptible even under meticulous inspection; possible minimal discrepancies in color are not due to incorrect color selection but due to internal staining of the hard tooth substance or, in case of fissure sealing, due to diagnostic needs
A	Imperceptible transition from restoration to hard tooth substance at normal talking distance; signs of underfilled margins, overhangs, roughness, or ditching; no visible or explorable discontinuities at the tooth-restoration interface; imperfections are readily improved through corrective measures	No marginal discoloration perceptible at normal talking distance; scattered slight discoloration when inspected carefully	Color, opacity, and/or translucency (possibly after stain/discoloration removal) match acceptably with the surrounding hard tooth substance; the restoration is not perceptible at normal talking distance; possible slight discrepancies in color are not due to incorrect selection of color, but due to internal staining of the hard tooth substance or, in case of fissure sealing, due to diagnostic needs
B	Perceptible transition from restoration to hard tooth substance; underfilled margins, steps, or ditches at the tooth-restoration interface; discontinuities are detectable with a fine probe; locally increased caries risk	Marginal discoloration perceptible at normal talking distance; scattered, marked discoloration when inspected carefully; locally increased caries risk	Color, opacity, and/or translucency (possibly after stain/discoloration) differ clearly from the surrounding hard tooth substance, due to incorrect selection of color or to change of restoration color; the restoration is perceptible at normal talking distance
C	Perceptible transition from restoration to hard tooth substance; marginal openings, defects, and/or fractures; the preservation of the hard tooth substance is threatened	Obvious, intense marginal discoloration; localized caries	The restoration markedly spoils esthetics given wrong color, opacity, and/or translucency

[†]Not caused by extant discoloration of hard tooth substance.
[‡]Assessment of restoration imperceptiveness according to restoration grade 3.

Restoration surface	Restoration–esthetics	Preventive and maintenance care	Self-care of the patient	Patient satisfaction
Enamel-like smooth restoration surface	The tooth-colored restoration is imperceptible even when inspected meticulously	The patient is cared for regularly within an adequate recall program including restoration maintenance	Self-care of patient is very good; risk of caries and periodontitis is low or medium	The patient is satisfied in all repects with the dental service received
Slightly rough restoration surface, albeit not enhancing plaque formation; repolishing is readily possible	The tooth-colored restoration is perceptible when inspected carefully; imperceptible at normal talking distance	The patient is dentally checked once a year; professional tooth cleaning and/or restoration maintenance is sporadic and/or only partly adequate	Self-care of patient is consistent and sufficient; risk of caries and periodontitis is low or medium	The patient is satisfied with the dental service provided
Obviously rough, not finishable/polishable surface that enhances plaque formation	The tooth-colored restoration is perceptible at normal talking distance	There are no regular dental checkups; no restoration maintenance	Self-care of patient is inconsistent and partly insufficient; risk of caries and/or periodontitis is high	The patient complains about certain objectively verifiable shortcomings of the dental service rendered
Obviously rough, fractured, defect surface that enhances plaque formation; damage to hard tooth substance and/or periodontium is to be expected	The tooth-colored restoration is conspicuous at normal speaking distance and is objectively unacceptable	No dental care at all	No dental awareness and generally insufficient self-care of patient; high risk of caries and/or periodontitis	The patient regards the dental service provided unacceptable because of objectively verifiable shortcomings

Table 17-3 Assessment of category I restorations*

Levels	Caries	Postoperative sensitivity	Pulp vitality	Anatomic form and wear	Occlusion	Marginal quality	Marginal discoloration	Color match	Restoration surface	Restoration esthetics	Preventive and maintenance care	Patient self-care	Patient satisfaction
	01	02	03	04	05	06	07	08	09	10	11	12	13
A+													
A													
B													
C													

■ = Excellent (E)   ■ = Insufficient (I)

□ = Good or sufficient (G)   ■ = Unacceptable or unbearable (U)

*Based on criteria 1 through 10; criterion 11 in the sense of process quality.

Category III
• Amalgam substitutes: Box-shaped, stress-bearing direct restorations, and direct Class V restorations

Category IV
• Metallic restoratives (amalgam and gold): Direct and indirect box-shaped, stress-bearing restorations
• Non-adhesive, non-tooth-colored restoratives: Direct and indirect restorations

In each restorative category, every level within each evaluation criterion must be assigned to one of the four restoration qualities "excellent," "good or sufficient," "insufficient," and "unacceptable or unbearable," respectively, resulting in four different assessment tables.

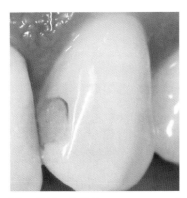

Fig 17-1a Initial appearance of anterior restoration.

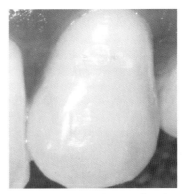

Fig 17-1b Adhesive tooth-colored restoration after 18 months of clinical service.

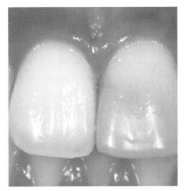

Fig 17-2a Initial appearance of direct addition.

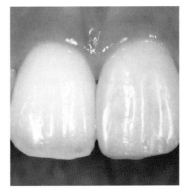

Fig 17-2b Completed direct addition in conjunction with additional bleaching after 12 months of clinical service.

Category I

With category I, regarding initial quality for an "excellent" restoration, the rating table (Table 17-3) depicts that all criteria must be in the A+ level. If one or more criteria fall in the A level, the restoration is rated as "good or sufficient." If one or more criteria fall in the B level, the restoration is rated "insufficient." If one or more criteria fall in the C level, the restoration is rated as "unaccept-

able or unbearable." The rating table for category I restorations is stringent, either because it is rather easy to attain this high quality standard or because there is no tolerance regarding esthetic considerations. This holds for anterior restorations (Figs 17-1a and 17-1b), additions (Figs 17-2a, 17-2b, 17-3a, and 17-3b) and veneers (Figs 17-4a and 17-4b), Class V restorations (Figs 17-5a and 17-5b) and Class I adhesive restorations (Figs 17-6a and 17-6b).

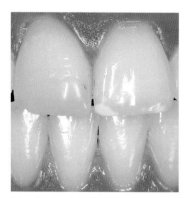

Fig 17-3a Initial appearance of indirect addition.

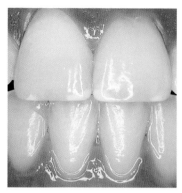

Fig 17-3b Indirect addition after 12 months of clinical service.

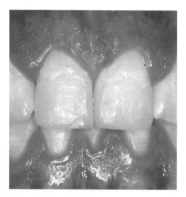

Fig 17-4a Initial appearance of veneers.

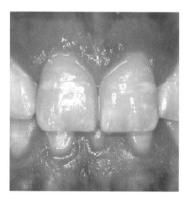

Fig 17-4b Veneers after 12 months of clinical service.

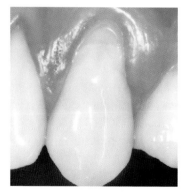

Fig 17-5a V-shaped cervical lesion.

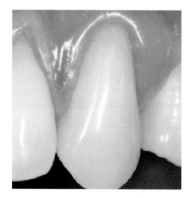

Fig 17-5b Adhesive Class V restoration.

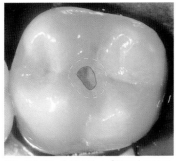

Fig 17-6a Adhesive Class I restoration: cavity preparation, well-preserved enamel shell, excavation of carious dentin.

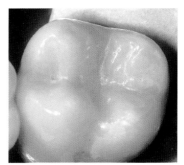

Fig 17-6b Completed adhesive Class I restoration.

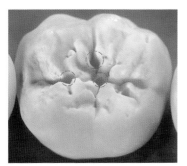

Fig 17-7a Extended fissure sealing: explorative mini access drillings toward the assumed dentinal caries, etched fissure system.

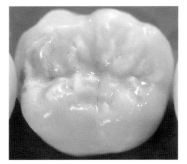

Fig 17-7b Completed extended fissure sealing.

Alternatively, as with fissure sealing and extended fissure sealing (Figs 17-7a and 17-7b), there is no tolerance regarding operative precision, otherwise there is an increased risk of caries, which this is unacceptable. For performance quality, the envisaged service time for direct restorations is 8 years; that is, no criterion must fall in the B or C level within 8 years of restoration placement. For indirect restorations (additions and veneers), the time period is 10 years. If a B level grading occurs, the restoration must be repaired or replaced if the preservation of the tooth structure or form and function of the restoration are compromised. If the B level criterion involves the esthetic appearance of the restoration, the patient decides whether the restoration has to be repaired or replaced. If a C level grading occurs, restoration replacement is unavoidable and urgent.

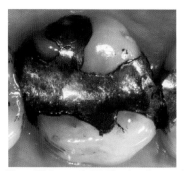 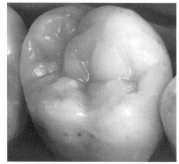

Figs 17-8a and 17-8b Amalgam alternative: composite restorations after 12 months of clinical service.

Category II

Category II covers amalgam alternatives; that is, stress-bearing direct and indirect tooth-colored restorations (Figs 17-8a and 17-8b). In this category, several criteria may be in the A level of initial quality in an "excellent" restoration (Table 17-4). However, the rating is stringent for the criteria "caries," "postoperative sensitivity," "pulp vitality," and "recall program and maintenance care." For the restoration assessment, criteria 12 and 13 are not included. However, it is noteworthy that, for amalgam alternatives, a high level of self-care is important. Because amalgam alternatives can be partly considered "want dentistry," patient satisfaction should also be in the A+ level. The rating of the listed types of restorations using amalgam alternatives must have some tolerance given that the necessary operative procedures are very demanding. Minor shortcomings are irrelevant as long as restoration grade 3 is attained. This includes preservation of

tooth structure, restoration of tooth form and function, and imperceptible appearance. If one or more of criteria 1, 2, 3, and 11 fall in the A level, the restoration is rated as "good or sufficient." If one or more criteria fall in the B level, the restoration is rated "insufficient." If one or more criteria fall in the C level, the restoration is rated as "unacceptable or unbearable." Regarding performance quality, the envisaged service time is 8 years for fillings and 10 years for inlays and overlays. This implies that no criterion must fall in the B or C level within 8 or 10 years, respectively, after restoration placement. If one criterion is in the B level, the restoration must be repaired or replaced if preservation of the tooth structure or form and function of the restoration are compromised. If the B level criterion comprises the esthetic appearance of the restoration, the patient decides whether the restoration must be repaired or replaced. If one criterion falls in the D level, restoration replacement is unavoidable and urgent.

Table 17-4 Assessment of category II restorations*

Levels		Caries	Postoperative sensitivity	Pulp vitality	Anatomic form and wear	Occlusion	Marginal quality	Marginal discoloration	Color match	Restoration surface	Restoration esthetics	Preventive and maintenance care	Patient self-care	Patient satisfaction
		01	02	03	04	05	06	07	08	09	10	11	12	13
	A+	E	E	E	E	E	E	E	E	E	E	E	E	E
	A	G	G	G	E	E	E	E	E	E	E	G	G	G
	B	I	I	I	I	I	I	I	I	I	I	I	I	I
	C	U	U	U	U	U	U	U	U	U	U	U	U	U

= Excellent (E) = Insufficient (I)
= Good or sufficient (G) = Unacceptable or unbearable (U)

*Based on criteria 1 through 10; criterion 11 in the sense of process quality.

Category III

Category III covers amalgam substitutes. The rating table (Table 17-5) is identical to that for amalgam alternatives, except that color match (criterion 8) and restoration esthetics (criterion 10) are not rated and do not count so long as they do not fall in the C level. Again, it is noteworthy that for amalgam substitutes (Fig 17-9), self-care should be high. This is because restorations placed using amalgam substitutes have open margins and the risk of secondary caries is relatively high. Whether patient satisfaction for amalgam substitutes should be in the A+ level or just in the A level remains questionable. The rating of the listed types of restorations using amalgam substitutes must also have some tol-

319

Table 17-5 Assessment of category III restorations*

Levels		01 Caries	02 Postoperative sensitivity	03 Pulp vitality	04 Anatomic form and wear	05 Occlusion	06 Marginal quality	07 Marginal discoloration	08 Color match	09 Restoration surface	10 Restoration esthetics	11 Preventive and maintenance care	12 Patient self-care	13 Patient satisfaction
	A+								Tooth-colored		Tooth-colored			
	A													
	B													
	C													

■ = Excellent (E) ▢ = Good or sufficient (G) ▨ = Insufficient (I) ▩ = Unacceptable or unbearable (U)

*Based on criteria 1 through 10; criterion 11 in the sense of process quality.

erance. This is not because the necessary operative procedures are very demanding, but because the restoration placement is challenging given the allotted treatment time and costs. Again, minor shortcomings are irrelevant so long as restoration grade 2 is attained. This includes preservation of tooth structure and restoration of tooth form and function. Although amalgam substitutes are preferably tooth-col-ored, esthetic consideration is not a rating factor. If one or more of criteria 1, 2, 3, and 11 fall in the A level, the restoration is rated as "good or sufficient." If one or more criteria fall in the B level, the restoration is rated "insufficient." If one or more criteria fall in the C level, the restoration is rated as "unacceptable or unbearable." A C level grading in criterion 8 or 10 means that the appearance of the restoration is so awful

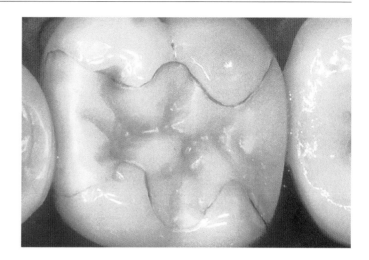

Fig 17-9 Amalgam substitute: compomer restoration after 18 months of clinical service. Marginal openings visualized by marginal discolorations.

that it is unbearable. However, in this respect, the final decision rests with the patient, so long as restoration grade 2 is attained. Regarding performance quality, the envisaged service time for these restorations is 8 years. This implies that no criterion must fall in the B or C level within 8 years after restoration placement. If a B level grading occurs, the restoration must be repaired or replaced. There is no patient option, because with amalgam substitutes, a B level grading automatically compromises either preservation or form and function. If a C level grading occurs, restoration replacement is unavoidable and urgent.

Category IV

Category IV covers metallic, nonadhesive and non–tooth-colored restoratives. The rating table (Table 17-6) is identical to the one for amalgam substitutes. However, color match (criterion 8) and restoration esthetics (criterion 10) are not rated at all.

With amalgam restorations (Figs 17-10a and 17-10b), criteria 11, 12, and 13 may be in the A level; with gold restorations, the same criteria should have an A+ rating. Conventionally, cemented gold restorations have a margin morphology totally different from that of adhesive restorations. Consequently, it is not rated so long as there is no B or C level quality. Regarding performance quality, the envisaged service time for these fillings is 8 years. For gold restorations it is 15 years, in accordance with the quality standard for crown and bridge work. Again, that means that no criterion must fall in the B or C level within 8 or 15 years, respectively, after restoration placement. If a B level grading occurs, the restoration must be repaired or replaced. As in category III, there is no patient option because with metallic, nonadhesive, non–tooth-colored restorations, a B level grading automatically compromises either preservation or form and function. If a C level grading occurs, restoration replacement is unavoidable and urgent.

Table 17-6 Assessment of category IV restorations*

Levels	Caries 01	Postoperative sensitivity 02	Pulp vitality 03	Anatomic form and wear 04	Occlusion 05	Marginal quality 06	Marginal discoloration 07	Color match 08	Restoration surface 09	Restoration esthetics 10	Preventive and maintenance care 11	Patient self-care 12	Patient satisfaction 13
A+						Gold							
A						Gold					Gold	Gold	Gold
B													
C													

= Excellent (E)
= Good or sufficient (G)
= Insufficient (I)
= Unacceptable or unbearable (U)

*Based on criteria 1 through 10; criterium 11 in the sense of process quality.

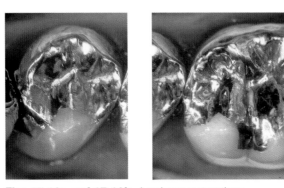

Figs 17-10a and 17-10b Amalgam restorations.

Quality Guidelines—
A Toothless Tiger?

The question as to whether quality guidelines are merely a waste of paper, a voluntary exercise, or a duty is clearly answered. In European health policy, quality standards in medicine are increasingly being adopted, and an increasing number of countries have passed relevant legislation. This is also true for Switzerland. The enactment of quality guidelines is therefore inevitable. However, the assumption that quality guidelines will lead to the creation of "health police" is ill-founded. In dentistry, from a legal standpoint, two conditions are relevant. First, the agreement between clinician and patient and, second, the product liability. Recently another factor has come into play. This is the warranty, which is based on medical device directives and on quality guidelines.

The professional activity of a dentist is legally based on an agreement, usually verbal, between the dentist and the patient. Decades ago, the goal of the mandate and/or agreement involved the construction and placement of an item of work. Currently, the goal is oral health in the realm of "need dentistry." In the future, the goal of the mandate will probably be increased quality of life based on oral health and esthetics in the realm of "want dentistry." In the scope of the agreement, any claim for damage can only be entered into if a fault has occurred.[16]

The product liability takes effect if there is a faulty product specifically threatening either security or health. Legal claims can be entered into if damage has occurred; a contractual relationship is not a prerequisite. The manufacturer is liable for replacement and damage induced by a defective product and this is unconditionally independent of any fault.[5]

With the warranty, the goal is to ensure restoration quality in accordance with the quality guidelines and for the envisaged service time. Four parties are involved with a warranty in operative dentistry: the clinician for restoration quality and dental care; the product manufacturer through the restorative; the patient for self-care and cooperation in the scope of preventive and maintenance care; and the professional authority who recommended the applied operative concept and appraised it as conforming to the quality guidelines. Legal claims can be entered into if shortcomings are evident or damage has occurred. In addition, the existence of a contractual relationship is a prerequisite. Liability, which covers replacement and damage induced by the defective dental work, can only be established if a fault has occurred. Consequently, a warranty clearly differs from a guarantee. Furthermore, if a warranty is not fulfilled, the reason for the fault occurring must be found among the four involved parties. Potential plaintiffs or initiators of lawsuits may be either patients, based on the quality guidelines or the medical device directives, or the profession itself, the dental industry, and/or the supervisory authority, based on the medical device directives.

Transparency in the Information Age

Restorations are products that are part luxury in nature. Dental clients are not just patients, but increasingly consumers. The right to have a say in dental care is uncontested, particularly if the patient/consumer

323

is largely or exclusively responsible for payment. A translation of the standards and quality assessment criteria for the nonprofessional is thus essential. The proven fourfold evaluation system comprising "excellent," "good or sufficient," "insufficient," and "unacceptable or unbearable" restorations could be converted to a two-part positive/negative evaluation system for the layman. Such a manual would allow the patient to recognize newly placed restorations that are unambiguously of poor quality or defective in terms of the prescribed quality standards. Moreover, the patient would have the chance to recognize or acknowledge the need for a replacement restoration before further consequential damage can occur. Furthermore, it would be prudent for the profession to edit these lay standards to ensure that they are correct, objective, and fair. The extant guidelines for dental patients published by patient advisory groups, and the unregulated dental information provided by the Internet, clearly show the urgency of such matters.[17]

Consequences of Quality Guidelines

In an increasing number of European countries, medical quality assessment has become compulsory by law. Consequently, the dental profession will also be obliged to present such definitions and descriptions for all forms of dental care, not just for operative dentistry. In Switzerland, for instance, this became compulsory during the year 2000. This is a fair recompense for the currently valid generous time-based, quality-compatible fee regulations for dentistry, which in

Switzerland is 90% privately financed. In other countries, the point may be to rehabilitate dentistry to become a profession that is meaningful and can simultaneously be economically viable. Furthermore, trust in the profession may also be restored.

The consequences for dentistry in a country that defines quality guidelines and makes them mandatory would be as follows:

- Above all, it would induce a reorientation of the clinician. According to the Swiss guidance to dentists on professional and personal conduct, the maintenance of primary oral health has priority. The presented guidelines would ensure that secondary oral health would be pursued effectively in operative dentistry.
- Practicing dentists will have to live up to these standards and quality requirements. They will have to master and routinely use operative techniques and materials that allow targets to be achieved in accordance with the standards. Simultaneously, minimum quality will be guaranteed. A time-based, fee-for-service regulation would thus be justified and allow high-quality dental care.
- Patients will become increasingly well-informed through readily available computerized information. To a certain extent, they also will be able to assess the quality of their dental services, and this high standard of information will provide a stimulus toward quality and contribute to quality assurance. In the future, patients may feel more present in the realm of dentistry. This should considerably improve the patient-dentist relationship, and enhance both trust in dentistry and the dentist's image.[10,17,23]

- Secondary oral health will become quantifiable. In this way health policy goals can be more accurately defined and priced.
- Health insurance systems in the future will also have to respect quality. In operative dentistry, underpayment for dental work has always resulted in an increased production of low-quality restorations.
- Research, for its part, will focus on standards, resulting in better targeting of areas that truly benefit patients.[17] At the launch of all new products, evidence must be presented that standards for the intended indications can be attained. Consequently, the practitioner can no longer be abused as a tester and the patient as a paying disposable commodity. Science will then clearly come before marketing.[19]
- Basic training, postgraduate education, and continuing education would also have to be subject to the standards. Proof of performance would have to be provided for all clinical concepts put forward. Simplified operative techniques, as published in the dental tabloids for treating patients, would no longer be tenable. "State of the art" would then no longer be what is fashionable or appealing, but would be based on how and with what materials the standards can be achieved.

Conclusion

Dentistry is increasingly a luxury service, and therefore may rightly be considered, at least in part, as a business. It will only develop as a highly respected, rewarding, and viable profession so long as the patient-dentist relationship is based on unreserved trust and consumers are content with the dental care practiced and offered. Quality guidelines have the potential to help generate trust in the profession and in this way, restorative dentistry would become true to its calling. A further improvement in oral health could be expected without additional costs and not at the expense of the practitioner.

References

1. Addy M, Adriaens P. Epidemiology and etiology of periodontal diseases and the role of plaque control in dental caries. In: Lang NP, Attström R, Löe H (eds). Proceedings of the European Workshop on Mechanical Plaque Control. Berlin: Quintessenz, 1998:98–101.

2. American Academy of Pediatric Dentistry. Quality assurance criteria: Section IV: Pediatric restorative dentistry. J Am Acad Pediatr Dent 2000;22(special issue):110–112.

3. Anderson R, Treasure ET, Whitehouse NH. Oral health systems in Europe. Part I: Finance and entitlement to care. Community Dent Health 1998;15:145–149.

4. Anderson R, Treasure ET, Whitehouse NH. Oral health systems in Europe. Part II: The dental workforce. Community Dent Health 1998;15:213–217.

5. Edelmann M. Leitfaden zur Medizinprodukte-verordnung. St. Gallen: Eigenverlag, 1998.

6. Elderton RJ. Ist Zahnmedizin schlecht für die Zähne. Phillip J 1997;14:287–291.

7. Evans BO. Dental economics and its effect on the quality of care. Oper Dent 1996;21:133.

8. Kenneth ER, Entwistle N, Gordon E, McLean J, Rear St, Seel D. Self Assessment Manual and Standards. London: Royal College of Surgeons of England, 1991.

9. Kersten S, Lutz F, Besek M. Zahnfarbene adhä-sive Füllungen im Seitenzahnbereich. Zürich: Eigenverlag PPK, 1999.

10. Kocher G. Rationierung in der Medizin—Um-denken in der Qualitätsförderung. Schweiz Ärztez 1997;78:748–750.

11. Lutz F, Krejci I, Besek M. Konservierende Zahn-heilkunde—Restaurationen für wen? Schweiz Monatsschr Zahnmed 1998;108:19–26.

12. Lutz F, Krejci I, Besek M. Operative dentistry: The missing clinical standards. Pract Periodontics Aesthet Dent 1997;9:541–548.

13. Meskin LH. Patients first and always. J Am Dent Assoc 1997;128:138–140.

14. Mueller CD, Schur CL, Paramore LC. Access to dental care in the United States. J Am Dent Assoc 1998;129:429–437.

15. Prange H. Qualitätsmanagement in der Zahn-arztpraxis. Phillip J 1997;14:225–235.

16. Raschein R. Die rechtliche Stellung des Zahn-arztes. Schweiz Monatsschr Zahnmed 1991; 101:1033–1036.

17. Reekie D. The future of dentistry—The evidence revolution. Br Dent J 1998;184:262–263.

18. Reford M. Dentist-patient interactions in treat-ment decision-making: A qualitative study. J Dent Educ 1997;61:16–21.

19. Robbins JW. Evidence-based dentistry: What is it, and what does it have to do with practice? Quintessence Int 1998;29:796–799.

20. Ryge G. Clinical criteria. Int Dent 1981;30: 347–358.

21. Schweizerische Zahnärztegesellschaft SSO. Qualitätsstandards in der Restaurativen Zahn-medizin. In: Qualitätsleitlinien in der Zahnmedizin. Bern: Eigenverlag SSO, 2000:75–103.

22. Schweizerische Zahnärztegesellschaft SSO. Zahnmedizinische Versorgung Schweiz. In: Berufsbild Zahnarzt 2010. Bern: Eigenverlag SSO, 1997:7–10.

23. Watts T. The large signpost in the background. Br Dent J 1999;187:61–62.

24. Wilson RD. Standards, parameters, and taking care of people. Int J Periodontics Restorative Dent 1998;18:4–5.

Index